Electrospun and Electrosprayed Formulations for Drug Delivery

Electrospun and Electrosprayed Formulations for Drug Delivery

Special Issue Editors

Ian S. Blagbrough
Gareth R. Williams

MDPI • Basel • Beijing • Wuhan • Barcelona • Belgrade

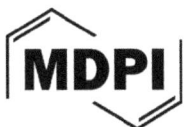

MDPI

Special Issue Editors

Ian S. Blagbrough
University of Bath
UK

Gareth R. Williams
University College London
UK

Editorial Office
MDPI
St. Alban-Anlage 66
4052 Basel, Switzerland

This is a reprint of articles from the Special Issue published online in the open access journal *Pharmaceutics* (ISSN 1999-4923) from 2018 to 2019 (available at: https://www.mdpi.com/journal/pharmaceutics/special_issues/drug_release_electrospinning_process)

For citation purposes, cite each article independently as indicated on the article page online and as indicated below:

LastName, A.A.; LastName, B.B.; LastName, C.C. Article Title. *Journal Name* **Year**, *Article Number, Page Range*.

ISBN 978-3-03897-912-8 (Pbk)
ISBN 978-3-03897-913-5 (PDF)

Cover image courtesy of G. R. Williams.

Contents

About the Special Issue Editors

Ian S. Blagbrough obtained his BSc (Hons) in Chemistry and his PhD (in general synthetic methods in Organic Chemistry, with Prof G Pattenden FRS) from the University of Nottingham in 1980 and 1983, respectively. He then undertook an NIH PDRF with Prof A I Scott FRS and Prof N E MacKenzie at Texas A&M University (1983–1985). He was a Senior Research Fellow in the School of Pharmacy, University of Nottingham working with Prof B W Bycroft and Prof P N R Usherwood (1985–1990). He was then appointed Lecturer and promoted to Senior Lecturer in the School of Pharmacy and Pharmacology, University of Bath where he leads an international research group of six PhD students working on a range of natural product and pharmaceutical analysis topics in molecular pharmaceutics and pharmaceutical research. He has co-authored over 110 refereed papers, 25 book chapters, 3 patents, and over 300 conference abstracts. He has successfully supervised 30 PhD students. He holds the Conference Science Medal (RPSGB) and won the Excellence in Doctoral Supervision Award (University of Bath, 2016).

Gareth R. Williams received an MChem (Hons) from the University of Oxford in 2002. He remained in Oxford for a DPhil in Materials Chemistry, with Prof D O'Hare, which was awarded in 2005. Gareth then spent three years working in science programme management for the UK Government, before returning to Oxford to take up a post-doctoral position in 2009. In September 2010, he joined London Metropolitan University as a Senior Lecturer in Pharmaceutical Science, and in November 2012 was appointed to the UCL School of Pharmacy as a Lecturer in Pharmaceutics. He was promoted to Senior Lecturer (Associate Professor) in 2016 and recognized as a Fellow of the Royal Society of Chemistry in 2017 and as a Fellow of the UK Academy of Pharmaceutical Sciences in 2018. Gareth leads a group of around 20 researchers working on a range of topics in drug delivery and vaccine formulation. He has co-authored over 100 refereed papers and a recent book on electrospinning entitled Nanofibres in Drug Delivery (UCL Press, 2018). His research group is particularly interested in using polymer-based nanomaterials (particles and fibres) prepared by electrohydrodynamic approaches for improving the efficacy of vaccines, targeted drug delivery, and theranostics.

Preface to "Electrospun and Electrosprayed Formulations for Drug Delivery"

Electrospinning and electrospraying have, in recent years, attracted increasing attention in the pharmaceutical sector. The use of electrical energy for solution solidification in these techniques is attractive because it obviates the need to apply heat, and thus does not damage thermally labile active pharmaceutical ingredients (APIs). Research in this area has advanced rapidly. It is now possible to prepare extremely complex systems using multi-fluid processes and to increase production rates to an industrial scale. Electrospun formulations such as the Rivelin Patch are now produced under GMP conditions and are in clinical trials.

In this volume derived from our Special Issue, a range of topics around electrospinning and electrospraying in drug delivery are explored. The volume begins with a review of cyclodextrin-containing nanofibers in drug delivery from Topuz and Uyar. Next, Bhattarai et al. review the potential of electrospun fibers in biomedical applications, with an emphasis on nanoparticle-impregnated nanofibers in drug delivery. De Mohac and colleagues review the use of electrospinning to prepare amorphous systems and thus improve the dissolution rate and solubility of poorly soluble active ingredients. The reviews section finishes with a comprehensive evaluation of electrospinning nanofibers and the potential applications of such novel materials in the tissue engineering field from Ye, Mo and co-workers.

We then present six original research papers. The first, from Burgess et al. investigates the effect of molecular properties on active ingredient release from Eudragit-based electrospun fibers. Huang and co-workers then report electrospun solid dispersions of ferulic acid and probe their ability to accelerate dissolution of this poorly soluble drug. Next, work undertaken by Martínez-Ortega and colleagues uses electrospinning as a route to develop medicines for the treatment of psoriasis. This is followed by work from Fülöp et al. in which electrospinning is scaled up and used to produce low-dose tablets. The penultimate paper comes from Faralli et al. and concerns the transepithelial permeation of drugs released from electrospun xanthan nanofibers using the Caco-2 cell-line model. The volume closes with an elegant study by Park and co-workers into gold nanocage-loaded fibers for the synergistic chemophotothermal treatment of cancer.

We hope that this collection of papers will be of use to colleagues working in the fields of electrospinning, controlled drug delivery, and pharmaceutical technology. We are grateful for the extensive efforts of those contributing to the Special Issue, to the many peer reviewers for their timely work, and to the editorial team at *Pharmaceutics*; we take this opportunity to extend our thanks to all of them.

Ian S. Blagbrough, Gareth R. Williams
Special Issue Editors

pharmaceutics

MDPI

Review

Electrospinning of Cyclodextrin Functional Nanofibers for Drug Delivery Applications

Fuat Topuz * and Tamer Uyar *

Institute of Materials Science & Nanotechnology, UNAM-National Nanotechnology Research Center, Bilkent University, 06800 Ankara, Turkey
* Correspondence: fuat.topuz@rwth-aachen.de (F.T.); tamer@unam.bilkent.edu.tr (T.U.);
  Tel.: +90-312-290-8987 (T.U.)

Received: 11 July 2018; Accepted: 24 August 2018; Published: 24 December 2018

Abstract: Electrospun nanofibers have sparked tremendous attention in drug delivery since they can offer high specific surface area, tailored release of drugs, controlled surface chemistry for preferred protein adsorption, and tunable porosity. Several functional motifs were incorporated into electrospun nanofibers to greatly expand their drug loading capacity or to provide the sustained release of the embedded drug molecules. In this regard, cyclodextrins (CyD) are considered as ideal drug carrier molecules as they are natural, edible, and biocompatible compounds with a truncated cone-shape with a relatively hydrophobic cavity interior for complexation with hydrophobic drugs and a hydrophilic exterior to increase the water-solubility of drugs. Further, the formation of CyD-drug inclusion complexes can protect drug molecules from physiological degradation, or elimination and thus increases the stability and bioavailability of drugs, of which the release takes place with time, accompanied by fiber degradation. In this review, we summarize studies related to CyD-functional electrospun nanofibers for drug delivery applications. The review begins with an introductory description of electrospinning; the structure, properties, and toxicology of CyD; and CyD-drug complexation. Thereafter, the release of various drug molecules from CyD-functional electrospun nanofibers is provided in subsequent sections. The review concludes with a summary and outlook on material strategies.

Keywords: cyclodextrin; electrospinning; drug delivery; nanofibers; cyclodextrin-inclusion complexes; essential oils; electrospun nanofibers; poly-cyclodextrin; antibacterial; antibiotics

---

1. Introduction

Electrospun nanofibers of synthetic, natural, and hybrid systems have been widely exploited as drug delivery materials due to their high specific surface area, which allows enhanced drug loading and ability to modulate release profiles by structural tuning [1–11]. They can be engineered in various shapes, textures, and sizes with diameters down to a few nanometers. Further, the fiber surface can be modified with specific functional ligands or molecules to hinder them from the nonspecific adsorption of proteins or make them cell adhesive via decoration with cell binding ligands [3,12,13]. Drugs can be loaded into electrospun nanofibers by blending prior to electrospinning or using specific chemistry for the controlled release of drugs from the fiber matrix [14,15]. Although there are many pros of electrospun nanofibers for drug delivery applications, they cannot serve as injectable drug reservoirs. On the other hand, the drug-loaded nanowebs or fiber-deposited meshes are quite promising as wound dressing materials [11,12]. Apart from their physical protection to the injured tissue, they can provide the sustained release of the entrapped drugs to achieve wound debridement and wound healing simultaneously [16]. In this regard, comprehensive reviews on the use of electrospun nanofibers for wound healing are available [16,17]. Likewise, the use of CyD-based hydrogel materials for wound dressing has been reviewed in detail [18]. As most drugs are hydrophobic compounds and thus not intrinsically water soluble, the incorporation of a considerable amount of drug molecules into electrospun nanofibers while maintaining their activity can be problematic. In this context, the use of CyD enhances the solubility of the embedded drugs while keeping them stable and bioavailable for enhanced therapy results. The drug release can take place as CyD/drug ICs, if CyD are not chemically attached to the material, or by altering the surrounding conditions that lead to entropically unfavorable inclusion complexation.

The use of drug-loaded electrospun mats as implant materials has taken considerable interest in wound healing. The release of the embedded drugs can take place with the degradation of nanofibers. With that, the entrapped drug molecules can be released from the fiber matrix. Particularly, the use of some specific drugs can accelerate wound healing process and reduce pain. Furthermore, the drug release can be tuned by the structure of the fiber components: sustained drug release can be obtained for the electrospun fibers made by hydrophobic polymers or structurally tuned fiber systems. In one example, core-sheath structured nanofibers with core-loading of hydroxycamptothecin (HCPT) were used on mice via intratumoral implantation [19]. The use of hydroxypropyl β-CyD (HP-β-CyD) molecules as an additive significantly fastened the HCPT release and allowed the higher degradation of emulsion electrospun fibers. The higher release of the loaded HCPT was ascribed to the distribution pattern of HP-β-CyD and HCPT within the fibers. In another example, CyD inclusion complexes (CyD:ICs) with perfluoroperhydrophenanthrene (PFP) as oxygen carriers to cells seeded on the electrospun scaffolds of poly(carbonate urethane) (PCU) and polycaprolactone (PCL) [20]. The ICs of PFP and CyD significantly increased the amount of the dissolved oxygen. Such a concept can be exploited in in vivo applications to fasten the healing of wounded tissues.

In the electrospinning, the texture, size, and structure of nanofibers can be tailored over electrospinning parameters and polymer formulation [21]. Such control on the fiber structure endows them with enhanced performance in drug loading and allows the sustained release of the embedded drug molecules. In this regard, several polymer-based fiber systems were implemented in drug delivery applications [1,22]. Particularly, biocompatible polymers are preferably chosen since they do not release any toxic products during their use. In this regard, polycaprolactone (PCL), poly-L-lactic acid (PLLA), and polycaprolactone/poly(ethylene oxide) (PCL/PEO) are the most widely used polymeric materials [23–26]. The degradation of such nanofibers takes place over hydrolysis, starting from the surface to the core through surface erosion without leaving any toxic byproducts [27]. Along with the fiber degradation, the entrapped drug molecules are released from the fiber matrix. The sustained drug release from such polymers is greatly influenced by the structural features of polymers (e.g., hydrophobicity and glass-transition temperature (T_g)) and the type of the used spinneret system. In this context, a comprehensive review on the sustained release of drugs from electrospun nanofibers was reported by Chou et al., in which the release from uniaxial and coaxial nanofibers from various polymers was deliberately discussed [28]. When hydrophilic electrospun nanofibers are used, the degradation mostly follows bulk erosion with the breakage of hydrolytically labile bonds. In other words, the bulk erosion takes place once the water diffusion is much faster than the scaffold degradation, followed by mass loss throughout the bulk of the material [29].

The crucial problems in drug delivery applications are (i) uncontrolled release of drug molecules (i.e., burst release), (ii) unsustainable drug delivery, (iii) low drug loading, and (iv) low stability and bioavailability of drugs. In this regard, the electrospinning can minimize these problems to some extent because of its unique features, including easy to use with tailored-made fiber properties and applicability to a wide range of materials, such as polymers, composites, and ceramics with fiber sizes ranging from nanometer to micrometer. Further, the functionalization of electrospun nanofibers with pharmaceutical excipients, such as CyD, improves their performance in drug delivery applications. CyD comprise unique features that are often desired in drug delivery carriers. For instance, drug molecules can be entrapped into the hydrophobic molecular-environment of CyD by inclusion-complexation, which dramatically increases the stability of drug molecules under harsh conditions, e.g., high temperature, sunlight, and pH [30]. Further, such complexation remarkably increases their water solubility since many drugs are hydrophobic molecules. Most importantly, for a drug molecule to be pharmacologically active, it should have significant water solubility and lipophilicity to be able to permeate biological membranes through passive diffusion so that no accumulation occurs that can give rise to toxicity. In this regard, lipophilic CyD may assist them in crossing the biological membranes through component extraction or fluidization and can minimize the immunogenic response of body [31]. Further, the surface of the electrospun nanofibers becomes crucial for their in vivo applications since the biocompatibility of the nanofibers and their interactions with the immune system are greatly defined by their surface chemistry. Undesired protein adsorption may occur rapidly when the material is implanted. The adsorbed proteins can denature on hydrophobic surfaces and thus affect the immune system and wound healing. Hence, the surface chemistry becomes a highly critical factor when the fiber mats are intended to be used in in vivo drug delivery.

CyD-functional electrospun nanofibers have been engineered using different approaches. Although most research has been focused on CyD/drug inclusion-complexes (ICs)-embedded polymeric electrospun nanofibers, the recent decade has witnessed significant advances in the polymer-free electrospinning of CyD and their use in drug delivery applications. Functional electrospun nanofibers were also produced using poly-cyclodextrin (polyCyD) molecules in the fiber matrix. In this regard, various active agents either with anticancer, antibacterial, antioxidant or anthelmintic properties have been incorporated into such nanofibers and exploited in drug delivery systems. In the first part of this review, some of the intriguing features of CyD and the mechanism of inclusion-complexation and drug solubility/stability are given. Afterward, several approaches based on CyD-functional nanofibers for drug delivery applications are discussed. The review ends with a future outlook and concluding remarks.

2. Electrospinning

Electrospinning is a versatile process that relies on the jetting of a viscous solution or polymer melt under an electrical field [32]. With the evaporation of solvent molecules, the solidified jet is directed to a collector by electrical forces. During the electrospinning, the fiber is subjected to many different forces, including aerodynamic, inertial, gravitational, rheological, and tensile forces [33,34]. Once an electrical voltage is applied, free charges in the solution lead to the movement and rapidly transfer a force to the electrospinning solution to flow. In this regard, the surface tension, viscoelasticity, and charge density of electrospinning solutions are the key factors for the formation of electrospun nanofibers. The texture, morphology, and size of the nanofibers depend on the processing parameters and solution properties. Mostly, polymeric solutions were used to produce continuous electrospun fibers due to their high viscosity and the presence of intra- and intermolecular interactions. Sometimes, because of the instability of the jet of polymer solutions, the formation of beaded fibers can be observed [35–37]. However, with increasing viscosity or tailoring other solution parameters, bead-free electrospun nanofibers can be obtained [37]. Further, various additives can be incorporated in the electrospinning solution to produce functional nanofibers.

The fiber stability can be provided using either hydrophobic molecules or cross-linking approaches to attain water-insoluble fiber meshes. The main advantages of the electrospinning process are as follows: (i) easy to operate, (ii) adaptability to various polymeric systems, and (iii) suitability to prepare the nanofibers with various diameters, textures, and structures. Figure 1 shows a general representation of an electrospinning setup together with some important processing parameters and nanofibers in various forms. The presence of additives can lead to nanofibers with different morphologies. Various nanoparticles can be loaded in the electrospinning solutions by blending to yield hybrid fibers, or the thermal treatment of nanofibers impregnated with inorganic or metallic precursors. Using different spinneret systems, hollow, core-shell, and triaxial fiber structures can be obtained. Particularly, the co-axial fibers show better sustained release profiles than uniaxial fiber systems as the outer shell acts as a molecular gate in the transport of drug molecules. The fiber size can simply be adapted by the electrospinning parameters or solution conductivity while the solution properties allow the fabrication of ultrafine fibers having diameters in the nanoscale with different morphologies and textures (Figure 1). In general, increasing the polymer concentration, and flow rate causes the formation of larger nanofibers [38]. On the other hand, the fiber diameter decreases with increasing distance between the needle and collector and solution conductivity [38]. In this regard, the addition of salts is a common approach to produce thinner nanofibers for various polymeric systems [39].

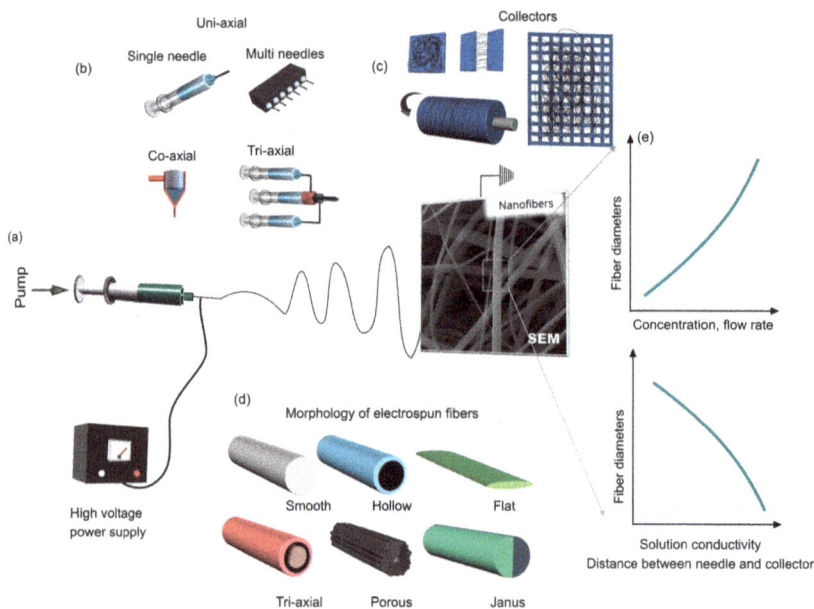

Figure 1. An electrospinning setup with important parameters is shown. (**a**) A cartoon scheme of an electrospinning system with the scanning electron micrograph of electrospun fibers, (**b**) common spinneret systems used in electrospinning, (**c**) collector types, (**d**) the morphology of electrospun fibers, and (**e**) diagrams showing the influence of electrospinning process parameters and solution properties on the electrospun fibers.

3. Cyclodextrins

Cyclodextrins (CyD) are cyclic oligosaccharides of glucopyranose formed during enzyme-catalyzed degradation of starch by glucosyltransferase over chain splitting and intramolecular rearrangement [40]. The molecular structure of CyD resembles a torus-like molecular ring, of which the interior is partially hydrophobic, while the exterior is hydrophilic because of many hydroxyl groups [41]. The inner cavity of CyD accommodates small hydrophobic molecules or portions of large compounds that can fit into their cavities [42]. Owing to their complexation with a wide spectrum of lipophilic molecules, CyD have been implemented in diverse applications, including solubilization enhancers, drug delivery, textile and food industry, tissue engineering, and allied applications [41].

CyD molecules do not elicit an immune response, have low toxicity, and hence are extensively used in bio-related fields, particularly to improve the bioavailability of drugs. In the following section, brief information is provided on the structure, properties, and toxicology of CyD and their inclusion-complexation with guest molecules.

3.1. Structure and Properties of Cyclodextrins

Due to the $^4C_1$ chair conformation (all equatorial groups in $^4C_1$ become axial and vice versa) of each glucopyranose unit, CyD have a shape of a hollow truncated cone, of which the cavity interior has a partial hydrophobic character because of hydrogen atoms of C-3, C-5, and the oxygen atoms of the glycosidic link [43]. Whereas the exterior of CyD is hydrophilic owing to the presence of several hydroxyl groups. Although the existence of numerous CyD with various ring sizes in the class of cycloamyloses, the most common ones are glucose hexamer, heptamer and octamer, which respectively have 6, 7, and 8 glucopyranose units (i.e., α-CyD, β-CyD, and γ-CyD) (Figure 2). The first reference to CyD was published in 1891 as the byproduct of bacterial digestion of starch, and at that time it was named as cellulosine [44]. After the exploration of their 3D structure in 1942 by X-ray analysis, they have been considered as complex-forming molecules, and to date, CyD have become common excipients for a diverse range of applications, including pharmaceuticals, foods, agrochemicals, and fragrances [45–48]. Figure 2 shows the molecular structure of a native CyD molecule. The interior size rises from ~5 to ~8 Å with increasing glucopyranose units from 6 to 8. Even though all CyD have an identical cavity height of ~7.9 Å, the cavity volume shows significant variations from 174 to 427 Å^3 with increasing the number of glucopyranose units from 6 to 8.

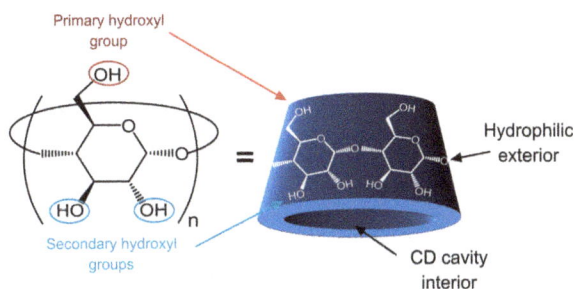

	α-CyD	β-CyD	γ-CyD
Number of glucose	6	7	8
Molecular weight (g/mol)	973	1135	1297
Water solubility (g/L)	145	18.5	232
Internal diameter (Å)	4.7-5.3	6.0-6.5	7.5-8.3
External diameter (Å)	14.6	15.4	17.5
Cavity volume (Å³)	174	262	427
Height (Å)	7.9	7.9	7.9

Figure 2. The chemical structure and the representative cartoon illustration of a native cyclodextrin (CyD) molecule in the 3D form. The general characteristics of CyD are given in the inset table [49].

Due to intermolecular hydrogen bonds, native CyD are not very water-soluble compounds. Particularly, β-CyD molecule has very limited water solubility (~18.5 g/L) while α-CyD and γ-CyD molecules have better water solubility at 145 and 232 g/L, respectively. The poor solubility of β-CyD is originated by the formation of a hydrogen-bond network between the secondary hydroxyl groups [50]. To enhance the water-solubility of the native CyD, they have been chemically modified with different functional groups via amination, esterification, or etherification to break 2-OH-3-OH hydrogen bonds. This also causes the loss of crystallization due to the formation of a statistically substituted material that is made up of many isomeric components with the resultant amorphous, highly soluble end-product. The relatively hydrophobic character of the cavity interior makes CyD ideal molecular carriers of numerous hydrophobic molecules, whose size should be small enough to fit into the cavity. In this context, CyD can form host-guest complexes with a diverse range of organic molecules, inorganic ions, rare gases, and coordination compounds [51–54]. For interested readers, comprehensive reviews on all aspects of CyD and their applications in drug delivery are available [40,55,56].

3.2. Toxicological Issues of Cyclodextrins

For their bio-related applications, CyD must possess some critical conditions, such as biocompatibility and biodegradation. CyD are biocompatible pharmaceutical excipients and have found a wide spectrum of biological use. Even though they have many applications, there are some critical remarks that must be taken into account in their in vivo use. CyD are relatively stable molecules against degradation by human enzymes, and, in this regard, it was reported that after intravenous uptake of CyD by humans, they are excreted intact via the kidney. On the other hand, CyD can be degraded by bacterial and fungal enzymes (i.e., amylases), and hence, in the body, CyD are metabolized in the colon before excretion. The toxicity of CyD arises from their administration route; for instance, for mice exposed to CyD intravenously, the dose that causes 50% death (LD_{50}) is 1.0 g/kg, 0.79 g/kg, and more than 4.0 g/kg for α-CyD, β-CyD, and γ-CyD, respectively [57,58]. Particularly, the uptake of high β-CyD content caused toxicity because of its low water solubility (i.e., 18.5 g/L) [59]. The poor water solubility of β-CyD led to microcrystalline precipitation in the kidney. Further, β-CyD altered the cell membrane permeability by leading hemolysis because of the binding and extraction of cholesterol through inclusion-complexation [60]. Likewise, Zimmer et al. reported that HP-β-CyD interact with cholesterol crystals and dissolve them, which enhance oxysterol production and promote the anti-inflammatory reprogramming of macrophages [61]. Moreover, β-CyD damage renal cells by the extraction of cholesterol from kidney membrane and lead to nephrotoxicity [62]. In vivo studies showed the insignificant amount of CyD adsorbed from the intestinal tract in intact form. The major part of orally administered CyD is metabolized in the colon, and the primary metabolites are further metabolized to CO_2 and H_2O. Because of structural differences between native CyD and CyD derivatives, the adsorption, distribution, and excretion of CyD might have different profiles. Even though the oral administration of CyD did not reveal any significant toxicity, some studies reported their adverse effects on long-term parenteral administration. In this regard, Kantner et al. reported subcutaneous long-term administration of HP-β-CyD with a daily dose of 200 mg/kg resulted in increased bone resorption and bone loss [63]. Even at low dosages (50 mg/kg), minor changes in bone metabolism were also observed. The 2-hydroxypropylation of β-CyD minimizes these toxic effects due to high water solubility of the resultant compound with the condition of less than 1.5% unmodified β-CyD presence. The native β-CyD have been approved in the USA as Generally Recognized as Safe (GRAS) [64]. Likewise, the modified CyD, particularly hydroxypropyl (HP) β-CyD and sulfobutyl ether (SBE) β-CyD, are also included in the FDA (Food and Drug Administration) list as approved chemicals for human use [65]. The metabolism of CyD inclusion complexes (ICs) on oral administration of CyD-ICs, they rapidly dissociate, and the guest molecule leaves the cavity [66]. Thereafter, CyD and guest molecules are involved in the normal biological pathway to be metabolized and excreted from the body. Overall, CyD are generally non-toxic chemicals and can potentially be used for many different biological applications.

3.3. Mechanism of Cyclodextrin Inclusion-Complexation and Drug Solubility

Many drug molecules are poorly soluble molecules in water and, hence, have affinity to complex with CyD. As the inner cavity of CyD molecules has partial hydrophobic character, they can accommodate small lipophilic molecules into their cavities and significantly enhance their water-solubility via inclusion-complexation. The main driving force of the inclusion-complexation relies on hydrophobic interactions between guest molecules and the CyD cavity. Further, other forces, such as van der Waals and dipole-dipole interactions may also be involved in the inclusion-complexation [67,68]. The outer surface of CyD forms hydrogen bonds with water to make them water-soluble. In the inclusion-complexation, intermolecular interactions occur between

CyD and guest molecules as partial or the complete penetration of a guest molecule into the CyD cavity. Figure 3a depicts a guest molecule entrapped in the CyD cavity, driven by inclusion-complexation. The inclusion-complexation may also occur in diverse ways as shown in Figure 3a. Depending on the conditions, one guest molecule can complex with two CyD molecules or vice versa (i.e., two guest molecules with one CyD). The interaction between CyD and guest molecule is in an equilibrium directed by an equilibrium constant (K_c). Figure 3b displays the phase solubility plot for guest molecules, where the increased solubility is associated with the CyD concentration. Each line highlights the type of inclusion-complex (IC) formed, as well as its stoichiometry. Linear line (shown in pink color (i)) represents the formation of soluble IC, while the line in orange color (ii) depicts the formation of IC with limited solubility.

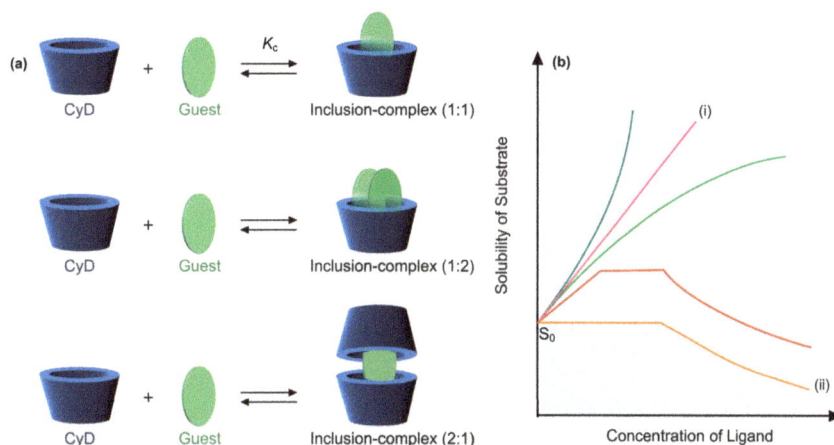

Figure 3. (**a**) The inclusion complex formation between CyD and guest molecules at various stoichiometries. (**b**) The plot shows a phase solubility of guest molecules; (i) represents the formation of soluble inclusion-complex (IC), and (ii) denotes the formation of IC with limited solubility.

Many studies have reported that the inclusion-complexation is governed by van der Waals, electrostatic forces, hydrophobic interactions, hydrogen bonding, and the release of conformational strain [43,69–71]. Some parameters define the strength and relative stability of the complexation. Particularly, the size of cavity and guest molecule, the presence of modified groups in the CyD structure, polarity, and substitution groups on the guest molecule, and environmental conditions, such as medium, ionic strength, and temperature, are prominent factors that can affect the relative strength of inclusion-complexation [72,73]. Normally, a CyD molecule exists in a hydrated form in water—that is, CyD cavity accommodates many water molecules. In the presence of a guest molecule, the replacement between high-energy water molecules and a hydrophobic guest is favored because of an energetically unfavored state of water molecules in the hydrophobic cavity, [41,74]. In general, α-CyD forms complexes with aliphatic chains and molecules (e.g., PCL and poly(ethylene glycol) (PEG)) [75–77], whereas larger cavity of the β-CyD allows host-guest complexes with aromatic rings, such as polycyclic aromatic hydrocarbons (PAHs) [78,79] and essential oils [80,81].

3.4. Drug Stability and Release from Cyclodextrin Inclusion Complexes

One of the currently important issues in drug delivery is the stability of drug molecules on exposure to some harsh conditions. Particularly, biological drugs are sensitive because of their limited stability upon oral administration and during subsequent circulation. They have low bioavailability and short therapeutic half-lives [82]. In this regard, the CyD cavity is enrolled as a shield to protect them from degradation and increase their bioavailability. CyD are stable molecules and can maintain their torus-like molecular structure even at basic pH values [83]. Further, the pyrolysis of CyD molecules starts over 300 °C, implying their thermal stability at high temperature conditions [84]. The inner cavity of CyD molecules accommodates various hydrophobic small molecules and increases their thermal stability. In this regard, various volatile substances (e.g., essential oils) were treated with CyD molecules to form inclusion-complexes for extending their shelf-lives [85,86]. Major benefits of CyD in their drug delivery are (i) increasing the water solubility, stability and bioavailability, (ii) reducing the evaporation of volatile active agents, (iii) low degree of hemolysis, and (iv) avoiding admixture incompatibilities [50].

Hydrophobic and van der Waals interactions are the main dominant driving forces for inclusion-complexation [87]. Therefore, the stability of CyD-ICs is highly dependent on the surrounding conditions that influence these interactions: if pH, ionic strength and temperature of the medium change, guest molecules may leave the CyD cavity because of an energetically unfavored state [72]. This can also be achieved by altering other conditions, making CyD-IC thermodynamically unfavorable.

4. Cyclodextrin Functional Electrospun Nanofibers for Drug Delivery Systems

Various CyD-functional electrospun nanofiber-based materials have been reported as drug delivery systems. These include the blending of polymers with CyD/drug ICs and using CyD-based polymers with drugs. Further, the electrospun nanofibers of only CyD/drug ICs were also performed without the requirement of a polymeric carrier. Due to the absence of a polymeric component, such nanostructured materials present high loading of active agents complexed with CyD for their use in drug delivery. In the following sections, we subcategorize CyD-functional electrospun nanofibers by means of their route of preparation.

4.1. Cyclodextrin-Drug Encapsulated Electrospun Polymeric Nanofibers for Drug Delivery Applications

This is the simplest method to engineer drug-encapsulated electrospun nanofibers through the blending of components (i.e., CyD, drug and polymeric matrix). Generally, CyD and drug are mixed to form inclusion complexes (ICs), and then, blended with the polymer solution, of which the electrospinning produces drug-encapsulated nanofibers. The inclusion-complexation with CyD motifs significantly enhances the water solubility of drug molecules so that high loading capacities can be achieved. In this regard, the Uyar research group reported naproxen (NAP)-CyD ICs loaded PCL nanofibers [88]. Naproxen (NAP), a non-steroidal anti-inflammatory drug, is used in the treatment of pain, inflammation, and fever [89,90]. Due to its lipophilic nature, it is practically insoluble in water at low pH, while it becomes soluble at high pH. To make them water-soluble under mild conditions, their ICs were prepared by slowly adding β-CyD into the aqueous solution of NAP, and the solution was stirred overnight in water until it became cloudy. Thereafter, the solution was freeze-dried, and IC powder was obtained. The complexation between CyD and NAP significantly enhanced the water solubility of NAP. The ICs were mixed with PCL solution and electrospun to form nanofibers. The mean diameter of PCL nanofibers slightly increased from ~335 to ~390 nm with the incorporation of NAP-β-CyD ICs. The release studies showed enhanced release of NAP from NAP-β-CyD ICs encapsulated PCL nanofibers when compared to the pristine NAP-loaded PCL nanofibers prepared in the absence of CyD. Likewise, Akduman et al. reported naproxen-CyD embedded polyurethane nanofibers and observed that the complete release of NAP from the only polyurethane fiber matrix took 120 h while the use of β-CyD or HP-β-CyD reduced the delivery time for NAP to ~36 and 5 h, respectively [91]. The difference in the release profiles from both CyD was due to the solubility difference of β-CyD and HP-β-CyD; HP-β-CyD has much higher water solubility than the unsubstituted β-CyD.

The Uyar research group also reported hydroxypropyl cellulose (HPC) nanofibers impregnated with sulfisoxazole/CyD ICs [92]. Sulfisoxazole (SFS) is a sulfonamide drug with antibiotic properties [93]. Because of its low water solubility (i.e., <0.1 g per 100 mL), it was mixed with HP-β-CyD to form inclusion-complexation, which significantly increased the water solubility of SFS for enhanced therapy results. Thereafter, ICs were mixed with HPC, and the resultant mixture was electrospun to obtain ultrafine nanofibers. The IC-loaded nanofibers had a mean fiber diameter of 60 ± 25 nm, while sole SFS-loaded nanofibers (i.e., produced in the absence of CyD) sized 90 ± 40 nm, suggesting the use of ICs as an additive reduced the fiber diameter. However, the incorporation of IC did not make any significant impact on the fiber morphology. Although the initial release of SFS from the fiber matrix was fast, the complete release process took 12 h. The inclusion-complexation increased the release rate of SFS than those released from the HPC fiber matrix in the absence of CyD. Further, a sandwich-like fiber system was engineered by placing HPC/SFS/HP-β-CyD-IC nanofibers between PCL nanowebs. This nanofiber system slowed the release rate of SFS than the fiber prepared without PCL nanofibers. Tonglairoum et al. reported clotrimazole (CZ) loaded nanofibers through electrospinning [94]. A multicomponent fiber system containing CZ-loaded polyvinylpyrrolidone (PVP)/hydroxypropyl-β-cyclodextrin (HP-β-CyD) was prepared, and the fiber surface was coated with chitosan-cysteine (CS-SH)/poly(vinyl alcohol) (PVA) to increase the mucoadhesive properties and achieve the sustained release of CZ from the nanofibers. CZ-loaded nanofibers were successful in killing *Candida* significantly faster than the commercially used CZ lozenges at 5, 15, and 30 min and were safe for 2 h incubation. The release profiles of the embedded CZ did not show significant variations, and 80–90% release was observed after 480 min. Overall, the nanofibers showed promising results in the treatment of oral candidiasis.

Voriconazole (VRC) is a triazole antifungal agent loaded as ICs with HP-β-CyD into poly(vinyl alcohol) (PVA) nanofibers and used for ophthalmic delivery [95]. The VRC-loading capacity could be enhanced with increasing CyD content. The total release of VRC took about 8 h from the nanofibers. Ocular irritation tests were performed on rabbit samples, and the Draize eye test results revealed that there was no ocular discomfort after the administration of the VRC nanofibers and VRC solution, suggesting that VRC-loaded PVA/HP-β-CyD composite nanofibers are promising non-irritant materials. Siafaka et al. reported voriconazole-loaded PCL nanofibers in the presence of β-CyD [96]. The ICs of VRC and β-CyD were mixed with PCL solution and electrospun to form nanofibers. VRC with various concentrations (5–20 wt.%) were loaded into nanofibers. All nanofibers showed an initial burst release of the VRC over 80%. The burst release was decreased with increasing VRC content. The nanofibers showed antifungal properties with the inhibition of *Candida albicans*. Opanasopit and co-workers reported fast releasing polyvinylpyrrolidone (PVP)/CyD composite nanofibers for the taste-masked meloxicam [97]. Meloxicam (MX) is a nonsteroidal anti-inflammatory drug molecule that is intended to be used in treating rheumatoid arthritis [98]. CyD molecules were blended to improve the fiber stability. MX was mixed with the CyD, and then PVP solution, of which the electrospinning led to nanofibers. In another CyD-based drug delivery system, electrospun mats were developed using PVP and HP-β-CyD/MX ICs [99]. MX was mixed with CyD molecules and electrospun in the presence of PVP in different solvent systems (dimethylformamide (DMF) and ethyl alcohol (EtOH)). HP-β-CyD molecules significantly improved the solubility of MX. A fast disintegration time and the burst release of MX were observed in an EtOH-based system. Furthermore, EtOH-based fiber system rapidly dissolved in the mouth. Cytotoxicity tests showed that the EtOH-system was much safer than the DMF-based system. Overall, the study showed a composite fiber of PVP and HP-β-CyD is ideal for fast-dissolving drug delivery to increase palatability of dosage forms.

Recently, Monteiro et al. reported tetracycline/β-CyD IC loaded PCL nanofibers [100]. Tetracycline (TCN) is a common drug used for periodontal disease treatment [101]. After the preparation of TCN/β-CyD ICs, they were incorporated in PCL solution and electrospun to form nanofibers. The half of the embedded-TCN released as a burst from the matrix and then a slow release profile was observed. Total release of the entrapped TCN took 350 min. The nanofibers showed antimicrobial activity against *Aggregatibacter actinomycetemcomitans* and *Porphyromonas gingivalis*. TCN was also released in a sustained manner from CyD-free electrospun fibers of PCL/Zein [102,103] and PCL/poly(ethylene-*co*-vinyl acetate) (PEVA) [104,105]. The incorporation of PCL into the zein fibers slowed the release rate of TCN. TCN release could also be tuned by multi-layered electrospun fibrous mats. In this regard, Alhusein et al. showed that the sustained release of TCN from triple-layered fibers of PCL and PEVA when TCN loaded PEVA fibers were used in the middle covered by TCN-free PCL fibers from both sides [105]. This dramatically reduced the burst release of TCN, demonstrating the importance of drug localization on the release profile. In this context, a detailed review on the controlled release of drugs, including TCN, from PCL-based fibers was reported by Blagbrough and colleagues [106]. Chen and coworkers used silk-fibroin based electrospun nanofibers impregnated with HP-β-CyD as the carrier of Tamoxifen [107]. Tamoxifen (TAM) is a selective estrogen receptor modulator and acts as antiestrogen by binding to the estrogen receptors to inhibit the growth of the malignant mammary tumors in some tissues [108]. It is also effective in patients with ER-positive metastatic breast cancer [109]. TAM was mixed with HP-β-CyD molecules to form ICs to make it water-soluble. Thereafter, the solution was mixed with silk-fibroin and electrospun to form composite fibers. The inclusion-complexation significantly decreased the fiber diameter. The effective loading of TAM was confirmed by the Raman analysis of the fibers. The release results showed that the TAM first dissociated from the ICs, and then, was subsequently released from the fiber matrix. The release occurs slowly, and 50% release was observed after two weeks of incubation, suggesting that the presented concept can be intended as a promising local drug delivery system for breast cancer therapy. Souza et al. recently reported PCL nanofibers impregnated with β-CyD-silver sulfadiazine ICs [110]. Silver sulfadiazine (SAg) pertains to a sulfanilamide class of chemicals and is known for its topical antimicrobial properties, and is commonly used for the treatment of infected burns [111]. After inclusion-complexation with β-CyD, the solution was electrospun in acetic acid to form fibers, whose diameters showed great variations depending on the components; the solution of 15 wt.% PCL led to nanofibers with a mean diameter 358 nm, while IC-loaded PCL nanofibers possessed a mean diameter of 892 nm, suggesting the IC incorporation led to a dramatic increase in the fiber diameter. The release studies showed that, after one day, ca. 80% of SAg was released from CyD-free PCL fibers, while the respective value was 66% from the IC-loaded PCL fibers. The nanofibers demonstrated antibacterial properties against *S. aureus* and *E. coli*.

Core-shell electrospun nanofibers impregnated with CyD functionalities have also been investigated in drug delivery applications. Generally, co-axial nanofibers promoted the sustained release of the entrapped drugs than the uniaxial fibers. In this regard, the Uyar research group reported the preparation of the core-shell nanofibers of curcumin/CyD IC and polylactic acid (PLA) [112]. The core of the nanofibers was IC of CyD and curcumin (CUR), while the shell layer was PLA. The formation of core-shell fiber structure was confirmed by TEM analysis with a contrast difference on the fibers. The slow release of CUR was achieved by core-shell nanofiber structure and the inclusion-complexation of CUR with HP-β-CyD provided high solubility. The embedded CUR showed antioxidant activity on the scavenging of 2,2-diphenyl-1-picrylhydrazyl (DPPH) radicals. CUR was also loaded into poly(vinyl alcohol) (PVA) nanofibers in a form of their complexes with CyD molecules [113]. The in vitro studies showed rapid diffusion of curcumin in the first hour followed by slower release. The nanofibers with low CUR loads showed faster release profiles. Another curcumin-loaded nanofiber system with multifunctional additives was developed using poly (L-lactic acid-*co*-ε-caprolactone) (PLACL) and Aloe Vera (AV), MgO nanoparticles, curcumin and β-CyD as a candidate material for breast cancer therapy [114]. These multifunctional nanofibers were tested with Michigan Cancer Foundation-7 (MCF-7) breast cancer cells. Depending on the fiber constituents, the proliferation of MCF-7 cells showed a clear decrease by 66% in PLACL/AV/MgO/CUR with respect to PLACL/AV/MgO nanofibrous scaffolds on day 9. The results demonstrated that 1% CUR interacting with MgO nanoparticles exhibited higher inhibition of MCF-7 cells among all other nanofibrous scaffolds, demonstrating their effectiveness for breast cancer therapy. Another PLLA-based nanofibers with CyD functionalities were prepared for the release of hydroxycamptothecin (HCPT) [115]. HCPT is an antitumor drug with poor water solubility, which restricts its use in clinical applications. The solution of PLLA and PEG was mixed with HP-β-CyD and HCPT and electrospun into nanofibers whose diameters slightly decreased from 780 to 700 nm in contrast to those nanofibers prepared in the absence of CyD and HCPT. The homogenous distribution of HCPT in the fiber matrix was confirmed by confocal analysis. The release studies revealed the initial burst release of ca. 15%, followed by a gradual release over 20 days. Increasing the HCPT content boosted the release percentage while the addition of higher CyD content minimized the burst release of HCPT. Recently, Masoumi et al. reported ciprofloxacin/CyD-encapsulated PCL nanofibers [116]. Ciprofloxacin (CIP) is an antibiotic drug molecule with poor water solubility and low dissolution rate, which limit its bioavailability [117]. CIP was mixed with α-CyD or β-CyD to form ICs and thereafter added to PCL solution. The electrospinning of these composite mixtures led to bead-free electrospun nanofibers loaded with CIP. The release tests were performed at pH = 7.2, and the released CIP content showed variations depending on the CyD-type and the preparation route of ICs; sonication-driven IC-loaded PCL fiber showed better release rate than those prepared without sonication. This can be ascribed to a higher amount of CIP entrapped in the CyD cavity under sonic energy.

The ICs of antifungal drug griseofulvin (GSV) [118], antipsychotic drug (aripiprazole) [119] and phytochemical (asiaticoside) [120] with CyD were also mixed with various polymeric matrices and electrospun to form drug-loaded nanofibers. The Uyar research group reported allyl isothiocyanate loaded PVA nanofibers and investigated their antibacterial properties [121]. The ICs of antibacterial agent allyl isocyanate (AITC) and β-CyD were loaded into the electrospun nanofibers of PVA. CyD molecules significantly stabilized AITC during the electrospinning because of inclusion-complexation. The release experiments were performed at three different temperatures (30, 50 and 75 °C) in gas phase, and the release was dramatically increased with higher temperature. The nanofibers showed antibacterial properties with the significant inhibition of *E. coli* and *S. aureus*. AITC/CyD ICs were also embedded in the electrospun nanofibers of soy protein isolate (SPI), PEO or PLLA [122]. Fiber morphologies were affected by the AITC concentration used. The AITC release was negligible under dry conditions but increased dramatically as relative humidity rose. Luo et al. reported CyD functional polymeric nanofibers for sequential release of vascular disrupting and chemotherapeutic agents from electrospun nanofibers [123]. Combretastatin A-4 (CA4) and hydroxycamptothecin (HCPT) were loaded in the nanofibers of poly(ethylene glycol)-polylactide (PELA) in the presence of HP-β-CyD. The sequential release of CA4 and HCPT could achieve a sequential killing of endothelial and tumor cells. Anthelmintic drugs were also released from CyD functional electrospun fibers. In this context, Vigh et al. reported flubendazole/HP-β-CyD IC embedded PVP nanofiber webs with enhanced oral bioavailability [124]. A forty milligram could be released in 15 min, and the administration of the nanofiber system led to an increased plasma concentration profile in rats in contrast to the practically non-absorbable crystalline flubendazole. This can be ascribed to the effect of the embedded CyD, which prevented the crystallization of flubendazole. Doxorubicin (DOX), a chemotherapy medicine, was released from the PLLA nanofibers in the form of their ICs with methylated-β-CyD in parallel to their release from CyD-free PLLA fibers [125]. The results showed that the use of CyD molecules led to controlled release, and 17% decrease in the burst release was observed, followed by a quantifiable sustained release up to two days. Metoclopramide hydrochloride (MH), a drug molecule that has been used to treat nausea and vomiting, was incorporated into HP-β-CyD functional PVA nanofibers, and the release of MA was performed in a phosphate buffer (pH = 6.8) at 37 °C [126]. 90% Release of MA took place in 1 min due to burst release of MA. CyD-functional electrospun nanofibers were also used for the delivery of proteins. In one example, β-lactamase BlaP protein was mixed with the solution of chitosan/PEO containing CyD molecules, and the resultant mixture was electrospun into fibers [127]. CyD were used to increase the protein stability. In the absence of protein, spindle-shaped fibers were formed. However, the protein addition gave rise to smooth, bead-free nanofibers. The activity of the β-lactamase tested over the hydrolysis of nitrocefin, and enhanced hydrolysis was observed for the CyD functional nanofibers, demonstrating that the embedded CyD stabilized the protein in the fiber matrix.

A blending method was also applied for the preparation of essential oil loaded CyD functional electrospun fibers. Essential oils are plant-derived phytochemicals with antibacterial and antimicrobial properties [128,129]. They have also shown antimutagenic and antifungal activities [130]. Opanasopit and colleagues reported plai oil/HP-β-CyD IC [131] and herbal oil/ HP-β-CyD IC [132] loaded PVP nanofibers and monitored release profiles of the oil from the fiber matrix. The release of plai oil from the fiber matrix demonstrated burst release and subsequent sustained release over 24 h. The release rate changed between 10 and 30% in 24 h depending upon the oil load in the fiber. The release of herbal oil took less than one minute. Lin et al. reported cinnamon essential oil (CEO)/CyD loaded PEO nanofibers [133]. In this regard, first CEO/β-CyD proteoliposomes were prepared by using a thin-lipid film evaporation-ultrasonic hydration-freeze and thaw technique. Afterwards, they mixed with PEO and electrospun to form bead-free nanofibers (Figure 4A). The CEO release studies were performed in ethanol, and the amount of CEO released from the fiber matrix was measured by GC-MS. In the presence of *Bacillus cereus*, the release of CEO was significantly enhanced. The CEO release from the nanofibers was about 30% in 96 h, whereas this increased to 80% in the presence of *B. cereus*. A similar effect was observed at higher temperature, which enhanced the release rate of CEO (Figure 4C). The resultant nanofibers showed significant inhibition against the growth of *B. cereus* due to the antibacterial property of CEO.

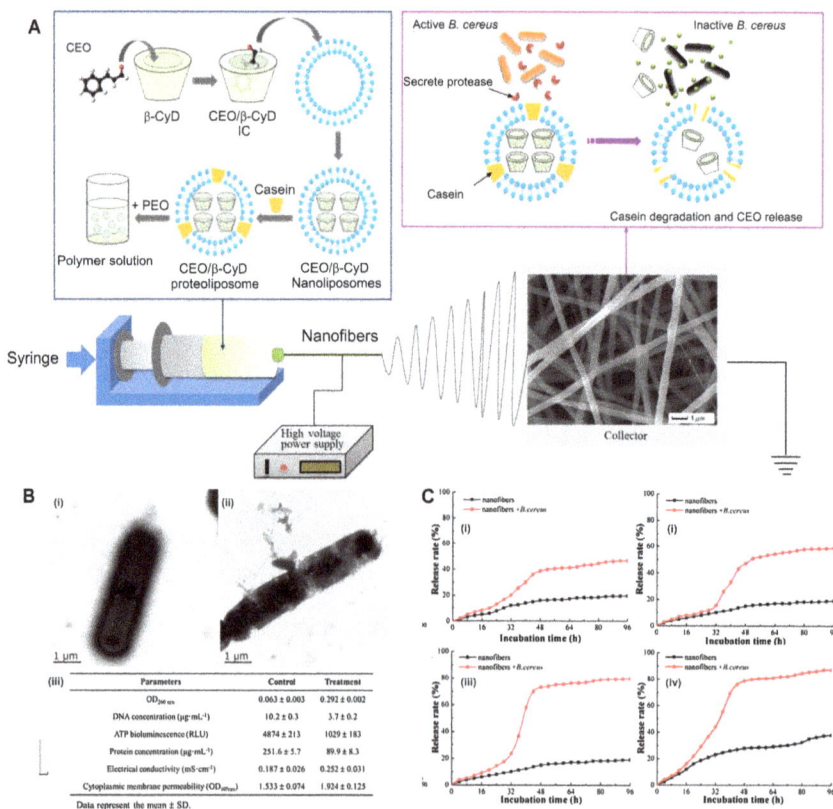

Figure 4. (**A**) Cartoon schemes of the production of CEO/β-CyD proteoliposomes incorporated poly(ethylene oxide) (PEO) fibers and *B. cereus* proteinase triggered cinnamon essential oil (CEO) delivery from CEO/β-CyD proteoliposomes. (**B**) TEM images of *B. cereus* before (i) and after the treatment (ii) of CEO/β-CyD proteoliposomes. (iii) The respective analysis results on the release of *B. cereus* cell constituents and the cell membrane permeability before and after proteoliposomes treatment. (**C**) The release rate of CEO/β-CyD proteoliposomes nanofibers stored at different temperatures 4 °C (i), 12 °C (ii), 25 °C (iii), and 37 °C (iv) for 4 days. The figure was reproduced from [133] with the permission of Elsevier, 2017.

The cinnamon essential oil (CEO) was also encapsulated in PVA/β-CyD nanofibers, and in this context, the ICs of cinnamon and β-CyD were mixed with PVA solutions and electrospun to form nanofibers with a mean diameter of 240 ± 40 nm [134]. CyD molecules notably increased the thermal stability of CEO after complexation. Due to the intrinsic antimicrobial property of CEO, the nanofibers exhibited strong antimicrobial activity against *E. coli* and *S. aureus*. Furthermore, the entrapment in fiber systems prolonged the shelf-life of CEO. Cinnamon/β-CyD ICs were also loaded into PLLA fibers, and the nanofibers showed antimicrobial properties [135]. The same research group also reported an identical fiber system using lysozyme as an additive and observed the enhancement of the antimicrobial activity of cinnamon essential oil-loaded electrospun nanofilm by the incorporation of lysozyme [136]. Recently, Munhuweyi et al. reported that cinnamon and oregano essential oils–loaded PVA-CyD nanofibers [137]. The ICs of essential oils with β-CyD molecules were prepared and mixed PVA solutions, of which the electrospinning led to nanofibers varying between 120 and 180 nm in diameter depending on essential oil loading. Liu et al. reported cinnamaldehyde/CyD loaded PLLA fibers via electrospinning [138]. Cinnamaldehyde (CA) pertains to the class of essential oils and is known for its antibacterial and antioxidant properties [139]. The ICs of the β-CyD and CA were mixed with PLA and electrospun into fibers of 4–6 μm depending on the IC loading. Increasing IC content in the PLLA fiber decreased water contact angle because of many OH groups. Increasing IC content led to high release percent of the embedded CA. In the first 20 h, a significant increase of CA was observed, but afterwards, almost no change on the release profile was monitored. The CA-loaded fibers showed antibacterial properties against *E. coli* and *S. aureus*. Likewise, ultrafine nanofibers from zein impregnated with the ICs of eucalyptus essential oil (EEO) and β-CyD were produced by electrospinning [140]. The ICs of EEO and β-CyD were prepared by co-precipitation technique and added to aqueous ethanol solutions of zein. The electrospinning of the mixtures led to the formation of bead-free nanofibers. The IC-loaded zein nanofibers showed 24% greater reduction of growth than pure zein fibers. For *Listeria monocytogenes*, the growth reduction was 28.5%, and for *Staphylococcus aureus*, it was 24.3%.

PLLA was also used as a carrier of gallic acid (GA)/CyD ICs [141]. The IC of GA with HP-β-CyD molecules was prepared and mixed with PLLA solutions whose electrospinning led to bead-free nanofibers. The release studies were performed in aqueous solution of EtOH and increased GA release was observed with increasing EtOH content. The release came to equilibrium after 4 h. The nanofibers showed antioxidant activity in the scavenging of DPPH radicals. Mascheroni et al. reported perillaldehyde-loaded pullulan nanofibers functionalized with β-CyD [142]. The blending of pullulan and β-CyD with embedded perillaldehyde was performed and electrospun. The release of volatile perillaldehyde showed a profound effect of RH on the release profile.

The Uyar research group has reported several studies related to the encapsulation of CyD ICs of volatile active agents such as essential oils (e.g., eugenol [85], geraniol [86]) or fragrance/flavor molecules (e.g., menthol [143–145], vanillin [146]) into electrospun polymeric nanofibers in order to enhance the temperature stability and shelf-life of such volatile active agents. Likewise, hexanal, a naturally occurring volatile compound, released from CyD-functional xanthan fibers. The CyD-functional xanthan fibers showed faster release of hexanal than pure xanthan fibers [147]. Moreover, a type of vitamin E (α-tocopherol), an antioxidant, was incorporated into PLLA nanofibers after its complexation with γ-CyD molecules [148]. The PLLA/α-tocopherol/γ-CyD nanofibers showed antioxidant properties. The Uyar research group has also reported β-CyD/quercetin ICs loaded poly(acrylic acid) (PAA) nanofibers [149]. The electrospinning of the mixture of PAA, β-CyD and quercetin led to well-tuned nanofibers with a mean diameter of 270 nm. The nanofibers showed a burst release of almost all quercetin molecules. The nanofibers showed antioxidant activity due to the embedded quercetin. Kingshott and colleagues reported retinyl acetate (RA) release from β-CyD functional PVA nanofibers [150]. The ICs of β-CyD and RA were incorporated into PVA nanofibers to enhance the shelf-life and thermal stability of RA. The release of RA was very slow, reaching 90% after 3 months. The general overview of the CyD/drug ICs loaded polymeric electrospun nanofibers was summarized in Table 1, where the composition of the fiber matrix and drug molecules were given, along with release data.

Table 1. General overview of CyD/drug ICs embedded polymeric electrospun nanofibers used in drug delivery.

CyD Type	Polymer Additive	Active Molecule	Release Data	Ref
β-CyD	PCL	Naproxen (NAP)	Higher NAP release with CyD	[88]
β-CyD, HP-β-CyD	Pellethane (TPU)	Naproxen (NAP)	10 h (NAP-TPU), 32 h (NAP/β-CyD/TPU), 120 h (NAP, HP-β-CyD/TPU)	[91]
HP-β-CyD	Hydroxypropyl cellulose (HPC)	Sulfisoxazole (SFS)	720 min (PCL-PCL-HPC/SFS/HP-β-CyD-IC-NF), >720 min (HPC/SFS/HP-β-CyD-IC-NF)	[92]
HP-β-CyD	PVP, PVA, Thiolated chitosan (CS-SH)	Clotrimazole (CZ)	For all nanofibers 80% in 480 min	[94]
HP-β-CyD	PVA	Voriconazole (VRC)	8 h for 100% release	[95]
β-CyD, HP-β-CyD	PVP	Meloxicam (MX)	For all nanofibers, 20 min for 100% release	[97]
HP-β-CyD	PVP	Meloxicam (MX)	Rapid release (<10 min)	[99]
β-CyD	PCL	Tetracycline (TCN)	Drug release occurred up to 2 weeks	[100]
HP-β-CyD	Silk fibroin (SF)	Tamoxifen (TAM)	10% in 22 days in PBS, 50–60% in PBS-EtOH (30%) in 22 days)	[107]
β-CyD	PCL	Silver sulfadiazine (SAg)	80% release from PCL/SAg, 66% release from PCL/SAg/β-CyD	[110]
HP-β-CyD	PLLA	Curcumin (CUR)	Higher release at pH of 1. CyD increased drug release.	[112]
β-CyD	PVA	Curcumin (CUR)	Higher drug content increased the release rate.	[113]
β-CyD	Poly (L-lactic acid-co-ε-caprolactone) (PLACL)	Curcumin (CUR)	1% CUR interacting with MgO nanoparticles showed higher inhibition of breast cancer cells.	[114]
HP-β-CyD	Poly(DL-lactic acid)–poly(ethylene glycol) (PELA)	Hydroxycamptothecin (HCPT)	Higher CyD content increased release rate. The release was slow and took many weeks.	[115]
α-CyD and β-CyD	PCL	Ciprofloxacin	Higher release with initial higher drug loading	[116]
SBE-β-CyD	PEO	Aripiprazole (ARP)	Rapid release in 2 min	[119]
HP-β-CyD	Cellulose acetate	Asiaticoside (AC)	Higher release with CyD and initial burst release within 300 min	[120]
β-CyD	PVA	Allyl isothiocyanate (AITC)	Higher release at 75 °C and followed by 50 and 30 °C.	[121]
β-CyD	PEO	Allyl isothiocyanate (AITC)	Higher release with increasing relative humidity	[122]
HP-β-CyD	Poly(ethylene glycol)-polylactide (PELA)	Combretastatin A-4 (CA4) and hydroxycamptothecin (HCPT)	Sustained release of CA4 over 30 days, fibers showed significant antitumor efficacy and tumor vasculature destruction	[123]
HP-β-CyD	PVP	Flubendazole	The release of a dose of 40 mg in 15 min	[124]
M-β-CyD	PLLA	Doxorubicin (DOX)	17% Decrease in the burst release was observed and followed by a quantifiable sustained release up to 2 days.	[125]
HP-β-CyD	PVA	Metoclopramide hydrochloride (MH)	Burst release: 90% release in 2 min	[126]

Table 1. *Cont.*

CyD Type	Polymer Additive	Active Molecule	Release Data	Ref
β-CyD derivative	Chitosan	β-Lactamase BlaP protein	CyD increased the stability of the embedded protein	[127]
HP-β-CyD	PVP	Plai oil	The release rate ranged was in the order of 10% > 20%~30% plai oil within 24 h.	[131]
HP-β-CyD	PVP	Herbal oil	Very rapid release: 50% release in 1 min	[132]
β-CyD	PEO	Cinnamon (CEO)	Controlled release in nanofibers via bacterial protease.	[133]
β-CyD	PVA	Cinnamon (CEO)	Nanofibers showed excellent antimicrobial activity against *E. coli* and *S. aureus*.	[134]
β-CyD	PLA	Cinnamon (CEO)	High antimicrobial activity due to released CEO	[135]
β-CyD	PVA	Cinnamon (CEO)	Stronger antimicrobial activity with incorporated lysozyme	[136]
β-CyD	Chitosan and PVA	Oregano and cinnamon EOs	Lower release of Oregano EO than CEO	[137]
β-CyD	PLA	Cinnamaldehyde (CA)	Higher release with increasing CA content	[138]
β-CyD	Zein	Eucalyptus EO	Higher antimicrobial activity with increasing EEO content	[140]
HP-β-CyD	PLA	Gallic acid	Increasing release rate with CyD incorporation	[141]
β-CyD	Pullulan	Perillaldehyde	Higher release with increasing humidity	[142]
α-CyD	Xanthan	Hexanal	CyD increased the release rate	[147]
γ-CyD	PLA	α-Tocopherol (α-TC)	CyD increased higher release of α-TC.	[148]
β-CyD	PAA	Quercetin	Nanofibers showed enhanced release rate than the films	[149]
β-CyD	PVA	Retinyl acetate (RA)	Slower release with CyD incorporation	[150]

4.2. Poly-Cyclodextrin Functional Electrospun Nanofibers for Drug Delivery Systems

CyD can be cross-linked or polymerized in controlled or noncontrolled routes to form cyclodextrin based polymeric materials (poly-cyclodextrin (polyCyD)). Further, CyD can be functionalized with polymerizable groups to produce controlled CyD polymers. The poly-cyclodextrin (polyCyD) was also electrospun to form nanofibers to be used in drug delivery applications. In this regard, Oliveira et al. reported coaxial nanofibers based on polyCyD associated with poly(methacrylic acid) (PMAA) for the release of hydrophilic drug, propranolol hydrochloride (PROP) [151]. The nanofibers were cross-linked with thermal treatment at 170 °C for 48 h to obtain water-insoluble polyCyD nanofibers (Figure 5a–c). The biocompatibility of the nanofibers was explored over fibroblast cells, and high cell viability was observed. The interaction between CyD and drug molecules was explored and found to be spontaneous. The burst release of the encapsulated PROP could be modulated by coaxial electrospinning. Uniaxial nanofibers produced with PMAA/polyCyD (80:20 *w/w*) and (60:40 *w/w*) released 30% and 35% PROP in 8 h, while sole PMAA nanofibers released 100% dose in 15 min. Further, coaxial nanofibers made by polyCyD/PROP core and a shell of PMAA showed better sustained release. In another study, polyCyD was used for the release of fluconazole from the uniaxial nanofibers of polyCyD mixed with PCL and PVP [152]. The nanofibers were further coated with a hydrophobic poly(hexamethyldisiloxane) (polyHMDSO) for tailoring the fiber dissolution and the respective drug release rate. The coating process was performed under mild condition plasma polymerization. Unlike non-coated fibers, which rapidly released the drug payload, polyHMDSO-coated nanofibers prolonged drug releasing time to 24 h. The coated nanofibers were tested with bacteria, and the results showed that they could inhibit the in vitro growth of *Candida albicans*. Another polyCyD-based electrospun nanofiber system was developed using a polymer of HP-β-CyD/citric acid mixed with chitosan to obtain polyelectrolyte complexes [153]. Triclosan was mixed with polyHP-β-CyD to form ICs, and thereafter, chitosan was added to the solution. The nanofibers were cross-linked with a treatment at 90 °C for 4 h and demonstrated antimicrobial activity against the growth of *S. aureus* and *E. coli* for longer periods of time.

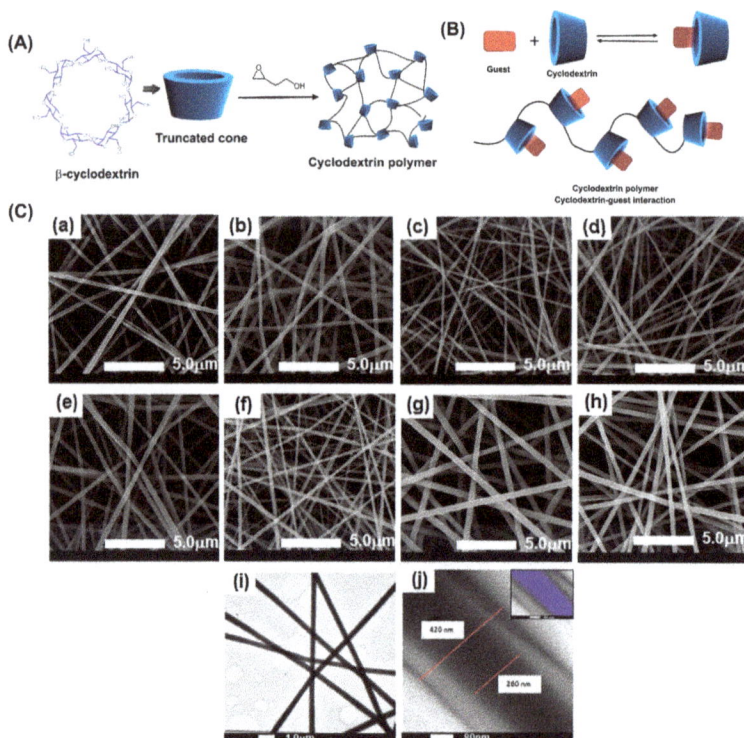

Figure 5. Cartoon schemes of (**A**) the synthesis pathway of CyD polymers and (**B**) their complexation with guest molecules. (**C**) scanning electron microscopy (SEM) and transmission electron microscopy (TEM) images of uni- and co-axial PMAA/polyCyD fibers: (**a**) SEM uniaxial–PMAA; (**b**) SEM uniaxial–PMAA + PROP; (**c**) SEM uniaxial PMAA/polyCyD (80:20); (**d**) SEM uniaxial PMAA/polyCyD (80:20) + PROP; (**e**) SEM uniaxial PMAA/polyCyD (60:40); (**f**) SEM uniaxial PMAA/polyCyD (60:40) + PROP; (**g**) SEM coaxial–shell (PMAA) and core (polyCyD); (**h**) SEM coaxial–shell (PMAA) and core (polyCyD + PROP); (**i**) TEM coaxial–shell (PMAA) and core (polyCyD + PROP); and (**j**) TEM coaxial–shell (PMAA) and core (polyCyD + PROP). The figure was reproduced from [151] with the permission of Elsevier, 2015.

Hydrophobic CyD-based polymers were also used for drug delivery applications. In this regard, Heydari et al. reported the controlled release of vitamin B2 from hydrophobic peracetyl-β-CyD polymer (Acβ-CyDP) based electrospun nanofibers [154]. Acβ-CyDP was synthesized by the acetylation of epichlorohydrin functional β-CyD polymer in the mixture of acetic acid and pyridine at 100 °C for 7 h. The electrospinning of Acβ-CyDP in the mixture of acetone and DMF (3:2, v/v) led to thin nanofibers, of which the diameters remained nearly stable even with increasing the polymer concentration from 8 to

25 wt.%, demonstrating no clear influence of CyD content on the diameters of the resultant fibers. The cumulative release of vitamin B2 from the fiber matrix was explored at two different pH values (1.2 and 7.4), and the results revealed enhanced release at pH = 1.2. The release of vitamin B2 gradually occurred, and 60 and 40% of the vitamin diffused out of the nanofibers after 170 h for the solutions having pH of 1.2 and 7.4, respectively. Nada et al. used a CyD cross-linked gelatin fiber matrix for the carrier of chloramphenicol [155]. Chloramphenicol is an antibiotic, which may lead to bone marrow suppression and influences red blood cells [156]. The oxidation of β-CyD led to polyaldehyde β-CyD, and it was used to cross-link gelatin. The nanofibers showed antimicrobial activities against *Staphylococcus aureus* (Gram positive) and *Pseudomonas aeruginosa* (Gram negative bacteria) and *Candida albicans*. After two days, the release was as ca. 90%. A water-insoluble anti-inflammatory drug atorvastatin was loaded in PCL fibers after its complexation with poly-amino-CyD molecules [157]. The quantity embedded was estimated (70–90 μg in 30 μm × 6 mm membrane) and the anti-inflammatory effect by cell contact-dependent release reached 60% inhibition for TNF-α and 80% for IL-6. Drug delivery electrospun nanofibers were also developed using PVA and carboxymethyl-β-CyD grafted chitosan [158]. The carboxymethyl-β-CyD was grafted on chitosan by 1-ethyl-3-(3-dimethylaminopropyl) carbodiimide (EDC) and *N*-hydroxysuccinimide (NHS) based coupling. Nanofibers between 130 and 210 nm in diameter were obtained. The presence of CyD molecules in the nanofibers slowed the release rate of salicylic acid (SA). After an initial burst release of SA, the release percentage reached over 80% after 24 h. CyD-functional fibers were also produced by the electrospinning of a CyD functional polymer and an antibiotic drug vancomycin [159]. The CyD-functional polymer was synthesized by poly(ethylene-vinyl alcohol) (pEVOH)/thiol-modified CyD and a bifunctional cross-linker *N*-(p-maleimidophenyl) isocyanate (PMPI). The fibers showed the sustained release of vancomycin. CyD-functional polymeric nanofibers were also used to the delivery of a common insect repellent, *N,N*-diethyl-3-toluamide (DEET) [160]. Micro-sized fibers with a diameter of 2.8 ± 0.8 μm were obtained by the electrospinning of a water-soluble β-CyD/pyromellitic dianhydride (PMDA) polymer and thereafter loaded with DEET in diethyl ether. The release data were obtained by TGA analysis, which revealed a sustained release of all DEET in two weeks. The details related to the polyCyD/drug nanofibers for drug delivery were summarized in Table 2.

Table 2. Overview of polyCyD/drug electrospun nanofibers used in drug delivery.

CyD Type	Polymer Additive	Active Molecule	Release Data	Ref
PolyCyD	PMAA	Propranolol hydrochloride (PROP)	40% Release (uniaxial PMAA:polyCyD (60:40, 80:20), 20% release from coaxial fibers	[151]
PolyCyD	PCL, PVP	Fluconazole	Burst release ((FLU-poly-α-CyD)-IC/PCL and (FLU-poly-β-CyD)-IC/PCL mats showed a burst of 85% in the first 15 min)	[152]
HP-β-CyD	Chitosan, citric acid (as cross-linker)	Triclosan	Higher release at lower pH (5.5), 80% release in 10 h	[153]
PolyCyD (peracetyl-β-CyD polymer)	-	Vitamin B2	60% (pH = 1.2) and 40% (pH = 7.4) release after 170 h	[154]
Poly aldehyde β-CyD (PA-β-CyD).	Gelatin	Chloramphenicol	Burst release for gelatin/drug (90% in 30 min), 90% release in 48 h for 7.5 and 10 wt.% PA-β-CyD	[155]
Poly-amino-β-CyD	PCL	Atorvastatin calcium trihydrate	TNF-α inhibition reached about 60% at 48 h (no dose effect), and up to 80% for IL-6, depending on the dose	[157]
Chitosan grafted carboxymethyl-β-CyD (CM β-CyD)	Chitosan	Salicylic acid	90% after 24 h at 37 °C, 84% after 24 h at 20 °C	[158]
Thiolated CyD	pEVOH/sH-CyD/PMDI	Vancomycin	Slow release	[159]
β-CyD	β-CyD/PMDA polymer	*N,N*-diethyl-3-toluamide (DEET)	Sustained release of all loaded DEET in 2 weeks.	[160]

4.3. Polymer-Free Cyclodextrin Electrospun Nanofibers for Drug Delivery Systems

Drug-loaded electrospun CyD nanofibers can also be prepared without using a polymeric carrier matrix. The electrospinning of polymer-free CyD/drug IC solutions can produce uniform nanofibers, which are solely based on CyD molecules and their ICs with drug molecules. As these electrospun nanofibers are mostly uncross-linked and hydrophilic, rapid release profiles were observed, along with the fast-dissolving fiber character. The electrospinning of CyD molecules takes place over their aggregates, which are governed by numerous hydrogen bonds. The Uyar research group has pioneered polymer-free electrospinning of nanofibers from CyD and CyD-IC based systems. The first paper was reported in 2010 [161], and it has been shown that highly concentrated (140–160 wt.%) solutions of methylated β-CyD (M-β-CyD) molecules either in water or dimethylformamide (DMF) form large aggregates driven by hydrogen bonds, which is the key factor for uniform fiber formation during electrospinning process [161]. In a later study, polymer-free nanofibers were successfully electrospun from three different CyD derivatives—HP-β-CyD, HP-γ-CyD and M-β-CyD—in three different solvent systems—water, DMF, and dimethylacetamide (DMAc) [162]. The polymer-free nanofibers from native CyD were also produced, in which electrospinning was carried out for α-CyD and β-CyD in alkaline aqueous systems [83], and γ-CyD nanofibers were electrospun from a dimethyl sulfoxide (DMSO)/water solvent system [163]. The Uyar research group has also shown that the electrospinning of uniform nanofibers could be produced from CyD-ICs without using a polymer carrier, in which triclosan/CyD ICs system was successfully electrospun into uniform and bead-free nanofibers [164]. In another study, antibacterial properties of electrospun nanofibers from triclosan/CyD IC using two different CyD derivatives (HP-β-CyD and HP-γ-CyD) were also reported [165]. Triclosan/CyD ICs electrospun nanofibers showed better antibacterial properties in the inhibition of growth of Gram-negative (*E. coli*) and Gram-positive (*S. aureus*) bacteria than pure triclosan.

Essential oils are widely implemented in medical, food, cosmetic, and allied applications due to their antibacterial, antiseptic, antifungal, and antioxidant properties [139]. The Uyar research group has made significant contributions in the fabrication of essential oil loaded CyD functional nanofibers, and several studies related to the polymer-free electrospinning of essential oils/CyD ICs were reported. Since the most of them are slightly water soluble, the use of CyD molecules in the nanofiber form can offer bulk materials loaded essential oils. Very recently, Celebioglu et al. has reported the electrospinning of CyD-camphor IC nanofibers [166]. Camphor-loaded CyD nanofibers rapidly dissolved in water because of their uncross-linked hydrophilic nature. Despite the fact that camphor is a volatile molecule, it can be preserved in the CyD cavity during electrospinning, and the molar ratio after electrospinning was calculated as ~1.00/0.65 and ~1.00/0.90 in HP-β-CyD/camphor-IC and HP-β-CyD/camphor-IC nanofibers, respectively. The camphor release from HP-β-CyD-IC and HP-γ-CyD-IC nanofibers in gas phase was monitored at two different temperatures (37 and 75 °C) using gas chromatography-mass spectrometry (GC-MS) for 4 h, where the higher temperature enhanced the release rate of camphor because of the diffusion coefficient increment of camphor molecules. Another important essential oil, eugenol, was complexed within CyD nanofibers [167]. The ICs of three cyclodextrin derivatives (HP-β-CyD, HP-γ-CyD, and M-β-CyD) with eugenol were prepared in water and electrospun to form nanofibers. Inclusion-complexation significantly enhanced water solubility and increased the thermal stability of volatile eugenol. Due to their hydrophilic and uncross-linked nature, CyD nanofibers rapidly dissolve in water. The eugenol-loaded CyD nanofibers showed a higher antioxidant capacity than eugenol itself, suggesting enhanced antioxidant activity of the fibers than the powder form of eugenol. Essential oils, *p*-cymene and cineole, were also embedded in polymer-free CyD nanofibers in the form of CyD-ICs [168]. Electrospun nanowebs were produced by the ICs of *p*-cymene and cineole with two modified cyclodextrins (HP-β-CyD and HP-γ-CyD). The thermal stability of both *p*-cymene and cineole increased with inclusion-complexation. On contact, the nanofibers rapidly dissolved in water. Linalool, a natural ingredient of many essential oils, was also loaded into CyD nanofibers as ICs through electrospinning [169]. Well-tuned nanofibers were obtained with antibacterial properties. Antibacterial limonene-loaded polymer-free CyD nanofibers were prepared by electrospinning [170]. Modified cyclodextrins (M-β-CyD, HP-β-CyD and HP-γ-CyD) and limonene were mixed to form ICs. The computational and experimental results revealed the molar ratio of the CyD-limonene was 1:1. The released limonene from M-β-CyD/limonene-IC was less than the nanofibers of HP-β-CyD/limonene-IC and HP-γ-CyD/limonene-IC due to the higher amount of the preserved limonene in the nanofiber. 25% limonene was released from M-β-CyD/limonene-IC nanofibers, whereas the nanofibers of HP-β-CyD/limonene-IC and HP-γ-CyD/limonene-IC released 51 and 88 wt.% limonene in 100 days, respectively. Inclusion-complexation significantly enhanced the thermal stability of the entrapped active molecules. The nanofibers significantly inhibited the growth of *S. aureus* and *E. coli* because of the antibacterial property of limonene. In addition, the nanofibers rapidly dissolved in water because of the polymer-free nature of hydrophilic CyD derivatives. Geraniol-CyD ICs-loaded nanofibers were also reported by the Uyar research group without the requirement of any polymer carrier [171]. Bead-free nanofibers were obtained using three different CyD types e.g., HP-β-CyD, M-β-CyD, and HP-γ-CyD. Even though geraniol is a volatile molecule, it could be preserved in the nanofibers in the range of ∼60–90% depending on formulation parameters. The release studies were either performed at room temperature or short term at high temperature (37, 50, and 75 °C), and the results revealed M-β-CyD /geraniol-IC complex loaded nanofibers released less geraniol than the nanofibers of HP-β-CyD/geraniol-IC and HP-γ-CyD/geraniol-IC, suggesting the strongest inclusion-complexation occurred between M-β-CyD and geraniol. The nanofibers showed antibacterial properties in the sense of the inhibition of growth of *E. coli* and *S. aureus* because of the released geraniol from the fiber matrix. Furthermore, the nanofibers showed enhanced antioxidant activity to those of pure geraniol because of its low water solubility. Likewise, thymol-loaded CyD nanofibers were prepared as ICs of CyD (M-β-CyD, HP-β-CyD, and HP-γ-CyD) [172]. Due to the volatile nature of thymol, it was entrapped in the CyD cavity to enhance its thermal stability. Thymol-loaded CyD nanofibers showed more rapid dissolution in water than hydrophobic thymol. Due to the antioxidant properties of thymol, the respective nanofibers were tested by DPPH radical scavenging, and high scavenging capacity was observed. Polymer-free CyD nanofibers were also electrospun from their ICs with volatile flavor agents e.g., menthol [173] and vanillin [174], and vitamins e.g., vitamin E [175] with enhanced solubility and prolonged shelf-life. Recently, Uyar and colleagues reported the polymer-free electrospinning of carvacrol/CyD ICs [176]. Carvacrol is a phenolic component of plant essential oils and has antioxidant and antimicrobial properties [177,178]. The ICs of carvacrol with HP-β-CyD or HP-β-CyD were electrospun into fibers. These fast dissolving fibers showed enhanced antioxidant activity with an increase content of carvacrol.

In order to develop a fast-dissolving drug/CyD IC nanofibrous system, the ICs of sulfisoxazole (SFS) and sulfobutyl ether β-CyD (SBE7-β-CyD) were prepared in water, and thereafter, electrospun into nanofibers in the form of self-standing flexible nanofibrous webs (Figure 6) [179]. In parallel, the ICs of SBE7-β-CyD and SFS were prepared as powder. On contact with water, the entrapped SFS was released from the polymer nanofibers, along with the disintegration of the fibers (Figure 7). The polymer-free nanofibers of SBE7-β-CyD-SFS ICs showed faster dissolution than the powder form of the SBE7-β-CyD-SFS ICs, and pure SFS was not soluble in water in the absence of CyD (Figure 7). These fast dissolving CyD functional fiber nanowebs can be implemented if the rapid release of water-insoluble drugs, as the case here with SFS, is desired.

Another fast-dissolving polymer-free fiber system loaded with poorly soluble diclofenac sodium was reported by Balogh et al. [180]. The fibers rapidly dissolved in water (within 2 min). Spironolactone, a diuretic drug with antiandrogenic properties, was complexed with CyD and electrospun into nanofibers without the requirement of any polymeric carrier [181]. The resultant nanofibers rapidly dissolved in water, and the system allowed high loading of lipophilic spironolactone. An interesting CyD based polymer-free fiber system for drug delivery applications was developed using modified γ-CyD molecules. Yu et al. modified γ-CyD with phenylacetic acid and performed electrospinning from the mixed solution of dichloromethane (DCM) and dimethylformamide (DMF) (8:2, *v/v*) to form fibers (Figure 8) [182]. The bead-free, water insoluble ultrafine fibers with a diameter range of 1–2 μm were obtained. Unlike other polymer-free CyD fibers, these fibers did not show rapid dissolution. In vitro cell tests revealed the fibers are biocompatible. Several drug molecules (doxorubicin, fluorescein isothiocyanate-dextran (FITC-dextran), recombinant human insulin (FITC-labeled insulin), and chlorin) were loaded by simply incubating the fibers in the solutions of the respective drug molecules. ~50% of Release of the entrapped drug molecules was observed from the fiber matrix in one month, demonstrating their slow release (Figure 8E). Chlorin-loaded fibers were also exploited for in vivo drug release in mice, and on day 28, the complete release of chlorin was observed because of the disappearance of its fluorescence signal. The general overview of polymer-free CD/drug ICs fibers for drug delivery was summarized in Table 3.

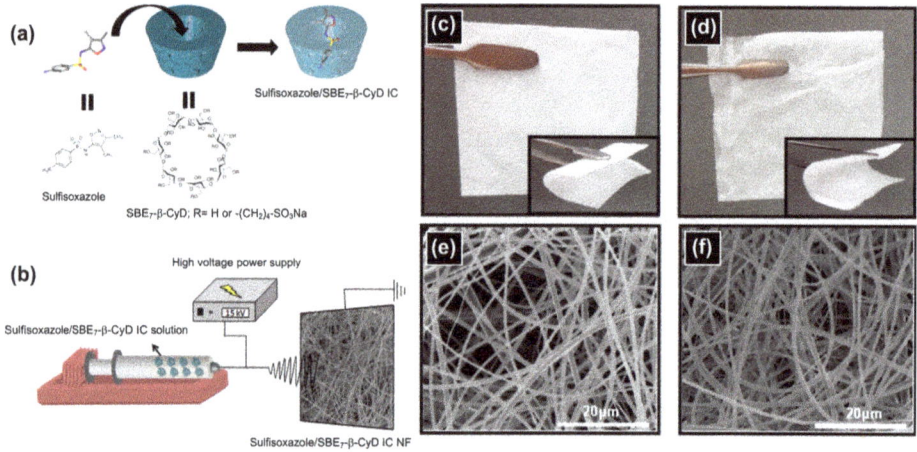

Figure 6. (a) Cartoon illustration of inclusion-complexation between CyD and sulfisoxazole (SFS). The chemical structure of sulfisoxazole and SBE_7-β-CyD with a schematic representation of sulfisoxazole, SBE_7-β-CyD and their IC, (b) schematic representation of the electrospinning of SFS/SBE_7-β-CyD-IC NF. Photographs of electrospun (c) SBE_7-β-CyD nanofibers, (d) SFS/SBE_7-β-CyD-IC nanofibers, and SEM images of (e) SBE_7-β-CyD NF, (f) SFS/SBE_7-β-CyD-IC nanofibers. The figure was reproduced from [179] with the permission of Elsevier, 2017.

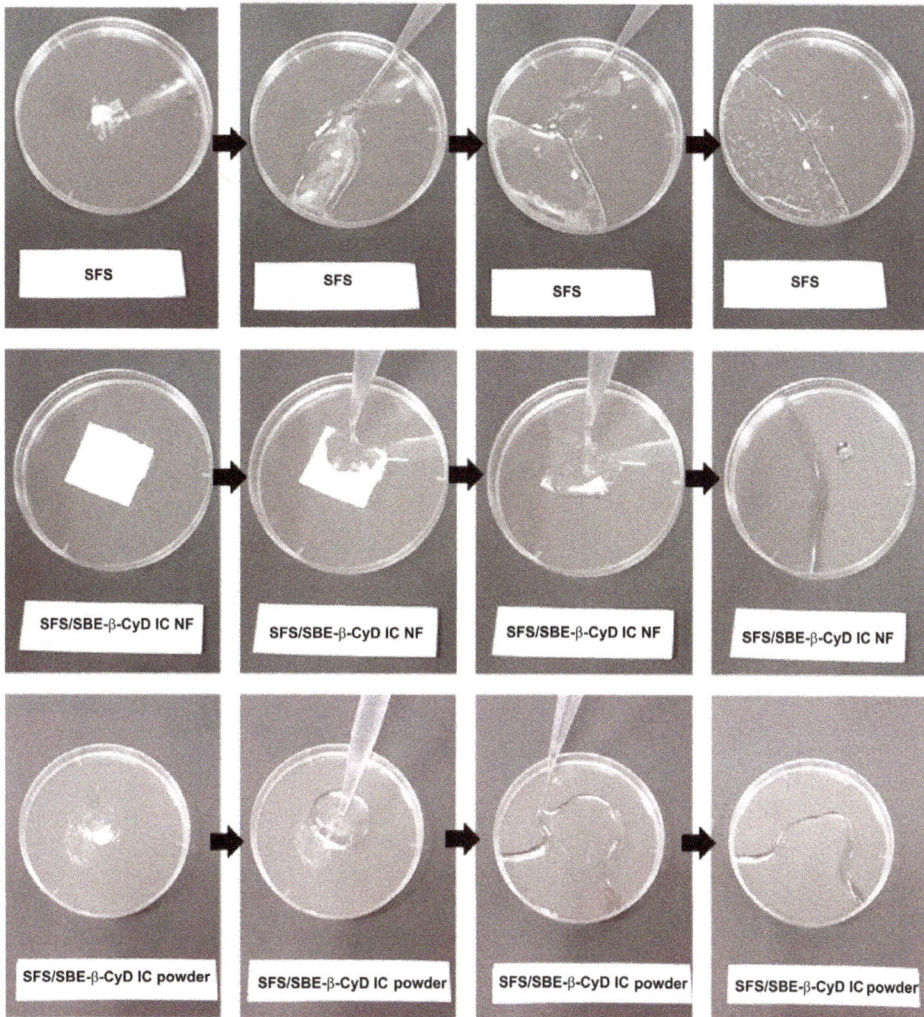

Figure 7. Typical water-solubility of the drug loaded polymer-free CyD fibers. The representative photos of the SFS and SFS/ SBE$_7$-β-CyD IC powder and SFS/ SBE$_7$-β-CyD IC nanofibers on exposure to water. The figure was reproduced from [179] with the permission of Elsevier, 2017.

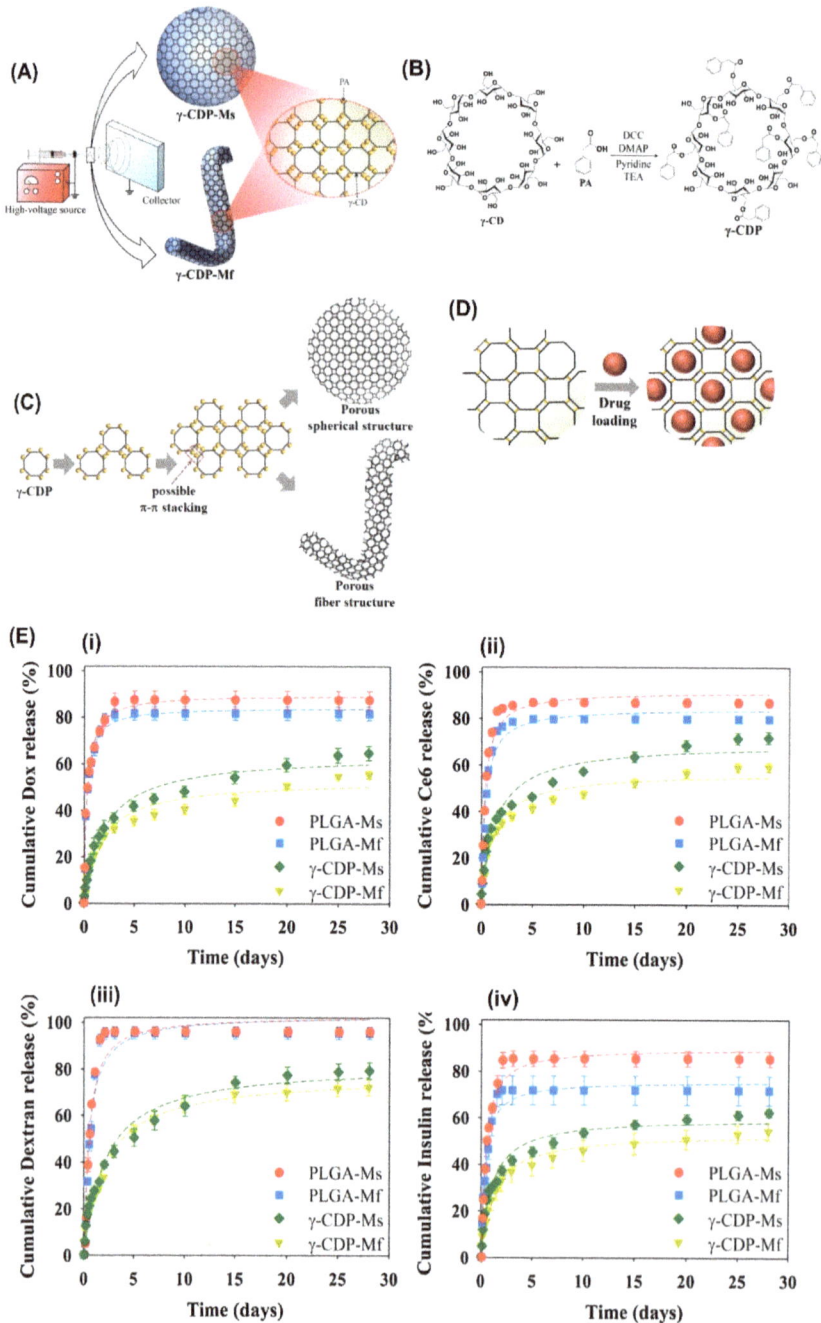

Figure 8. (**A**) A schematic representation of the electrospinning and electrospraying of γ-CyDPs. (**B**) The synthesis pathway of γ-CyDP. (**C**) Cartoon schemes of γ-CyDP-microspheres (Ms) or γ-CyDP microfibers (Mf) with porous structure and (**D**) their drug loading. (**E**) The cumulative molecule (**i**) Dox, (**ii**) Ce6, (**iii**) dextran, and (**iv**) insulin release (wt. %) from PLGA-Ms, PLGA-Mf, γ-CyDP-Ms, and γ-CyDP-Mf (*n* = 3). The figure was reproduced from [182] with the permission of Elsevier, 2018.

Table 3. Overview of polymer-free CyD/drug ICs electrospun nanofibers used in drug delivery.

CyD type	Active molecule	Release data	Ref
HP-β-CyD, HP-γ-CyD	Triclosan	Rapid release on contact with water and significant inhibition against *E. coli* and *S. aureus*	[165]
HP-β-CyD, HP-γ-CyD	Camphor	In gas phase, faster release at higher temp., faster for the HP-β-CyD system	[166]
HP-β-CyD, HP-γ-CyD, and M-β-CyD	Eugenol	Rapid release on contact with water, enhanced antioxidant activity than eugenol itself	[167]
HP-β-CyD, HP-γ-CyD	Cineole and *p*-cymene	Rapid release along with the fiber dissolution	[168]
HP-β-CyD, HP-γ-CyD, and M-β-CyD	Linalool	Rapid release, significant inhibition against the growth of *E. coli* and *S. aureus*	[169]
HP-β-CyD, HP-γ-CyD and M-β-CyD	Limonene	25% Release M-β-CyD/limonene-IC-NF, 51% release HP-β-CyD/limonene-IC-NF, 88% release HP-γ-CyD/limonene-IC-NF in 100 days	[170]
HP-β-CyD, HP-γ-CyD and M-β-CyD	Geraniol	Long-term stability of geraniol in gas phase	[171]
HP-β-CyD, HP-γ-CyD and M-β-CyD	Thymol	Immediately on contact with water	[172]
HP-β-CyD, HP-γ-CyD	Menthol	Rapid release along with the fiber dissolution	[173]
HP-β-CyD, HP-γ-CyD and M-β-CyD	Vanillin	Immediately on contact with water, enhanced antioxidant activity with nanofibers	[174]
HP-β-CyD	Vitamin E	Rapid and enhanced release, higher antioxidant activity with CyD	[175]
HP-β-CyD, HP-β-CyD	Carvacrol	Rapid release on contact with water	[176]
SBE$_7$-β-CyD	Sulfisoxazole	Rapid and enhanced release of sulfisoxazole on contact with water	[179]
HP-β-CyD	Diclofenac sodium	Release in few minutes	[180]
HP-β-CyD	Spironolactone	Total release in 1 h	[181]
Phenylacetic-β-CyD	Doxorubicin, fluorescein isothiocyanate-dextran (FITC-dextran), recombinant human insulin (FITC-labeled insulin) and chlorin e6	50% Release of drugs in vitro in 30 days, ~100% release of chlorin in vivo on day 28	[182]

5. Concluding Remarks and Future Outlook

Electrospinning has become a dynamic, rapidly changing field that can affect human lives in diverse ways. It allows for the production of electrospun nanofibers with tailored-made properties to address problems in the environment, biomedicine, textile, and food industries. High specific surface area, ease of operation, adaptability, tunable fiber texture, and a wide size spectrum make the electrospun nanofibers potential drug carriers with many intrinsic benefits, including enhanced drug loading, controlled release of drugs, and a short diffusion pathway. Further, processing parameters and structural modification allow tuning the fiber structure for the sustained release of drug molecules—for example, in the case of co-axial nanofibers with the drugs-embedded in the core. In this regard, various drug molecules with anticancer, antibiotic, antimicrobial, or antioxidant properties were incorporated into electrospun fibers, mostly using their ICs with CyD. The non-specific incorporation of such drug molecules can cause undesired release profiles, low drug loadings, activity loss of environmentally sensitive drugs, or other problems. In this regard, the incorporation of biocompatible nanocarriers into such systems allows the fabrication of high-performance drug delivery nanomaterials. Toward this goal, CyD molecules have found a large application area because of their unique 3D structure, which endows nanofibers with distinct features e.g., enhanced drug solubility, stability, and bioavailability useful in drug delivery applications. Furthermore, they do not provoke the immune system and have low toxicities to mammals. Hence, they have become important excipients in pharmaceutical applications. Native CyD, particularly β-CyD, have ideal cavity size related to complex with a wide range of chemicals but have significant issues related to the poor water solubility of native CyD. These drawbacks of β-CyD can be mitigated by chemical modifications to produce highly soluble derivatives, such as hydroxypropyl functional-CyD. CyD-functional electrospun nanofibers were prepared by either blending of CyD-drug complexes with polymers or using CyD polymers with another polymer carrier or standalone. CyD molecules could also be electrospun without the requirement of a carrier polymer. In the latter case, CyD and guest molecules were mixed to form ICs and their electrospinning produced polymer-free nanofibers with high drug loading. However, these fibers, on contact, rapidly dissolve in water and release the entrapped drug molecules in the form of CyD-drug ICs without any control on drug release. Tables 1–3 give the characteristics of some selected examples on CyD functional electrospun nanofibers used in drug delivery applications. All these fiber systems have their own pros and cons. Still, there is a growing interest to engineer CyD-functional drug delivery systems that deliver therapeutics in a safe, effective, and targeted fashion. The most of researches in this field concentrated on the blending of CyD-drug ICs with various polymers. This route produces CyD-drug IC loaded polymeric nanofibers with longer dissolution time depending on the structural properties of polymeric carrier in the fiber. The CyD-drug ICs can also be electrospun in the absence of a polymer. However, such fibers rapidly dissolve on contact with water, and drug molecules are released in the forms of CyD-drug ICs. In contrast to both methods, the polyCyD fibers can be engineered and used in drug delivery with a better control on release profiles. A schematic overview of the CyD-functional nanofibers was shown in Figure 9, where important parameters of the relevant synthesis routes are pointed out. Each preparation approach comprises different benefits. While polymer-free CyD nanofibers are simpler to produce, they suffer from the instant water solubility. However, in this context, hydrophobically-modified CyD can offer water-insoluble polymer-free fiber meshes. On the other hand, polyCyD functional nanofibers have certain difficulties in the synthesis of functional CyD derivatives and their polymers. Regardless of preparation route, the ability to tune fiber structure should facilitate the sustained release of drugs, such as through co-axial electrospinning.

The use of CyD in electrospun nanofibers for drug delivery systems are likely to find increasing interest in the coming years. Currently, there are significant advances in polyCyD electrospun nanofibers produced without the need of any additional polymeric carrier. These water insoluble nanofibers exhibited the efficient removal of water micropollutants, e.g., methylene blue, because of their high active CyD contents [183]. In the future, such nanofibers may find applications in drug delivery. Further, a stimulus can be applied for the release of drug molecules from the CyD cavity in a controllable fashion. Likewise, CyD-containing polymers, particularly those contain CyD as pendent motifs on the polymer backbone can offer promising results for the sustained release of drugs from the fiber matrix depending on the hydrophobicity of the polymer. In this regard, cross-linked nano-porous β-CyD polymers showed enhanced IC constant as high as 10^9 M^{-1} than those uncross-linked ones (native β-CyD, 10^3 M^{-1}) [184]. Beside their use in in vitro drug release applications, CyD-functional electrospun materials will find more applications as implant materials in tissue engineering. Unlike CyD-free electrospun fibers, the functionalization of electrospun fibers with CyD can improve their properties in terms of high drug loading, increased stability, and bioavailability of the payloads in the body.

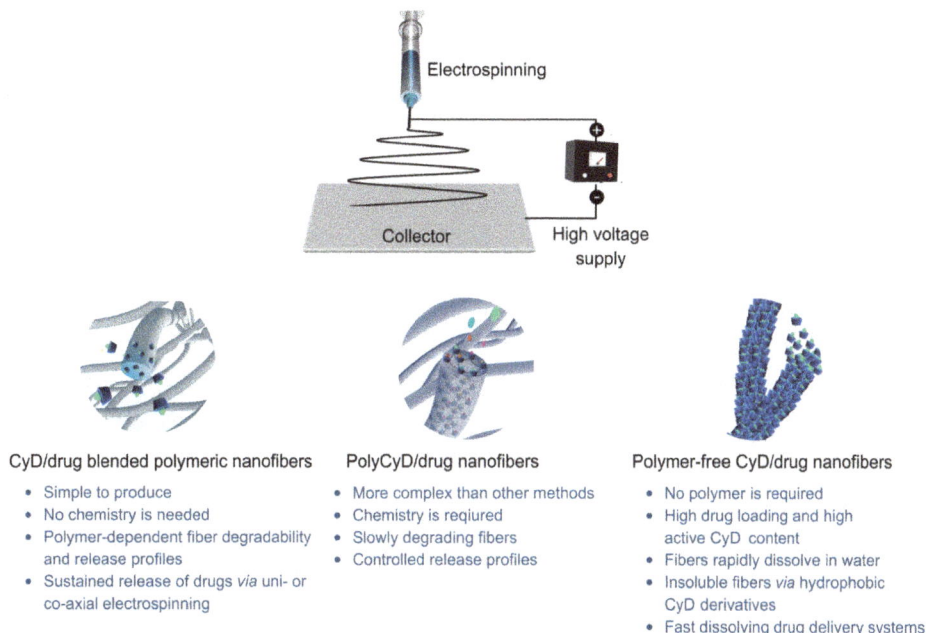

CyD/drug blended polymeric nanofibers	PolyCyD/drug nanofibers	Polymer-free CyD/drug nanofibers
• Simple to produce • No chemistry is needed • Polymer-dependent fiber degradability and release profiles • Sustained release of drugs *via* uni- or co-axial electrospinning	• More complex than other methods • Chemistry is reqiured • Slowly degrading fibers • Controlled release profiles	• No polymer is required • High drug loading and high active CyD content • Fibers rapidly dissolve in water • Insoluble fibers *via* hydrophobic CyD derivatives • Fast dissolving drug delivery systems

Figure 9. Cartoon illustration of CyD-functional electrospun nanofibers used for drug delivery applications.

To conclude, drug delivery is a dynamic and complex process and can be adapted to meet the needs of the targeted application. Advanced drug delivery therapy requires nontoxic pharmaceutical excipients to provide high drug loading and keeps the drugs stable, active, and accessible for bioavailability. In this regard, CyD-functional nanofibers would be one of the best material systems for drug delivery applications since they offer intrinsic features of both electrospun nanofibers and CyD possessing a hydrophobic molecular-environment for drug entrapment. CyD, thus, significantly increase water solubility of hydrophobic drug molecules (i.e., for high drug loading) and shield drug molecules from physiological degradation or elimination for bioavailability while nanofiber form offers high specific surface area, ease of operation, and further control on the nanofiber form for the sustained release of the entrapped drug molecules. As the electrospinning produces tailored nanostructured materials with further control mechanisms on drug release, the utilization of CyD-functional electrospun materials will increase to meet the demands of advanced drug delivery systems.

Author Contributions: F.T. and T.U. conceived the review. F.T. with the supervision of T.U. analyzed the references and wrote the manuscript. T.U. revised and reviewed the manuscript.

Conflicts of Interest: The authors have no conflicts of interest to declare.

Abbreviations

Ac-β-CyDP	Peracetyl-β-CyD polymer
AITC	Allyl isocyanate
AV	Aloe Vera
CEO	Cinnamon essential oil
CIP	Ciprofloxacin
CUR	Curcumin
CyD	Cyclodextrins
CZ	Clotrimazole
DDS	Drug Delivery System
DPPH	2,2-Diphenyl-1-picrylhydrazyl
E. coli	*Escherichia coli*
EEO	Eucalyptus essential oil
EtOH	Ethanol
FDA	Federal Drug Administration
GC-MS	Gas chromatograph mass spectrometry
HCPT	Hydroxycamptothecin
HPC	Hydroxypropyl cellulose
HP-β-CyD	Hydroxypropyl-β-cyclodextrin
IC	Inclusion-Complex
MX	Meloxicam
M-β-CyD	Methyl-β-Cyclodextrin
NAP	Naproxen
PCL	Polycaprolactone
PEG	Poly(ethylene glycol)
PEO	Poly(ethylene oxide)
PLACL	Poly (L-lactic acid-*co*-ε-caprolactone)
PLLA	Poly (L-lactic acid)
PMAA	Poly(methylacrylic acid)
PolyCyD	Polycyclodextrin
PROP	Propranolol hydrochloride
PS	Polystyrene
PVA	Poly(vinyl alcohol)
RA	Retinyl acetate
RH	Relative humidity
S. aureus	*Staphylococcus aureus*
SA	Salicylic acid
SAg	Silver sulfadiazine
SFS	Sulfisoxazole
TAM	Tamoxifen
TCN	Tetracycline
VRC	Voriconazole

References

1. Zeng, J.; Xu, X.; Chen, X.; Liang, Q.; Bian, X.; Yang, L.; Jing, X. Biodegradable electrospun fibers for drug delivery. *J. Control. Release* **2003**, *92*, 227–231. [CrossRef]
2. Sill, T.J.; von Recum, H.A. Electrospinning: Applications in drug delivery and tissue engineering. *Biomaterials* **2008**, *29*, 1989–2006. [CrossRef] [PubMed]
3. Yoo, H.S.; Kim, T.G.; Park, T.G. Surface-functionalized electrospun nanofibers for tissue engineering and drug delivery. *Adv. Drug Deliv. Rev.* **2009**, *61*, 1033–1042. [CrossRef] [PubMed]

4. Kenawy, E.-R.; Bowlin, G.L.; Mansfield, K.; Layman, J.; Simpson, D.G.; Sanders, E.H.; Wnek, G.E. Release of tetracycline hydrochloride from electrospun poly(ethylene-co-vinylacetate), poly(lactic acid), and a blend. *J. Control. Release* **2002**, *81*, 57–64. [CrossRef]

5. Zeng, J.; Yang, L.; Liang, Q.; Zhang, X.; Guan, H.; Xu, X.; Chen, X.; Jing, X. Influence of the drug compatibility with polymer solution on the release kinetics of electrospun fiber formulation. *J. Control. Release* **2005**, *105*, 43–51. [CrossRef] [PubMed]

6. Katti, D.S.; Robinson, K.W.; Ko, F.K.; Laurencin, C.T. Bioresorbable nanofiber-based systems for wound healing and drug delivery: Optimization of fabrication parameters. *J. Biomed. Mater. Res. Part B Appl. Biomater.* **2004**, *70B*, 286–296. [CrossRef] [PubMed]

7. Wenguo, C.; Yue, Z.; Jiang, C. Electrospun nanofibrous materials for tissue engineering and drug delivery. *Sci. Technol. Adv. Mater.* **2010**, *11*, 014108.

8. Deng-Guang, Y.; Xia-Xia, S.; Chris, B.-W.; Kenneth, W.; Li-Min, Z.; Bligh, S.W.A. Oral fast-dissolving drug delivery membranes prepared from electrospun polyvinylpyrrolidone ultrafine fibers. *Nanotechnology* **2009**, *20*, 055104.

9. Bognitzki, M.; Czado, W.; Frese, T.; Schaper, A.; Hellwig, M.; Steinhart, M.; Greiner, A.; Wendorff, J.H. Nanostructured fibers via electrospinning. *Adv. Mater.* **2001**, *13*, 70–72. [CrossRef]

10. He, C.L.; Huang, Z.M.; Han, X.J.; Liu, L.; Zhang, H.S.; Chen, L.S. Coaxial electrospun poly(L-lactic acid) ultrafine fibers for sustained drug delivery. *J. Macromol. Sci. Part B* **2006**, *45*, 515–524. [CrossRef]

11. Uyar, T.; Kny, E. *Electrospun Materials for Tissue Engineering and Biomedical Applications: Research, Design and Commercialization*; Elsevier: New York, NY, USA; Woodhead Publishing: Sawston/Cambridge, UK, 2017; ISBN 9780081010228.

12. Grafahrend, D.; Heffels, K.-H.; Beer, M.V.; Gasteier, P.; Möller, M.; Boehm, G.; Dalton, P.D.; Groll, J. Degradable polyester scaffolds with controlled surface chemistry combining minimal protein adsorption with specific bioactivation. *Nat. Mater.* **2010**, *10*, 67. [CrossRef] [PubMed]

13. Choi Ji, S.; Messersmith Phillip, B.; Yoo Hyuk, S. Decoration of electrospun nanofibers with monomeric catechols to facilitate cell adhesion. *Macromol. Biosci.* **2013**, *14*, 270–279. [CrossRef] [PubMed]

14. Pires, L.R. 9-electrospun fibers for drug and molecular delivery a2-guarino, vincenzo. In *Electrofluidodynamic Technologies (Efdts) for Biomaterials and Medical Devices*; Ambrosio, L., Ed.; Woodhead Publishing: Sawston/Cambridge, UK, 2018; pp. 157–177.

15. Yu, D.-G.; Li, X.-Y.; Wang, X.; Chian, W.; Liao, Y.-Z.; Li, Y. Zero-order drug release cellulose acetate nanofibers prepared using coaxial electrospinning. *Cellulose* **2013**, *20*, 379–389. [CrossRef]

16. Gizaw, M.; Thompson, J.; Faglie, A.; Lee, S.-Y.; Neuenschwander, P.; Chou, S.-F. Electrospun fibers as a dressing material for drug and biological agent delivery in wound healing applications. *Bioengineering* **2018**, *5*, 9. [CrossRef] [PubMed]

17. Liu, M.; Duan, X.-P.; Li, Y.-M.; Yang, D.-P.; Long, Y.-Z. Electrospun nanofibers for wound healing. *Mater. Sci. Eng. C* **2017**, *76*, 1413–1423. [CrossRef] [PubMed]

18. Pinho, E.; Grootveld, M.; Soares, G.; Henriques, M. Cyclodextrin-based hydrogels toward improved wound dressings. *Crit. Rev. Biotechnol.* **2014**, *34*, 328–337. [CrossRef] [PubMed]

19. Luo, X.; Xie, C.; Wang, H.; Liu, C.; Yan, S.; Li, X. Antitumor activities of emulsion electrospun fibers with core loading of hydroxycamptothccin via intratumoral implantation. *Int. J. Pharm.* **2012**, *425*, 19–28. [CrossRef] [PubMed]

20. Deluzio, T.G.B.; Penev, K.I.; Mequanint, K. Cyclodextrin inclusion complexes as potential oxygen delivery vehicles in tissue engineering. *J. Biomater. Tissue Eng.* **2014**, *4*, 957–966. [CrossRef]

21. Khajavi, R.; Abbasipour, M. Electrospinning as a versatile method for fabricating coreshell, hollow and porous nanofibers. *Sci. Iran.* **2012**, *19*, 2029–2034. [CrossRef]

22. Al-Enizi, A.; Zagho, M.; Elzatahry, A. Polymer-based electrospun nanofibers for biomedical applications. *Nanomaterials* **2018**, *8*, 259. [CrossRef]

23. Dash, T.K.; Konkimalla, V.B. Poly-e-caprolactone based formulations for drug delivery and tissue engineering: A review. *J. Control. Release* **2012**, *158*, 15–33. [CrossRef]

24. Yoon, H.; Kim, G. A three-dimensional polycaprolactone scaffold combined with a drug delivery system consisting of electrospun nanofibers. *J. Pharm. Sci.* **2011**, *100*, 424–430. [CrossRef]

25. Chen, S.C.; Huang, X.B.; Cai, X.M.; Lu, J.; Yuan, J.; Shen, J. The influence of fiber diameter of electrospun poly(lactic acid) on drug delivery. *Fibers Polym.* **2012**, *13*, 1120–1125. [CrossRef]

26. Repanas, A.; Glasmacher, B. Dipyridamole embedded in polycaprolactone fibers prepared by coaxial electrospinning as a novel drug delivery system. *J. Drug Deliv. Sci. Technol.* **2015**, *29*, 132–142. [CrossRef]

27. Schaub, N.J.; Le Beux, C.; Miao, J.; Linhardt, R.J.; Alauzun, J.G.; Laurencin, D.; Gilbert, R.J. The effect of surface modification of aligned poly-L-lactic acid electrospun fibers on fiber degradation and neurite extension. *PLoS ONE* **2015**, *10*, e0136780. [CrossRef] [PubMed]

28. Chou, S.-F.; Carson, D.; Woodrow, K.A. Current strategies for sustaining drug release from electrospun nanofibers. *J. Control. Release* **2015**, *220*, 584–591. [CrossRef]

29. Ulery, B.D.; Nair, L.S.; Laurencin, C.T. Biomedical applications of biodegradable polymers. *J. Polym. Sci. Part B Polym. Phys.* **2011**, *49*, 832–864. [CrossRef]

30. Otero-Espinar, F.J.; Torres-Labandeira, J.J.; Alvarez-Lorenzo, C.; Blanco-Méndez, J. Cyclodextrins in drug delivery systems. *J. Drug Deliv. Sci. Technol.* **2010**, *20*, 289–301. [CrossRef]

31. Loftsson, T.; Vogensen, S.B.; Brewster, M.E.; Konradsdottir, F. Effects of cyclodextrins on drug delivery through biological membranes. *J. Pharm. Sci.* **2007**, *96*, 2532–2546. [CrossRef]

32. Garg, K.; Bowlin, G.L. Electrospinning jets and nanofibrous structures. *Biomicrofluidics* **2011**, *5*, 013403. [CrossRef]

33. Darrell, H.R.; Iksoo, C. Nanometre diameter fibres of polymer, produced by electrospinning. *Nanotechnology* **1996**, *7*, 216.

34. Ziabicki, A. *Fundamentals of Fibre Formation*; Wiley-Interscience: New York, NY, USA, 1976.

35. Fong, H.; Chun, I.; Reneker, D.H. Beaded nanofibers formed during electrospinning. *Polymer* **1999**, *40*, 4585–4592. [CrossRef]

36. Lee, K.H.; Kim, H.Y.; Bang, H.J.; Jung, Y.H.; Lee, S.G. The change of bead morphology formed on electrospun polystyrene fibers. *Polymer* **2003**, *44*, 4029–4034. [CrossRef]

37. Uyar, T.; Besenbacher, F. Electrospinning of uniform polystyrene fibers: The effect of solvent conductivity. *Polymer* **2008**, *49*, 5336–5343. [CrossRef]

38. Li, Z.; Wang, C. Effects of working parameters on electrospinning. In *One-Dimensional Nanostructures: Electrospinning Technique and Unique Nanofibers*; Li, Z., Wang, C., Eds.; Springer: Berlin/Heidelberg, Germany, 2013; pp. 15–28.

39. Qin, X.H.; Yang, E.L.; Li, N.; Wang, S.Y. Effect of different salts on electrospinning of polyacrylonitrile (PAN) polymer solution. *J. Appl. Polym. Sci.* **2006**, *103*, 3865–3870. [CrossRef]

40. Loftsson, T.; Duchene, D. Cyclodextrins and their pharmaceutical applications. *Int. J. Pharm.* **2007**, *329*, 1–11. [CrossRef]

41. Crini, G. Review: A history of cyclodextrins. *Chem. Rev.* **2014**, *114*, 10940–10975. [CrossRef]

42. Morillo, E.; Sánchez-Trujillo, M.A.; Moyano, J.R.; Villaverde, J.; Gómez-Pantoja, M.E.; Pérez-Martínez, J.I. Enhanced solubilisation of six pahs by three synthetic cyclodextrins for remediation applications: Molecular modelling of the inclusion complexes. *PLoS ONE* **2012**, *7*, e44137. [CrossRef]

43. Song, L.X.; Bai, L.; Xu, X.M.; He, J.; Pan, S.Z. Inclusion complexation, encapsulation interaction and inclusion number in cyclodextrin chemistry. *Coord. Chem. Rev.* **2009**, *253*, 1276–1284. [CrossRef]

44. Villiers, A. Sur la fermentation de la fecule par l'action du ferment butyrique. *Compt. Rend. Acad. Sci.* **1891**, *112*, 536–538.

45. Lakkakula, J.R.; Krause, R.W.M. A vision for cyclodextrin nanoparticles in drug delivery systems and pharmaceutical applications. *Nanomedicine* **2014**, *9*, 877–894. [CrossRef] [PubMed]

46. Tiwari, G.; Tiwari, R.; Rai, A.K. Cyclodextrins in delivery systems: Applications. *J. Pharm. Bioallied Sci.* **2010**, *2*, 72–79. [CrossRef] [PubMed]

47. Shieh, W.J.; Hedges, A.R. Properties and applications of cyclodextrins. *J. Macromol. Sci. Part A* **1996**, *33*, 673–683. [CrossRef]

48. Singh, M.; Sharma, R.; Banerjee, U.C. Biotechnological applications of cyclodextrins. *Biotechnol. Adv.* **2002**, *20*, 341–359. [CrossRef]

49. Szejtli, J. Introduction and general overview of cyclodextrin chemistry. *Chem. Rev.* **1998**, *98*, 1743–1754. [CrossRef] [PubMed]

50. Davis, M.E.; Brewster, M.E. Cyclodextrin-based pharmaceutics: Past, present and future. *Nat. Rev. Drug Discov.* **2004**, *3*, 1023. [CrossRef]

51. Wolfram, S.; Mathias, N. Topographie der cyclodextrin-einschlußverbindungen, VII. Röntgenstrukturanalyse des α-cyclodextrin. Krypton-pentahydrats. Zum einschlußmechanismus des modell-enzyms. *Chem. Ber.* **1976**, *109*, 503–517.

52. Harata, K. Structural aspects of stereodifferentiation in the solid state. *Chem. Rev.* **1998**, *98*, 1803–1828. [CrossRef]

53. Sonoda, Y.; Hirayama, F.; Arima, H.; Yamaguchi, Y.; Saenger, W.; Uekama, K. Cyclodextrin-based isolation of ostwald's metastable polymorphs occurring during crystallization. *Chem. Commun.* **2006**, 517–519. [CrossRef] [PubMed]

54. Hapiot, F.; Tilloy, S.; Monflier, E. Cyclodextrins as supramolecular hosts for organometallic complexes. *Chem. Rev.* **2006**, *106*, 767–781. [CrossRef] [PubMed]

55. Loftsson, T.; Jarho, P.; Másson, M.; Järvinen, T. Cyclodextrins in drug delivery. *Expert Opin. Drug Deliv.* **2005**, *2*, 335–351. [CrossRef] [PubMed]

56. Uekama, K.; Hirayama, F.; Irie, T. Cyclodextrin drug carrier systems. *Chem. Rev.* **1998**, *98*, 2045–2076. [CrossRef] [PubMed]

57. Frank, D.W.; Gray, J.E.; Weaver, R.N. Cyclodextrin nephrosis in the rat. *Am. J. Pathol.* **1976**, *83*, 367–382. [PubMed]

58. Matsuda, K.; Mera, Y.; Segawa, Y. Acute toxicity study of γ-cyclodextrin (γ-CD) in mice and rats. *Pharmacometrics* **1983**, *26*, 287–291.

59. Irie, T.; Uekama, K. Pharmaceutical applications of cyclodextrins. Iii. Toxicological issues and safety evaluation. *J. Pharm. Sci.* **1997**, *86*, 147–162. [CrossRef]

60. Ohtani, Y.; Irie, T.; Uekama, K.; Fukunaga, K.; Pitha, J. Differential effects of α-, β- and γ-cyclodextrins on human erythrocytes. *Eur. J. Biochem.* **1989**, *186*, 17–22. [CrossRef]

61. Zimmer, S.; Grebe, A.; Bakke, S.S.; Bode, N.; Halvorsen, B.; Ulas, T.; Skjelland, M.; De Nardo, D.; Labzin, L.I.; Kerksiek, A.; et al. Cyclodextrin promotes atherosclerosis regression via macrophage reprogramming. *Sci. Transl. Med.* **2016**, *8*, 333ra350. [CrossRef]

62. Rajewski, R.A.; Traiger, G.; Bresnahan, J.; Jaberaboansar, P.; Stella, V.J.; Thompson, D.O. Preliminary safety evaluation of parenterally administered sulfoalkyl ether β-cyclodextrin derivatives. *J. Pharm. Sci.* **1995**, *84*, 927–932. [CrossRef]

63. Kantner, I.; Erben, R.G. Long-term parenteral administration of 2-hydroxypropyl-β-cyclodextrin causes bone loss. *Toxicol. Pathol.* **2012**, *40*, 742–750. [CrossRef]

64. Szente, L.; Szejtli, J. Cyclodextrins as food ingredients. *Trends Food Sci. Technol.* **2004**, *15*, 137–142. [CrossRef]

65. Stella, V.J.; He, Q. Cyclodextrins. *Toxicol. Pathol.* **2008**, *36*, 30–42. [CrossRef] [PubMed]

66. Frömming, K.-H.; Szejtli, J. Pharmacokinetics and toxicology of cyclodextrins. In *Cyclodextrins in Pharmacy*; Frömming, K.-H., Szejtli, J., Eds.; Springer: Dordrecht, The Netherlands, 1994; pp. 33–44.

67. Miranda, J.C.D.; Martins, T.E.A.; Veiga, F.; Ferraz, H.G. Cyclodextrins and ternary complexes: Technology to improve solubility of poorly soluble drugs. *Braz. J. Pharm. Sci.* **2011**, *47*, 665–681. [CrossRef]

68. Amiri, S. Introduction. In *Cyclodextrins: Properties and Industrial Applications*; Amiri, S., Ed.; Wiley: Hoboken, NY, USA, 2017; Volume 1, pp. 1–39.

69. Mohanty, J.; Bhasikuttan, A.C.; Nau, W.M.; Pal, H. Host−guest complexation of neutral red with macrocyclic host molecules: Contrasting pka shifts and binding affinities for cucurbit[7]uril and β-cyclodextrin. *J. Phys. Chem. B* **2006**, *110*, 5132–5138. [CrossRef] [PubMed]

70. Kim, H.; Jeong, K.; Park, H.; Jung, S. Preference prediction for the stable inclusion complexes between cyclodextrins and monocyclic insoluble chemicals based on monte carlo docking simulations. *J. Incl. Phenom. Macrocycl. Chem.* **2006**, *54*, 165–170. [CrossRef]

71. Li, S.; Purdy, W.C. Cyclodextrins and their applications in analytical chemistry. *Chem. Rev.* **1992**, *92*, 1457–1470. [CrossRef]

72. Al Omari, M.M.; Zughul, M.B.; Davies, J.E.D.; Badwan, A.A. Effect of buffer species on the complexation of basic drug terfenadine with β-cyclodextrin. *J. Incl. Phenom. Macrocycl. Chem.* **2007**, *58*, 227–235. [CrossRef]

73. Rekharsky, M.V.; Inoue, Y. Complexation thermodynamics of cyclodextrins. *Chem. Rev.* **1998**, *98*, 1875–1918. [CrossRef]

74. Dua, K.; Pabreja, K.; Ramana, M.V.; Lather, V. Dissolution behavior of β-cyclodextrin molecular inclusion complexes of aceclofenac. *J. Pharm. Bioallied Sci.* **2011**, *3*, 417–425. [CrossRef]

75. Shin, K.-M.; Dong, T.; He, Y.; Taguchi, Y.; Oishi, A.; Nishida, H.; Inoue, Y. Inclusion complex formation between α-cyclodextrin and biodegradable aliphatic polyesters. *Macromol. Biosci.* **2004**, *4*, 1075–1083. [CrossRef]

76. Oster, M.; Schlatter, G.; Gallet, S.; Baati, R.; Pollet, E.; Gaillard, C.; Averous, L.; Fajolles, C.; Hebraud, A. The study of the pseudo-polyrotaxane architecture as a route for mild surface functionalization by click chemistry of poly(ε-caprolactone)-based electrospun fibers. *J. Mater. Chem. B* **2017**, *5*, 2181–2189. [CrossRef]

77. Rusa, C.C.; Wei, M.; Bullions, T.A.; Rusa, M.; Gomez, M.A.; Porbeni, F.E.; Wang, X.; Shin, I.D.; Balik, C.M.; White, J.L.; et al. Controlling the polymorphic behaviors of semicrystalline polymers with cyclodextrins. *Cryst. Growth Design* **2004**, *4*, 1431–1441. [CrossRef]

78. Topuz, F.; Uyar, T. Cyclodextrin-functionalized mesostructured silica nanoparticles for removal of polycyclic aromatic hydrocarbons. *J. Colloid Interface Sci.* **2017**, *497*, 233–241. [CrossRef] [PubMed]

79. Topuz, F.; Uyar, T. Poly-cyclodextrin cryogels with aligned porous structure for removal of polycyclic aromatic hydrocarbons (PAHS) from water. *J. Hazard. Mater.* **2017**, *335*, 108–116. [CrossRef] [PubMed]

80. Kotronia, M.; Kavetsou, E.; Loupassaki, S.; Kikionis, S.; Vouyiouka, S.; Detsi, A. Encapsulation of oregano (*Origanum onites* L.) essential oil in β-cyclodextrin (β-CD): Synthesis and characterization of the inclusion complexes. *Bioengineering* **2017**, *4*, 74. [CrossRef] [PubMed]

81. Wadhwa, G.; Kumar, S.; Chhabra, L.; Mahant, S.; Rao, R. *Essential coil*–cyclodextrin complexes: An updated review. *J. Incl. Phenom. Macrocycl. Chem.* **2017**, *89*, 39–58. [CrossRef]

82. Zelikin, A.N.; Ehrhardt, C.; Healy, A.M. Materials and methods for delivery of biological drugs. *Nat. Chem.* **2016**, *8*, 997. [CrossRef] [PubMed]

83. Celebioglu, A.; Uyar, T. Electrospinning of nanofibers from non-polymeric systems: Electrospun nanofibers from native cyclodextrins. *J. Colloid Interface Sci.* **2013**, *404*, 1–7. [CrossRef] [PubMed]

84. Uyar, T.; El-Shafei, A.; Wang, X.; Hacaloglu, J.; Tonelli, A.E. The solid channel structure inclusion complex formed between guest styrene and host γ-cyclodextrin. *J. Incl. Phenom. Macrocycl. Chem.* **2006**, *55*, 109–121. [CrossRef]

85. Kayaci, F.; Ertas, Y.; Uyar, T. Enhanced thermal stability of eugenol by cyclodextrin inclusion complex encapsulated in electrospun polymeric nanofibers. *J. Agric. Food Chem.* **2013**, *61*, 8156–8165. [CrossRef]

86. Kayaci, F.; Sen, H.S.; Durgun, E.; Uyar, T. Functional electrospun polymeric nanofibers incorporating geraniol–cyclodextrin inclusion complexes: High thermal stability and enhanced durability of geraniol. *Food Res. Int.* **2014**, *62*, 424–431. [CrossRef]

87. Liu, L.; Guo, Q.-X. The driving forces in the inclusion complexation of cyclodextrins. *J. Incl. Phenom. Macrocycl. Chem.* **2002**, *42*, 1–14. [CrossRef]

88. Canbolat, M.F.; Celebioglu, A.; Uyar, T. Drug delivery system based on cyclodextrin-naproxen inclusion complex incorporated in electrospun polycaprolactone nanofibers. *Colloids Surf. B Biointerfaces* **2014**, *115*, 15–21. [CrossRef] [PubMed]

89. Sadlej-Sosnowska, N.; Kozerski, L.; Bednarek, E.; Sitkowski, J. Fluorometric and NMR studies of the naproxen–cyclodextrin inclusion complexes in aqueous solutions. *J. Incl. Phenom. Macrocycl. Chem.* **2000**, *37*, 383–394. [CrossRef]

90. Banik, A.; Gogoi, P.; Saikia, M.D. Interaction of naproxen with β-cyclodextrin and its derivatives/polymer: Experimental and molecular modeling studies. *J. Incl. Phenom. Macrocycl. Chem.* **2012**, *72*, 449–458. [CrossRef]

91. Akduman, C.; Ozguney, I.; Kumbasar, E.P. Electrospun thermoplastic polyurethane mats containing naproxen-cyclodextrin inclusion complex. *Autex Res. J.* **2014**, *14*, 239–246. [CrossRef]

92. Aytac, Z.; Sen, H.S.; Durgun, E.; Uyar, T. Sulfisoxazole/cyclodextrin inclusion complex incorporated in electrospun hydroxypropyl cellulose nanofibers as drug delivery system. *Colloids Surf. B. Biointerfaces* **2015**, *128*, 331–338. [CrossRef]

93. Connor, E.E. Sulfonamide antibiotics. *Prim. Care Update Ob Gyns* **1998**, *5*, 32–35. [CrossRef]

94. Tonglairoum, P.; Ngawhirunpat, T.; Rojanarata, T.; Panomsuk, S.; Kaomongkolgit, R.; Opanasopit, P. Fabrication of mucoadhesive chitosan coated polyvinylpyrrolidone/cyclodextrin/clotrimazole sandwich patches for oral candidiasis. *Carbohydr. Polym.* **2015**, *132*, 173–179. [CrossRef]

95. Sun, X.; Yu, Z.; Cai, Z.; Yu, L.; Lv, Y. Voriconazole composited polyvinyl alcohol/hydroxypropyl-β-cyclodextrin nanofibers for ophthalmic delivery. *PLoS ONE* **2016**, *11*, e0167961. [CrossRef]

96.	Siafaka, P.I.; Okur, N.U.; Mone, M.; Giannakopoulou, S.; Er, S.; Pavlidou, E.; Karavas, E.; Bikiaris, D.N. Two different approaches for oral administration of voriconazole loaded formulations: Electrospun fibers versus β-cyclodextrin complexes. *Int. J. Mol. Sci.* **2016**, *17*, 282. [CrossRef]

97.	Samprasit, W.; Akkaramongkolporn, P.; Ngawhirunpat, T.; Rojanarata, T.; Kaomongkolgit, R.; Opanasopit, P. Fast releasing oral electrospun PVP/CD nanofiber mats of taste-masked meloxicam. *Int. J. Pharm.* **2015**, *487*, 213–222. [CrossRef]

98.	Noble, S.; Balfour, J.A. Meloxicam. *Drugs* **1996**, *51*, 424–430. [CrossRef] [PubMed]

99.	Samprasit, W.; Akkaramongkolporn, P.; Kaomongkolgit, R.; Opanasopit, P. Cyclodextrin-based oral dissolving films formulation of taste-masked meloxicam. *Pharm. Dev. Technol.* **2018**, *23*, 530–539. [CrossRef]

100.	Monteiro, A.P.F.; Rocha, C.M.S.L.; Oliveira, M.F.; Gontijo, S.M.L.; Agudelo, R.R.; Sinisterra, R.D.; Cortés, M.E. Nanofibers containing tetracycline/β-cyclodextrin: Physico-chemical characterization and antimicrobial evaluation. *Carbohydr. Polym.* **2017**, *156*, 417–426. [CrossRef] [PubMed]

101.	Prakasam, A.; Elavarasu, S.S.; Natarajan, R.K. Antibiotics in the management of aggressive periodontitis. *J. Pharm. Bioallied Sci.* **2012**, *4*, S252–S255. [CrossRef] [PubMed]

102.	Alhusein, N.; Blagbrough, I.S.; Beeton, M.L.; Bolhuis, A.; De Bank, P.A. Electrospun zein/pcl fibrous matrices release tetracycline in a controlled manner, killing staphylococcus aureus both in biofilms and ex vivo on pig skin, and are compatible with human skin cells. *Pharm. Res.* **2016**, *33*, 237–246. [CrossRef] [PubMed]

103.	Alhusein, N.; Blagbrough, I.S.; De Bank, P.A. Zein/polycaprolactone electrospun matrices for localised controlled delivery of tetracycline. *Drug Deliv.Transl. Res.* **2013**, *3*, 542–550. [CrossRef] [PubMed]

104.	Alhusein, N.; De Bank, P.A.; Blagbrough, I.S.; Bolhuis, A. Killing bacteria within biofilms by sustained release of tetracycline from triple-layered electrospun micro/nanofibre matrices of polycaprolactone and poly(ethylene-co-vinyl acetate). *Drug Deliv. Transl. Res.* **2013**, *3*, 531–541. [CrossRef] [PubMed]

105.	Alhusein, N.; Blagbrough, I.S.; De Bank, P.A. Electrospun matrices for localised controlled drug delivery: Release of tetracycline hydrochloride from layers of polycaprolactone and poly(ethylene-co-vinyl acetate). *Drug Deliv. Transl. Res.* **2012**, *2*, 477–488. [CrossRef] [PubMed]

106.	Alhusein, N.; De Bank, P.; Blagbrough, I.S. Polycaprolactone electrospun nanofibers for controlled drug delivery. In *The Encyclopedia of Biomedical Polymers and Polymeric Biomaterials*; Mishra, M., Ed.; CRC Press: Boca Raton, FL, USA, 2015; Volume 7, pp. 5239–5249.

107.	Liu, W.; Wang, Y.; Yao, J.; Shao, Z.; Chen, X. Tamoxifen-loaded silk fibroin electrospun fibers. *Mater. Lett.* **2016**, *178*, 31–34. [CrossRef]

108.	Stygar, D.; Muravitskaya, N.; Eriksson, B.; Eriksson, H.; Sahlin, L. Effects of serm (selective estrogen receptor modulator) treatment on growth and proliferation in the rat uterus. *Reprod. Biol. Endocrinol.* **2003**, *1*, 40. [CrossRef] [PubMed]

109.	Osborne, C.K.; Zhao, H.; Fuqua, S.A.W. Selective estrogen receptor modulators: Structure, function, and clinical use. *J. Clin. Oncol.* **2000**, *18*, 3172–3186. [CrossRef] [PubMed]

110.	Souza, S.O.L.; Cotrim, M.A.P.; Oréfice, R.L.; Carvalho, S.G.; Dutra, J.A.P.; de Paula Careta, F.; Resende, J.A.; Villanova, J.C.O. Electrospun poly(ε-caprolactone) matrices containing silver sulfadiazine complexed with β-cyclodextrin as a new pharmaceutical dosage form to wound healing: Preliminary physicochemical and biological evaluation. *J. Mater. Sci. Mater. Med.* **2018**, *29*, 67. [CrossRef] [PubMed]

111	Muangman, P.; Pundee, C.; Opasanon, S.; Muangman, S. A prospective, randomized trial of silver containing hydrofiber dressing versus 1% silver sulfadiazine for the treatment of partial thickness burns. *Int. Wound J.* **2010**, *7*, 271–276. [CrossRef] [PubMed]

112.	Aytac, Z.; Uyar, T. Core-shell nanofibers of curcumin/cyclodextrin inclusion complex and polylactic acid: Enhanced water solubility and slow release of curcumin. *Int. J. Pharm.* **2017**, *518*, 177–184. [CrossRef] [PubMed]

113.	Sun, X.Z.; Williams, G.R.; Hou, X.X.; Zhu, L.M. Electrospun curcumin-loaded fibers with potential biomedical applications. *Carbohydr. Polym.* **2013**, *94*, 147–153. [CrossRef]

114.	Sudakaran, S.V.; Venugopal, J.R.; Vijayakumar, G.P.; Abisegapriyan, S.; Grace, A.N.; Ramakrishna, S. Sequel of MgO nanoparticles in PLACL nanofibers for anti-cancer therapy in synergy with curcumin/β-cyclodextrin. *Mater. Sci. Eng. C* **2017**, *71*, 620–628. [CrossRef]

115.	Xie, C.; Li, X.; Luo, X.; Yang, Y.; Cui, W.; Zou, J.; Zhou, S. Release modulation and cytotoxicity of hydroxycamptothecin-loaded electrospun fibers with 2-hydroxypropyl-β-cyclodextrin inoculations. *Int. J. Pharm.* **2010**, *391*, 55–64. [CrossRef]

116. Masoumi, S.; Amiri, S.; Bahrami, S.H. Pcl-based nanofibers loaded with ciprofloxacin/cyclodextrin containers. *J. Text. Inst.* **2018**, *109*, 1044–1053. [CrossRef]
117. Sousa, J.; Alves, G.; Oliveira, P.; Fortuna, A.; Falcão, A. Intranasal delivery of ciprofloxacin to rats: A topical approach using a thermoreversible in situ gel. *Eur. J. Pharm. Sci.* **2017**, *97*, 30–37. [CrossRef]
118. Zhou, J.; Wang, Q.; Lu, H.; Zhang, Q.; Lv, P.; Wei, Q. Preparation and characterization of electrospun polyvinyl alcoholstyrylpyridinium/β-cyclodextrin composite nanofibers: Release behavior and potential use for wound dressing. *Fibers Polym.* **2016**, *17*, 1835–1841. [CrossRef]
119. Borbás, E.; Balogh, A.; Bocz, K.; Müller, J.; Kiserdei, É.; Vigh, T.; Sinkó, B.; Marosi, A.; Halász, A.; Dohányos, Z.; et al. In vitro dissolution–permeation evaluation of an electrospun cyclodextrin-based formulation of aripiprazole using μflux™. *Int. J. Pharm.* **2015**, *491*, 180–189. [CrossRef] [PubMed]
120. Panichpakdee, J.; Pavasant, P.; Supaphol, P. Electrospinning of asiaticoside/2-hydroxypropyl-β-cyclodextrin inclusion complex-loaded cellulose acetate fiber mats: Release characteristics and potential for use as wound dressing. *Polymer* **2014**, *38*, 338–350. [CrossRef]
121. Aytac, Z.; Dogan, S.Y.; Tekinay, T.; Uyar, T. Release and antibacterial activity of allyl isothiocyanate/β-cyclodextrin complex encapsulated in electrospun nanofibers. *Colloids Surf. B Biointerfaces* **2014**, *120*, 125–131. [CrossRef] [PubMed]
122. Vega-Lugo, A.C.; Lim, L.T. Controlled release of allyl isothiocyanate using soy protein and poly(lactic acid) electrospun fibers. *Food Res. Int.* **2009**, *42*, 933–940. [CrossRef]
123. Luo, X.; Zhang, H.; Chen, M.; Wei, J.; Zhang, Y.; Li, X. Antimetastasis and antitumor efficacy promoted by sequential release of vascular disrupting and chemotherapeutic agents from electrospun fibers. *Int. J. Pharm.* **2014**, *475*, 438–449. [CrossRef] [PubMed]
124. Vigh, T.; Démuth, B.; Balogh, A.; Galata, D.L.; Van Assche, I.; Mackie, C.; Vialpando, M.; Van Hove, B.; Psathas, P.; Borbás, E.; et al. Oral bioavailability enhancement of flubendazole by developing nanofibrous solid dosage forms. *Drug Dev. Ind. Pharm.* **2017**, *43*, 1126–1133. [CrossRef]
125. Shastri, V.P.; Sy, J.C. Modulation of Drug Release Rate from Electrospun Fibers. U.S. Patent US20080220054A1, 11 September 2008.
126. Kazsoki, A.; Szabó, P.; Domján, A.; Balázs, A.; Bozó, T.; Kellermayer, M.; Farkas, A.; Balogh-Weiser, D.; Pinke, B.; Darcsi, A.; et al. Microstructural distinction of electrospun nanofibrous drug delivery systems formulated with different excipients. *Mol. Pharm.* **2018**. [CrossRef]
127. Filée, P.; Freichels, A.; Jéröme, C.; Aquil, A.; Colige, A.; Tateu, V.T. Chitosan-Based Biomimetic Scaffolds and Methods for Preparing the Same. U.S. Patent WO2011151225A1, 13 February 2011.
128. Puškárová, A.; Bučková, M.; Kraková, L.; Pangallo, D.; Kozics, K. The antibacterial and antifungal activity of six essential oils and their cyto/genotoxicity to human hel 12469 cells. *Sci. Rep.* **2017**, *7*, 8211. [CrossRef]
129. Finnemore, H. The essential oils. *Nature* **1927**, *119*, 920.
130. Toscano-Garibay, J.D.; Arriaga-Alba, M.; Sánchez-Navarrete, J.; Mendoza-García, M.; Flores-Estrada, J.J.; Moreno-Eutimio, M.A.; Espinosa-Aguirre, J.J.; González-Ávila, M.; Ruiz-Pérez, N.J. Antimutagenic and antioxidant activity of the essential oils of citrus sinensis and citrus latifolia. *Sci. Rep.* **2017**, *7*, 11479. [CrossRef] [PubMed]
131. Tonglairoum, P.; Chuchote, T.; Ngawhirunpat, T.; Rojanarata, T.; Opanasopit, P. Encapsulation of plai oil/2-hydroxypropyl-β-cyclodextrin inclusion complexes in polyvinylpyrrolidone (PVP) electrospun nanofibers for topical application. *Pharm. Dev. Technol.* **2014**, *19*, 430–437. [CrossRef] [PubMed]
132. Tonglairoum, P.; Ngawhirunpat, T.; Rojanarata, T.; Kaomongkolgit, R.; Opanasopit, P. Fabrication and evaluation of nanostructured herbal oil/hydroxypropyl-β-cyclodextrin/polyvinylpyrrolidone mats for denture stomatitis prevention and treatment. *AAPS Pharm. Sci. Tech.* **2016**, *17*, 1441–1449. [CrossRef] [PubMed]
133. Lin, L.; Dai, Y.; Cui, H. Antibacterial poly(ethylene oxide) electrospun nanofibers containing cinnamon essential oil/beta-cyclodextrin proteoliposomes. *Carbohydr. Polym.* **2017**, *178*, 131–140. [CrossRef] [PubMed]
134. Wen, P.; Zhu, D.H.; Wu, H.; Zong, M.H.; Jing, Y.R.; Han, S.Y. Encapsulation of cinnamon essential oil in electrospun nanofibrous film for active food packaging. *Food Control* **2016**, *59*, 366–376. [CrossRef]
135. Wen, P.; Zhu, D.H.; Feng, K.; Liu, F.J.; Lou, W.Y.; Li, N.; Zong, M.H.; Wu, H. Fabrication of electrospun polylactic acid nanofilm incorporating cinnamon essential oil/β-cyclodextrin inclusion complex for antimicrobial packaging. *Food Chem.* **2016**, *196*, 996–1004. [CrossRef] [PubMed]

136. Feng, K.; Wen, P.; Yang, H.; Li, N.; Lou, W.Y.; Zong, M.H.; Wu, H. Enhancement of the antimicrobial activity of cinnamon essential oil-loaded electrospun nanofilm by the incorporation of lysozyme. *RSC Adv.* **2017**, *7*, 1572–1580. [CrossRef]

137. Munhuweyi, K.; Caleb, O.J.; van Reenen, A.J.; Opara, U.L. Physical and antifungal properties of β-cyclodextrin microcapsules and nanofibre films containing cinnamon and oregano essential oils. *LWT Food Sci. Technol.* **2018**, *87*, 413–422. [CrossRef]

138. Liu, Y.; Liang, X.; Zhang, R.; Lan, W.; Qin, W. Fabrication of electrospun polylactic acid/cinnamaldehyde/β-cyclodextrin fibers as an antimicrobial wound dressing. *Polymers* **2017**, *9*, 464. [CrossRef]

139. Dhifi, W.; Bellili, S.; Jazi, S.; Bahloul, N.; Mnif, W. Essential oils' chemical characterization and investigation of some biological activities: A critical review. *Medicines* **2016**, *3*, 25. [CrossRef]

140. Dias Antunes, M.; da Silva Dannenberg, G.; Fiorentini, Â.M.; Pinto, V.Z.; Lim, L.T.; da Rosa Zavareze, E.; Dias, A.R.G. Antimicrobial electrospun ultrafine fibers from zein containing eucalyptus essential oil/cyclodextrin inclusion complex. *Int. J. Biol. Macromol.* **2017**, *104*, 874–882. [CrossRef] [PubMed]

141. Aytac, Z.; Kusku, S.I.; Durgun, E.; Uyar, T. Encapsulation of gallic acid/cyclodextrin inclusion complex in electrospun polylactic acid nanofibers: Release behavior and antioxidant activity of gallic acid. *Mater. Sci. Eng. C* **2016**, *63*, 231–239. [CrossRef]

142. Mascheroni, E.; Fuenmayor, C.A.; Cosio, M.S.; Di Silvestro, G.; Piergiovanni, L.; Mannino, S.; Schiraldi, A. Encapsulation of volatiles in nanofibrous polysaccharide membranes for humidity-triggered release. *Carbohydr. Polym.* **2013**, *98*, 17–25. [CrossRef]

143. Uyar, T.; Hacaloglu, J.; Besenbacher, F. Electrospun polystyrene fibers containing high temperature stable volatile fragrance/flavor facilitated by cyclodextrin inclusion complexes. *React. Funct. Polym.* **2009**, *69*, 145–150. [CrossRef]

144. Uyar, T.; Nur, Y.; Hacaloglu, J.; Besenbacher, F. Electrospinning of functional poly(methyl methacrylate) nanofibers containing cyclodextrin-menthol inclusion complexes. *Nanotechnology* **2009**, *20*, 125703. [CrossRef] [PubMed]

145. Uyar, T.; Hacaloglu, J.; Besenbacher, F. Electrospun polyethylene oxide (PEO) nanofibers containing cyclodextrin inclusion complex. *J. Nanosci. Nanotechnol.* **2011**, *11*, 3949–3958. [CrossRef] [PubMed]

146. Kayaci, F.; Uyar, T. Encapsulation of vanillin/cyclodextrin inclusion complex in electrospun polyvinyl alcohol (PVA) nanowebs: Prolonged shelf-life and high temperature stability of vanillin. *Food Chem.* **2012**, *133*, 641–649. [CrossRef]

147. Loong-Tak Lim, S.D.F.M.; Gopinadhan, P.; Jayasankar Subramanian, J. Alan Sullivan Encapsulation and Controlled Release of Volatile Organic Compounds. U.S. Patent US20160330952A1, 17 November 2016.

148. Aytac, Z.; Keskin, N.O.S.; Tekinay, T.; Uyar, T. Antioxidant α-tocopherol/γ-cyclodextrin–inclusion complex encapsulated poly(lactic acid) electrospun nanofibrous web for food packaging. *J. Appl. Polym. Sci.* **2017**, *134*, 44858. [CrossRef]

149. Aytac, Z.; Kusku, S.I.; Durgun, E.; Uyar, T. Quercetin/β-cyclodextrin inclusion complex embedded nanofibres: Slow release and high solubility. *Food Chem.* **2016**, *197*, 864–871. [CrossRef]

150. Lemma, S.M.; Scampicchio, M.; Mahon, P.J.; Sbarski, I.; Wang, J.; Kingshott, P. Controlled release of retinyl acetate from β-cyclodextrin functionalized poly(vinyl alcohol) electrospun nanofibers. *J. Agric. Food Chem.* **2015**, *63*, 3481–3488. [CrossRef]

151. Oliveira, M.F.; Suarez, D.; Rocha, J.C.B.; de Carvalho Teixeira, A.V.N.; Cortés, M.E.; De Sousa, F.B.; Sinisterra, R.D. Electrospun nanofibers of polycd/PMAA polymers and their potential application as drug delivery system. *Mater. Sci. Eng. C* **2015**, *54*, 252–261. [CrossRef] [PubMed]

152. Costoya, A.; Ballarin, F.M.; Llovo, J.; Concheiro, A.; Abraham, G.A.; Alvarez-Lorenzo, C. Hmdso-plasma coated electrospun fibers of poly(cyclodextrin)s for antifungal dressings. *Int. J. Pharm.* **2016**, *513*, 518–527. [CrossRef] [PubMed]

153. Ouerghemmi, S.; Degoutin, S.; Tabary, N.; Cazaux, F.; Maton, M.; Gaucher, V.; Janus, L.; Neut, C.; Chai, F.; Blanchemain, N.; et al. Triclosan loaded electrospun nanofibers based on a cyclodextrin polymer and chitosan polyelectrolyte complex. *Int. J. Pharm.* **2016**, *513*, 483–495. [CrossRef] [PubMed]

154. Heydari, A.; Mehrabi, F.; Shamspur, T.; Sheibani, H.; Mostafavi, A. Encapsulation and controlled release of vitamin b2 using peracetyl-β-cyclodextrin polymer-based electrospun nanofiber scaffold. *Pharm. Chem. J.* **2018**, *52*, 19–25. [CrossRef]

155. Nada, A.A.; Montaser, A.S.; Abdel Azeem, R.A.; Mounier, M.M. Eco-friendly gelatin-based electrospun fibers to control the release of chloramphenicol. *Fibers Polym.* **2016**, *17*, 1985–1994. [CrossRef]

156. Gross, B.J.; Branchflower, R.V.; Burke, T.R.; Lees, D.E.; Pohl, L.R. Bone marrow toxicity in vitro of chloramphenicol and its metabolites. *Toxicol. Appl. Pharmacol.* **1982**, *64*, 557–565. [CrossRef]

157. Schwinté, P.; Mariotte, A.; Anand, P.; Keller, L.; Idoux-Gillet, Y.; Huck, O.; Fioretti, F.; Tenenbaum, H.; Georgel, P.; Wenzel, W.; et al. Anti-inflammatory effect of active nanofibrous polymeric membrane bearing nanocontainers of atorvastatin complexes. *Nanomedicine* **2017**, *12*, 2651–2674. [CrossRef]

158. Bazhban, M.; Nouri, M.; Mokhtari, J. Electrospinning of cyclodextrin functionalized chitosan/pva nanofibers as a drug delivery system. *Chin. J. Polym. Sci.* **2013**, *31*, 1343–1351. [CrossRef]

159. Horst, A.; von Recum, T.T.; Julius, N.K.; Travis, S.; Iryna, M. Therapeutic Agent Delivery System and Method. U.S. Patent US20150010608A1, 8 January 2015.

160. Cecone, C.; Caldera, F.; Trotta, F.; Bracco, P.; Zanetti, M. Controlled release of deet loaded on fibrous mats from electrospun pmda/cyclodextrin polymer. *Molecules* **2018**, *23*, 1694. [CrossRef]

161. Celebioglu, A.; Uyar, T. Cyclodextrin nanofibers by electrospinning. *Chem. Commun.* **2010**, *46*, 6903–6905. [CrossRef]

162. Celebioglu, A.; Uyar, T. Electrospinning of nanofibers from non-polymeric systems: Polymer-free nanofibers from cyclodextrin derivatives. *Nanoscale* **2012**, *4*, 621–631. [CrossRef] [PubMed]

163. Celebioglu, A.; Uyar, T. Electrospun gamma-cyclodextrin ([gamma]-CD) nanofibers for the entrapment of volatile organic compounds. *RSC Adv.* **2013**, *3*, 22891–22895. [CrossRef]

164. Celebioglu, A.; Uyar, T. Electrospinning of polymer-free nanofibers from cyclodextrin inclusion complexes. *Langmuir* **2011**, *27*, 6218–6226. [CrossRef] [PubMed]

165. Celebioglu, A.; Umu, O.C.O.; Tekinay, T.; Uyar, T. Antibacterial electrospun nanofibers from triclosan/cyclodextrin inclusion complexes. *Colloids Surf. B Biointerfaces* **2014**, *116*, 612–619. [CrossRef] [PubMed]

166. Celebioglu, A.; Aytac, Z.; Kilic, M.E.; Durgun, E.; Uyar, T. Encapsulation of camphor in cyclodextrin inclusion complex nanofibers via polymer-free electrospinning: Enhanced water solubility, high temperature stability, and slow release of camphor. *J. Mater. Sci.* **2018**, *53*, 5436–5449. [CrossRef]

167. Celebioglu, A.; Yildiz, Z.I.; Uyar, T. Fabrication of electrospun eugenol/cyclodextrin inclusion complex nanofibrous webs for enhanced antioxidant property, water solubility, and high temperature stability. *J. Agric. Food Chem.* **2018**, *66*, 457–466. [CrossRef] [PubMed]

168. Celebioglu, A.; Yildiz, Z.I.; Uyar, T. Electrospun nanofibers from cyclodextrin inclusion complexes with cineole and p-cymene: Enhanced water solubility and thermal stability. *Int. J. Food Sci. Technol.* **2018**, *53*, 112–120. [CrossRef]

169. Aytac, Z.; Yildiz, Z.I.; Kayaci-Senirmak, F.; Tekinay, T.; Uyar, T. Electrospinning of cyclodextrin/linalool-inclusion complex nanofibers: Fast-dissolving nanofibrous web with prolonged release and antibacterial activity. *Food Chem.* **2017**, *231*, 192–201. [CrossRef]

170. Aytac, Z.; Yildiz, Z.I.; Kayaci-Senirmak, F.; San Keskin, N.O.; Kusku, S.I.; Durgun, E.; Tekinay, T.; Uyar, T. Fast-dissolving, prolonged release, and antibacterial cyclodextrin/limonene-inclusion complex nanofibrous webs via polymer-free electrospinning. *J. Agric. Food Chem.* **2016**, *64*, 7325–7334. [CrossRef]

171. Aytac, Z.; Yildiz, Z.I.; Kayaci-Senirmak, F.; San Keskin, N.O.; Tekinay, T.; Uyar, T. Electrospinning of polymer-free cyclodextrin/geraniol-inclusion complex nanofibers: Enhanced shelf-life of geraniol with antibacterial and antioxidant properties. *RSC Adv.* **2016**, *6*, 46089–46099. [CrossRef]

172. Celebioglu, A.; Yildiz, Z.I.; Uyar, T. Thymol/cyclodextrin inclusion complex nanofibrous webs: Enhanced water solubility, high thermal stability and antioxidant property of thymol. *Food Res. Int.* **2018**, *106*, 280–290. [CrossRef] [PubMed]

173. Yildiz, Z.I.; Celebioglu, A.; Kilic, M.E.; Durgun, E.; Uyar, T. Menthol/cyclodextrin inclusion complex nanofibers: Enhanced water-solubility and high-temperature stability of menthol. *J. Food Eng.* **2018**, *224*, 27–36. [CrossRef]

174. Celebioglu, A.; Kayaci-Senirmak, F.; Ipek, S.; Durgun, E.; Uyar, T. Polymer-free nanofibers from vanillin/cyclodextrin inclusion complexes: High thermal stability, enhanced solubility and antioxidant property. *Food Funct.* **2016**, *7*, 3141–3153. [CrossRef]

175. Celebioglu, A.; Uyar, T. Antioxidant vitamin e/cyclodextrin inclusion complex electrospun nanofibers: Enhanced water solubility, prolonged shelf life, and photostability of vitamin E. *J. Agric. Food Chem.* **2017**, *65*, 5404–5412. [CrossRef]

176. Yildiz, Z.I.; Celebioglu, A.; Kilic, M.E.; Durgun, E.; Uyar, T. Fast-dissolving carvacrol/cyclodextrin inclusion complex electrospun fibers with enhanced thermal stability, water solubility, and antioxidant activity. *J. Mater. Sci.* **2018**. [CrossRef]

177. Ultee, A.; Bennik, M.H.J.; Moezelaar, R. The phenolic hydroxyl group of carvacrol is essential for action against the food-borne pathogen bacillus cereus. *Appl. Environ. Microbiol.* **2002**, *68*, 1561–1568. [CrossRef] [PubMed]

178. Beena; Kumar, D.; Rawat, D.S. Synthesis and antioxidant activity of thymol and carvacrol based schiff bases. *Bioorg. Med. Chem. Lett.* **2013**, *23*, 641–645. [CrossRef]

179. Yildiz, Z.I.; Celebioglu, A.; Uyar, T. Polymer-free electrospun nanofibers from sulfobutyl ether7-beta-cyclodextrin (SBE7-β-CD) inclusion complex with sulfisoxazole: Fast-dissolving and enhanced water-solubility of sulfisoxazole. *Int. J. Pharm.* **2017**, *531*, 550–558. [CrossRef]

180. Balogh, A.; Horváthová, T.; Fülöp, Z.; Loftsson, T.; Harasztos, A.H.; Marosi, G.; Nagy, Z.K. Electroblowing and electrospinning of fibrous diclofenac sodium-cyclodextrin complex-based reconstitution injection. *J. Drug Deliv. Sci. Technol.* **2015**, *26*, 28–34. [CrossRef]

181. Vigh, T.; Horváthová, T.; Balogh, A.; Sóti, P.L.; Drávavölgyi, G.; Nagy, Z.K.; Marosi, G. Polymer-free and polyvinylpirrolidone-based electrospun solid dosage forms for drug dissolution enhancement. *Eur. J. Pharm. Sci.* **2013**, *49*, 595–602. [CrossRef]

182. Yu, H.S.; Lee, J.M.; Youn, Y.S.; Oh, K.T.; Na, K.; Lee, E.S. γ-cyclodextrin-phenylacetic acid mesh as a drug trap. *Carbohydr. Polym.* **2018**, *184*, 390–400. [CrossRef] [PubMed]

183. Celebioglu, A.; Yildiz, Z.I.; Uyar, T. Electrospun crosslinked poly-cyclodextrin nanofibers: Highly efficient molecular filtration thru host-guest inclusion complexation. *Sci. Rep.* **2017**, *7*, 7369. [CrossRef] [PubMed]

184. Ma, M.; Li, D. New organic nanoporous polymers and their inclusion complexes. *Chem. Mater.* **1999**, *11*, 872–874. [CrossRef]

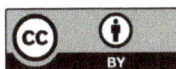

pharmaceutics

MDPI

Review

Biomedical Applications of Electrospun Nanofibers: Drug and Nanoparticle Delivery

Rajan Sharma Bhattarai [1], Rinda Devi Bachu [1], Sai H. S. Boddu [2,* and Sarit Bhaduri [3,4]

[1] College of Pharmacy and Pharmaceutical Sciences, The University of Toledo Health Science Campus, Toledo, OH 43614, USA; RajanSharma.Bhattarai@rockets.utoledo.edu (R.S.B.); RindaDevi.Bachu@rockets.utoledo.edu (R.D.B.)

[2] Department of Pharmaceutical Sciences, College of Pharmacy and Health Sciences, Ajman University, Ajman 2758, UAE

[3] Department of Mechanical, Industrial and Manufacturing Engineering, University of Toledo, Toledo, OH 43614, USA; Sarit.Bhaduri@utoledo.edu

[4] Department of Surgery (Dentistry), University of Toledo, Toledo, OH 43614, USA

* Correspondence: s.boddu@ajman.ac.ae; Tel.: +971-6-705-6345

Received: 20 September 2018; Accepted: 26 October 2018; Published: 24 December 2018

Abstract: The electrospinning process has gained popularity due to its ease of use, simplicity and diverse applications. The properties of electrospun fibers can be controlled by modifying either process variables (e.g., applied voltage, solution flow rate, and distance between charged capillary and collector) or polymeric solution properties (e.g., concentration, molecular weight, viscosity, surface tension, solvent volatility, conductivity, and surface charge density). However, many variables affecting electrospinning are interdependent. An optimized electrospinning process is one in which these parameters remain constant and continuously produce nanofibers consistent in physicochemical properties. In addition, nozzle configurations, such as single nozzle, coaxial, multi-jet electrospinning, have an impact on the fiber characteristics. The polymeric solution could be aqueous, a polymeric melt or an emulsion, which in turn leads to different types of nanofiber formation. Nanofiber properties can also be modified by polarity inversion and by varying the collector design. The active moiety is incorporated into polymeric fibers by blending, surface modification or emulsion formation. The nanofibers can be further modified to deliver multiple drugs, and multilayer polymer coating allows sustained release of the incorporated active moiety. Electrospun nanofibers prepared from polymers are used to deliver antibiotic and anticancer agents, DNA, RNA, proteins and growth factors. This review provides a compilation of studies involving the use of electrospun fibers in biomedical applications with emphasis on nanoparticle-impregnated nanofibers.

Keywords: electrospinning; parameters; drug delivery; applications

---

1. Electrospinning and Its History

Electrospinning is a process of forming micro/nanometer-sized polymeric fibers, either hollow or solid, with the application of the electric force on the polymeric solution at the tip of a conducting tube. It is one of the most commonly used techniques to obtain continuous fibers in the nanometer size range [1–3]. Electrospinning, also known as electrostatic spinning, has been used extensively for over three decades, and its usefulness in the fields of science and technology is still on the increase. Bose et al. first described the aerosols generated by the application of electric potential to the fluids in 1745 [4]. Further, Lord Rayleigh studied the amount of charge needed by the fluid to overcome the surface tension of a drop. Cooley and Morton patented the first device to spray the liquids under the influence of electrical charge in 1902 and 1903, and the fabrication of artificial silk was undertaken by Kiyohito et al. in 1929 [4]. Studies in the 1940s, 1950s and 1960s were limited and mainly focused on obtaining uniform-sized particle/fibers, decreasing the size, understanding and optimizing parameters, and designing the instruments [5,6]. In the 1990s, the process was finally taken up by educational institutions and, since then, many studies have been carried out on the versatility of manufacturing and the applications of the electrospun particles [2].

1.1. Process of Electrospinning

The electrospinning process involves the use of a very high voltage source (of either positive or negative polarity) to charge the polymer solution or melt, a grounded collector, and a syringe pump (Figure 1). It is advisable to perform the electrospinning process in a closed hood with minimal atmospheric influence, which serves as a safety measure for fibers and for the personnel. When a sufficient repulsive charge is accumulated and the repulsive force is equal to the surface tension, the drop surface on the conducting tube starts to form a cone called a Taylor cone. The conducting polymer solution/melt can exist in an equilibrium cone form under the influence of the electric field at an angle of 49.3° [7]. If the electric field is increased further, the repulsive force overcomes the surface tension. This results in the formation of a liquid jet from the Taylor cone when there is sufficient attraction between the molecules in the solution/melt. If the solution does not have sufficient cohesive attraction, the jets break and the resulting particles are sprayed onto a collector plate. The fiber originating from the Taylor cone travels through the air towards the collector plate, and during the process, the solvent evaporates, leading to a solid fiber deposit onto the collector plate [6,7]. The jet starts to experience instability after traveling through the air for a short distance and then starts to whip, thus increasing the path distance to the collector. This process assists in fiber thinning and solvent evaporation. There are multiple theories proposed on the reason behind jet instability. Some of the prominent theories include: repulsive interaction of charges in the polymer jet [8]; increase in charge density during jet thinning, thus increasing radial charge repulsion to cause jet splitting at a critical charge density [9]; and, "whipping" instability (spiraling loops) [10], causing the fiber to turn, bend [11] and/or splay [12]. Shin et al. have suggested the whipping stability concept based on the results obtained using high-speed photography, where a single strand of jet whipped very fast to give a cone-like appearance [11]. The "inverted cone" appearance had long been misunderstood as a splitting of the jet midway through its travel in the air.

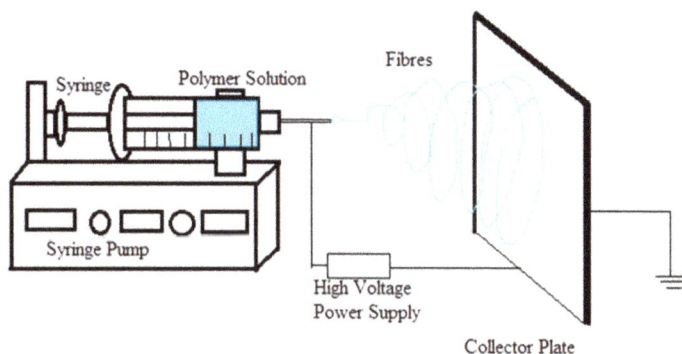

Figure 1. Schematic of electrospinning system. The system consists of polymer solution/melt in a syringe, mounted on a syringe pump, operating at a constant slow speed. High voltage direct current supply is connected to the needle of the syringe to charge the fluid. With sufficient voltage, the fluid forms a Taylor cone and then jet erupts from the cone towards the collector plate with whipping instability.

1.2. Physics of Electrospinning

When the electric field/voltage is increased gradually and the surface of the drop becomes convex at a certain voltage, V_c (critical voltage) is reached. At V_c, the jets (electrospinning) and sprays (electrospraying) begin, which are represented by Equation (1):

$$V_c = 4\frac{H^2}{L^2}\left(Ln\frac{2L}{R} - \frac{3}{2}\right)(0.117\pi\gamma R) \tag{1}$$

where H is the separation between capillary and the collector, L is the length of capillary, R is the radius of capillary and γ is the surface tension [7]. This relationship was identified by Taylor, and a similar relationship for the potential required for the electrospraying of charged pendant drops of solutions from the pendant in a capillary tube was established by Hendrick et al., in Equation (2) [13,14]:

$$V = 300\sqrt{20\pi\gamma r} \tag{2}$$

where, V is the required voltage, γ is the surface tension and r is the radius of the pendant drop. Even though viscosity and conductivity are vital in the electrospinning process, they are missing from the equation. The use of applied voltage and the surface tension gives a representative equation for slightly conducting, medium- to low-conductivity solutions [14].

2. Parameters of Electrospinning

The electrospinning process is simple and does not involve heavy machinery. The processing parameters and solution parameters affect the size, porosity and uniformity of the fibers. These parameters have been discussed individually; however, the observations made in any particular study by a team of researchers are not universal. The modification of a parameter in one polymer may produce a totally different result with another polymer. In addition, none of the parameters act independently during the electrospinning process, and the final fibers are the result of a combination of several parameters.

2.1. Process-Related Parameters of Electrospinning

2.1.1. Applied Voltage

The primary factor influencing the formation of fibers is the strength of the applied DC voltage. The size of the fiber, formation of beads and absence of jet formation are all dependent on the applied DC voltage. With an increase in the applied voltage of a polyethylene oxide (PEO)/water system, the originating site for the jet changes from the tip of the pendant drop to the tip of the capillary, and the volume of the pendant drop decreases gradually (Figure 2). When the fiber is formed from within the capillary, the bead defects in the fiber increase [6,15]. A reduction in voltage up to some range moves the splaying (instability) point towards the tip of the capillary (i.e., the jet becomes unstable earlier) [12]. A study by Reneker and Chun reported no significant change in the fiber diameter with a change in the electric field with PEO solution [16]. On the other hand, electrospun polyvinyl alcohol (PVA)/water solution exhibited a broad diameter distribution above 10 kV [17,18]. In another study, Megelski et al. observed an increase in fiber size of polystyrene with a decrease in spinning voltage and with no significant change in the pore formation in fibers [19].

Spinning solution leaving the blunt needle end

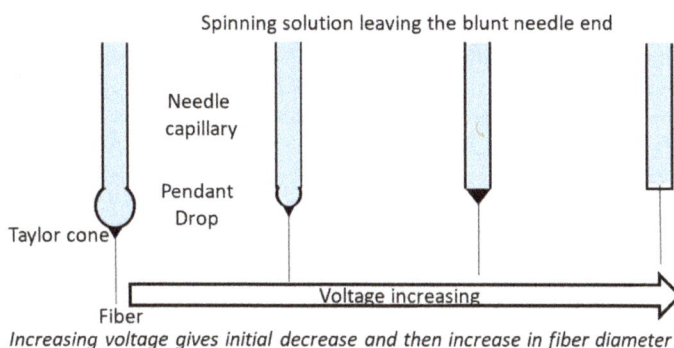

Increasing voltage gives initial decrease and then increase in fiber diameter

Figure 2. The effect of applied electric field on Taylor cone formation (dark colored tip). At low electric field, pendant drop is formed at the tip of the capillary and then a cone is formed on the tip. When the applied voltage is increased gradually, the drop size decreases until just a cone is formed at the tip of the capillary. If the voltage is further increased, fiber formation starts from within the needle without forming a visible Taylor cone on the blunt tip of the needle.

The fibers formed during the electrospinning process transport the charge to the grounded collector plate to close the circuit. This allows the electric current associated with the process to be measured; it is small (high voltage, 10–15 kV, high resistance and therefore very low current). When conductivity, dielectric constant and flow rate through the pump remain the same, an increase in current indicates an increase in the mass of the fibers formed. During the electrospinning process, the increase in current is gradual at first and then increases sharply from one voltage point, while sharp, steep increases are observed during electrospraying. The point of a sharp change in current could be indicative of the defect/change in the bead density [15].

Studies on the reversal of polarity obtained by grounding the solution in capillary and charging the collects resulted in inconsistent findings. Kilic et al. studied the effect of polarity on the electrospinning process of 7.5 wt% poly(vinyl alcohol)/water solution on production efficiency and nanofiber morphology. They concluded that due to the lack of columbic force acting on the polymer jet, the new reversed setup resulted in less nanofiber production. They also reported that the diameter and pore size of the web layer were much finer and more homogeneously distributed in the conventional setup [20]. On the other hand, Varesano et al. reported the production of good quality nanofibers with multi-jet electrospinning using both conventional and reverse polarity [21].

2.1.2. Flow Rate

The polymer flow rate has a direct impact on the size, shape and porosity of electrospun fibers. A study on polystyrene/tetrahydrofuran (THF) solutions by Megelski et al. reported an increased fiber diameter and pore size with flow rate. However, at high flow rates, bead defects and flat, ribbon-like structures were observed due to insufficient drying [19]. In a different study, a similar effect on fiber morphology was observed with a 20 wt% solution of nylon 6 in formic acid at a constant electric field of 20 kV at flow rates of 0.1, 0.5, 1 and 1.5 mL/h. An optimal flow rate of 0.5 mL/h resulted in fibers with the narrowest fiber diameter distribution and a stable Taylor cone. However, at a flow rate of 0.1 mL/h, the Taylor cone could not be maintained and reduced over time to obtain fiber from within the capillary tip. At flow rates of 1.0 mL/h and 1.5 mL/h, the electric field was not sufficient to spin all the solution, and only a few drops were sprayed as they broke off from the capillary due to the gravitational force [22].

2.1.3. Capillary–Collector Distance

The distance between the capillary and the collector is another factor which plays a significant role in controlling the size and morphology of the nanofibers [23]. This distance needs to be optimized as it might be the factor that distinguishes electrospraying and electrospinning. Typically a distance ranging from 10 to 20 cm is considered to be an effective spinning distance with the conventional method of electrospinning [24]. According to Doshi and Reneker, the larger the distance from the Taylor cone, the smaller the fiber diameter [9]. Jaeger et al. reported a decrease in fiber diameter (19 μm, 11 μm and 9 μm) with increasing distance (1 cm, 2 cm and 3.5 cm) from the orifice [12]. In another study investigating the electrospun polystyrene polymer fibers, decreasing the distance between the capillary and the collector from 35 cm to 30 cm did not change the diameter of the fibers significantly; however it led to the formation of non-homogeneous and elongated beads [19].

2.2. Solution-Related Parameters of Electrospinning

2.2.1. Concentration of Solution

Viscosity and surface tension, which determine the spinnability of a solution, should be taken into consideration in determining the concentration of solution/melt for electrospinning. Surface tension is a dominating factor in a low concentration solution (low viscosity, <1 poise), and at such concentration, drops will be formed instead of a continuous fiber. At a higher concentration (viscosity >20 poise), the flow of the solution cannot be controlled and maintained. In the PEO/water study discussed above in Section 2.1.1, a concentration range of 4–10 wt% with viscosity and surface tension ranging between 1–20 poise and 55–35 dynes/cm, respectively, were studied. At low concentrations of 4%, fibers were not sufficiently dry and formed fiber junctions and bundles. At higher concentrations, straight and cylindrical fibers with fewer fiber junctions and bundles were reported. The diameter of the electrospun PEO fibers increased with concentration, and a bimodal size distribution was observed above 7 wt% concentration. The average diameter of the fibers was reported to be related to solution concentration through the power law relationship, with an exponent of 0.5 [15]. A statistical study by Sukigara et al. on regenerated silk proved that the silk concentration was the most important parameter in producing uniform fibers of a diameter less than 100 nm [25]. Fong et al. investigated the effect of viscosity on morphology defects (bead formation) of electrospun nanofibers formed from PEO solutions. An increase in bead diameter and decrease in bead density was observed with solution viscosity. At higher viscosity, the shape of beads changed from spherical to spindle resulting in the formation of nanofibers with diminished morphology defects [26]. Solutions with low polymer concentration and high surface tension produced droplets as the viscoelastic forces could not overcome the repulsive forces of charge, resulting in the fragmentation of fiber jet into droplets. At higher concentrations, the viscoelastic forces are sufficient to prevent the fragmentation resulting in the formation of smooth nanofibers. Nanofibers of polyacrylonitrile solutions were formed in the viscosity range of 1.7 to 215 centipoise. With increase in viscosity, the fiber jet length and the nanofiber diameter increased and the drop at the capillary tip changed from hemispherical to conical shape [27]. In a different study, 15 and 20% w/v solutions of poly(desaminotyrosyl-tyrosine ethyl ester carbonate) (poly(DTE carbonate)) were electrospun at a voltage of 10 kV to 25 kV at 10 cm distance. Beaded fibers were observed during electrospinning at a lower concentration solution until the voltage reached 20 kV, and the density of beads decreased until the voltage reached 15 kV; average fiber diameter increased, while increasing the voltage from 20 kV to 25 kV. At higher solution concentrations, the smooth fibers obtained showed an increasing diameter and decreasing fiber density with the increase in the electric field from 10 kV to 25 kV [28].

2.2.2. Molecular Weight

The molecular weight of polymer influences the solution viscosity and thus has an important effect on fiber morphology. For example, decreasing the molecular weight of poly(vinyl alcohol) while maintaining other parameters constant resulted in the formation of bead-like structures. On the other hand, higher molecular weight resulted in smooth fibers initially followed by ribbon-like fibers upon further increase in molecular weight [29]. Ultra-high molecular weight polymers, such as polyacrylamide (molecular weight 9×10^6 g/mol), exhibited a variety of fiber morphologies even with a minute change in the concentration within the range 0.3–3.0 wt%. Beaded and smooth fibers were formed at concentrations between 0.3 to 0.7 wt%, whereas smooth fibers with ribbons coexisted at 0.7 to 2 wt%. Above 2.0 wt%, only ribbons were formed, which were either helical or zigzag with triangular beads on them [30]. Additionally, a study on the melts of polypropylene with varying molecular weights showed an increase in the fiber diameter with molecular weight. High molecular weight polymers show the highest degree of entanglement and pose difficulties for the electric field to pull on individual polymer chains to obtain a thin fiber [31].

2.2.3. Solution Viscosity

Viscosity determines the solution's ability to form fibers. Smooth continuous fibers can be obtained at optimum viscosity for a particular polymer solvent combination. The viscosity, molecular weight of the polymer and polymer concentration are interrelated, and one cannot be independently judged. Low viscosity fails to form the fibers, while high viscosity requires a higher electric field for electrospinning, making it hard to operate [25,32]. Baumgarten observed the formation of fine droplets at a lower viscosity and with incomplete drying. At higher viscosity, the droplets bumped into each other in mid-air due to incomplete drying with acrylic polymer [27]. When a solution has low viscosity, surface tension dominates the process of fiber formation, but at optimum concentration, it is the combined effect of both parameters [29,33–36]. Yang et al. suggested a mixed solvent system of dimethylformamide (DMF) and ethanol (50:50) for obtaining the best electrospun fibers of poly(vinyl pyrrolidone) and attributed the success to the combined effect of solution viscosity and charge density [10].

2.2.4. Surface Tension of the Solution

Surface tension is the measure of cohesive forces between the molecules in solution form and is dependent upon the solution composition, polymer and solvent(s) used. Yang et al. studied the influence of solvents on the formation of nanofibers with poly(vinyl pyrrolidone) and concluded that lower surface tension with high viscosity formed smooth nanofibers with ethanol as the solvent. They proposed the use of a multi-solvent system to obtain optimum surface tension and viscosity parameters for better electrospun fibers [10]. Like viscosity, surface tension can define the range of solvents and concentrations to be used in the electrospinning process [18].

2.2.5. Conductivity and Surface Charge Density

The impact of conductivity and surface charge density of solution also plays an important role in the process of electrospinning. It is important to have high conductivity for a greater charge-carrying capacity. A highly conductive solution experiences a stronger tensile force in an electric field compared to the less conductive solution, making the former preferable for electrospinning. An increase in the conductivity of the solution causes a substantial decrease in the diameter of the nanofibers. The radius of the fiber jet varies inversely as the cube root of the conductivity of solution [37]. For preparation of acrylic microfibers, Baumgarten reported that the jet radius is dependent on the inverse cube root of electric conductivity [27]. Natural polymers, being polyelectrolytic, have better charge-carrying ability and lead to poor fiber formation compared to synthetic polymers [38]. Hayati et al. observed that stable jets could be obtained by semi-conducting liquids by applying sufficient voltage. Due to insufficient free charges, the insulating liquids, such as paraffin oil, could not build an electrostatic charge on the surface, while highly conducting water produced an unstable stream and sparking at higher electric fields. Consequently, insulating liquids and semiconducting liquids could produce stable fibers [39]. Yet another study on poly(vinyl alcohol) solution showed that the addition of a small amount of sodium chloride drastically increased the conductivity and decreased the fiber diameter [17]. The addition of sodium chloride has an effect on decreasing the occurrence of beads in PEO solution [26]. Sodium phosphate [38], potassium phosphate [38], ammonium chloride [26], and lithium chloride [26] are also used to obtain better fibers by changing the conductivity of solutions. Huang et al. used compounds soluble in organic solvents, such as pyridine, that react with formic acid in solution to form a salt. Pyridine improves the conductivity and can easily be removed to obtain dry fibers. The addition of 0.4 wt% of pyridine doubled the electrical conductivity of 2% nylon-4,6 in formic acid [40].

2.2.6. Solvent Volatility

The distance between the tip of the capillary and the collector is only a few centimeters (typically 10–15 cm), and the path taken by the jet to reach the collector is a few folds more. The fibers formed during the process are porous and dry fast, depending on the choice of the solvent used for solubilization of the polymer. The insufficiently dried fiber may attach to itself mid-air [27], form ribbon-like fibers [19] or attach to itself after depositing on the collector. A study on polystyrene fibers showed that the use of more volatile tetrahydrofuran (THF) as a solvent produced high-density pores and increased the surface area of fibers by up to 40%. The same polymer in DMF lost the microtexture completely. A combination of these solvents in different ratios gave different morphology profiles as the volatility of the mixture varied [19].

3. Types of Electrospinning

The type of electrospinning process can have a significant impact on fiber formation in addition to the process and solution parameters. Two main aspects to deal with in the type of electrospinning are solution vs. melt electrospinning and nozzle configuration [6].

3.1. Solution vs. Melt vs. Emulsion Electrospinning

Electrospun fibers are generally obtained from polymer solutions or melts or emulsions. Melt spinning has high-throughput rate and process safety; solutions have the advantage of using a large variety of polymeric materials, lower energy consumption and superior mechanical, optical and electrical properties of prepared fibers. Emulsion electrospinning is needed for high melting polymers to prepare flame-retardant fibers. A comparison of different spinning methods using poly(lactic acid) (PLA) as a model polymer has been reported by Gupta et al. [41].

The melt of the polymer with other additives is extruded through the capillary, resulting in a thin fiber that cools and solidifies rapidly during its time in the air before depositing onto the collector [41]. Take-up speed, drawing temperature and draw ratio define the structural and tensile properties of the fiber. Draw ratio is the amount of stretching that the material undergoes during the drawing stage of electrospinning. The increase in draw ratio [42] and take-up speed [43] increases the molecular chain orientation along the fiber axis as well as the overall crystallinity of fibers formed from the melt. A higher entanglement of polymer fibers amongst themselves gives sub-par fibers compared to the solution of the same polymer.

The solution spinning method is ideal for polymers or blends of polymers that are thermally unstable or degrade upon melting. Based on how the solvent used for preparing the polymer solution is removed from the fibers, this method can be divided into two different types, namely, dry spinning and wet spinning. The dry spinning process uses hot air or inert gas on the polymer jet to facilitate the solvent's evaporation and fiber solidification. For example, Postema et al. used a solvent combination of chloroform and toluene to produce PLA fibers of high strength by using dry spinning and hot-drawing processes. They were able to obtain an optimal tensile strength of 2.2 GPa by electrospinning at 25 °C [44]. The wet-spinning process involves the use of a viscous coagulation bath containing the liquid, which is miscible with the spinning solvent but not with the polymer. The interaction between the polymer solvent and non-solvent leads to phase separation and then solvent removal from the jet.

This process is known to show fiber defects that can, to some extent, be limited by using 3–5 mm of air gap before the non-solvent, as this allows for stress relaxation of the polymeric chain [41].

In the emulsion electrospinning process, finely ground polymers, insoluble and non-melting, are mixed with another polymer solution with a catalyst and emulsifying agents. The formed emulsion is then electrospun by either the dry or the wet spinning method. This technique has been used in preparing fibers from fluorocarbons with high melting points, ceramics, and polymer blends with flame-retardant properties [45]. Persano et al. have discussed in detail the methods and their industrial application in their review [45].

3.2. Nozzle Configuration

Nozzle configuration relates to the number and the arrangement of capillary tubes from which the jets of fibers emerge. A single nozzle configuration is the simplest and most common configuration, wherein the charged solution flows through a single capillary (Figure 1). This particular configuration has been used to electrospin different polymeric fibers either singly [46,47] or in combination [48] or solvent systems [10]. Co-electrospinning of polymer blends in the same solvent or a mixture was the first and most common modification in the process. Zhou et al. mixed polyaniline with poly(ethylene oxide) in chloroform to obtain nanofibers of a size below 30 nm [49]. Sometimes polymer blends are used to obtain the final properties of fibers. If the polymers are not miscible in a common solvent, or when a homogeneous solution of polymers cannot be obtained, thermodynamic and kinetic aspects should be considered for electrospinning. One way around that problem is to modify the nozzle configuration, where different polymer solutions are electrospun from different capillaries, side-by-side. In this type of configuration, two polymer solutions pass through separate capillaries arranged side-by-side, which are connected to a high voltage supply and never come into contact until they reach the end of the capillary. A single Taylor cone is formed, which ejects the jet with a non-uniform mixture of both polymer solutions and, after drying, is deposited in the collector (Figure 3). The side-by-side technique yields Janus fibers having two different materials on either side of the fiber. The special morphology obtained provides combinational properties of two different polymers and allows several post electrospinning modifications [50]. For this type of configuration to work, it is necessary that both the polymeric solutions have similar conductivity for them to form a single Taylor cone and eject as a mixture. A bicomponent system consisting of poly(vinyl chloride)/segmented polyurethane and poly(vinyl chloride)/poly(vinyl fluoride) was studied [51].

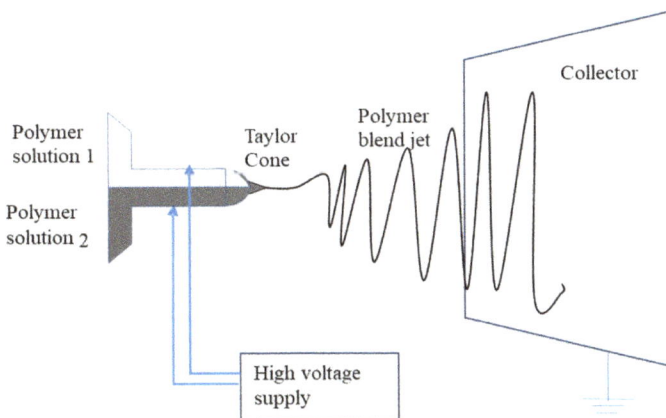

Figure 3. Side-by-side electrospinning schematic diagram: Polymer solutions 1 and 2 pass through separate capillaries, which are connected to the same high voltage supply, at either the same or different rates. A single Taylor cone is formed, which ejects the jet with non-uniform mixture of both the polymer solutions and, after drying, is deposited on the collector.

A second type of nozzle configuration that has recently been introduced is coaxial configuration. Two separate polymer solutions flow through two different capillaries, where the small capillary is within the larger capillary. This configuration can easily encapsulate a small fiber within a larger fiber, forming core-shell morphology (Figure 4). In one study, living cells were encapsulated in poly(dimethylsiloxane) fiber with high cell viability (67.6 ± 1.9%) compared to the control cells (70.6 ± 5.0%). Though the initial viability was comparable, over time, issues with cell morphology and growth rate were observed. This was the first study of its kind, and authors noted the need for further research to obtain the best possible results for encapsulation of living cells [52]. Encapsulation of a model protein, fluorescein isothiocyanate conjugated bovine serum albumin (BSA), with poly(ethylene glycol) in poly(epsilon-caprolactone), was able to sustain the release of the drug, defining its use in drug delivery. Coaxial fibers of proteins, such as fibrinogen [53], BSA, and lysozyme [54] and growth factors, such as bone morphogenetic protein2 (BMP-2) [55], bFGF [56], PDGF [57], VEGF [58], and EGF [59] have been reported. Apart from the regular parameters that affect the quality of fibers being produced by coaxial electrospinning, the relative flow rate of the core and the shell solutions (ratios between 5:1 and 6:1) is important in determining the encapsulation efficiency [60]. At a lower flow rate, the core phase is not continuous, which results in breaking up of the core, whereas a higher flow rate causes the formation of pendent droplets. Wang and co-workers reported that at an optimal flow rate, the core diameter could be easily controlled. Also, the flow rate is related to the core diameter by scaling laws of $d_f \sim Q_c^{0.18}$ where d_f represents the inner diameter of the fiber and Q_c represents the flow rate of core solution [61] This method is widely used in tissue engineering to achieve sustained, local and efficient gene and growth factor delivery to the cells [60,62,63]. Coaxial fibers of different non-steroidal anti-inflammatory drugs such as ketprofen [64], flurbiprofen axetil [65], and ibuprofen [64] and antibiotics such as levofloxacin, tetracycline hydrochloride, ciprofloxacin, moxifloxacin, and fusidic acid [66] were prepared and investigated. Though this method is now widely used, it still has the drawbacks of complexity of design and precise control of spinning parameters e.g., interfacial tension, viscoelasticity of the polymers or two different solutions used.

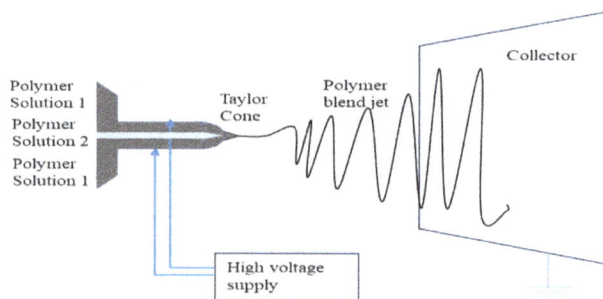

Figure 4. Coaxial electrospinning schematic diagram: Polymer solution 2 is passed through the inner capillary tube, while polymer solution 1 is passed through the outer capillary tube. The Taylor cone is formed where the inner solution (polymer solution 2) is surrounded by the outer solution. The jet erupts from the Taylor cone, and during that process, the polymer in the inner layer is coated with the polymer in the outer layer. The dried fiber with a core-shell design is then deposited on the collector.

The multi-jet electrospinning based on multiple capillaries arranged in circular geometry is yet another modification of the nozzle that can both increase the throughput and facilitate scale up and commercialization. This modification increases the mat thickness, deposits in a larger area and can mix fibers of different materials for better strength and versatility of use [21,67]. In the study by Varesano et al., the morphology of PEO fibers was found to be acceptable in both polarities applied in standard and reverse configuration [21]. The main drawback of the multi-capillary method is the alteration of the electric field due to the presence of other electrospinning jets in the vicinity [68].

This can be overcome by using an auxiliary electrode of any polarity [69] or by using a secondary electrode [70]. Hong et al. fabricated an elastic, fibrous, composite sheet with biodegradable poly(ester urethane) urea (PEUU) and poly(lactide-co-glycolide) (PLGA) using a two-stream electrospinning setup with a rotating metal rod as the collector [71]. Such composite sheets possessed better breaking strains, tensile strength and suture retention capacity. In a review article, Persano et al. discussed different multi-jet configurations and the further possibilities of syringe-free approaches to multi-jet electrospinning [45].

3.3. Collector Modification

The collector plate can be configured based on the application of polymeric fibers. Commercially, the most common collectors are stationary plates (or aluminum foil) and rotating plates. Both these types of collectors can be subdivided further into continual or patterned. A continual collector is simple and can be used to obtain fibers with a random internal structure on a stationary type, while some degree of directional control can be gained with the higher speed of a rotating collector. The patterned collectors have thin conductive wires separated from one another by an air gap. During the process, the fibers are deposited either between or perpendicular to the wires, individually, achieving some degree of alignment. Properly aligned polymer fibers are mostly useful in tissue engineering. In the rotating type of patterned collector, operation at lower speeds deposits fibers between the conductive wires, while deposits at the higher speed are dependent on electrostatic and mechanical forces increasing the degree of alignment. For research purposes, different designs of collectors have been used, including: mesh [72], pin [73], grids [74], liquid bath [75,76], rotating rods [77], rotating cylinder [78], parallel bars [77], rotating drum with wire wound on it [79], and disc [34,80].

4. Methods of Incorporating Drugs

Electrospinning is easy and cost effective, and it offers great flexibility in selecting materials, high loading capacity and high encapsulation efficiency, which makes it suitable for medical and drug-related research. There are various methods of drug loading in the polymeric solution for electrospinning.

4.1. Blending

Blending is the primary method for incorporating drugs into the polymer solution by dissolving or dispersing the drug and then subsequently electrospinning. Though this method is simple and easy, the physicochemical properties of the drug and the polymer need to be precisely considered, as these affect the encapsulation efficiency, the drug distribution in the fiber and the kinetics of the drug release. Lipophilic drugs (e.g., paclitaxel) should be dissolved in a lipophilic polymer and hydrophilic drugs (e.g., doxorubicin hydrochloride) in a hydrophilic polymer for better encapsulation. When the drug is not dissolved properly in the polymer solution, a dispersion is obtained, which might lead to burst release if the drug migrates to the fiber surface [81]. To obtain a sustained release of the drug from the electrospun fibers, in order to enhance the drug-loading efficiency and to reduce the burst release, different combinations of the mixtures of hydrophilic and hydrophobic polymers are used [82–84]. This process was modified by Ma et al. to obtain highly porous chitosan nanofibers by electrospinning chitosan/polyethylene oxide (PEO) blend solutions and then removing PEO with water [85]. They then soaked the porous nanofibers in 0.1 wt% paclitaxel solution to load the drug, and then into 4 wt% hyaluronic acid for encapsulation. Mickova et al. have compared electrospinning of a liposome by blending and by coaxial electrospinning and have reported that blend electrospinning could not conserve intact nanofibers [86].

4.2. Surface Modification

Surface modification is the technique in which the therapeutic agent is bound or conjugated to the fiber surface to make it structurally and biochemically similar to the tissue. The drug release in this case will be attenuated, and the functionality of the biomolecules will be protected [87]. The burst release and short-term release will be mitigated with this strategy, making it highly applicable for slow and prolonged delivery of gene or growth factors. Incorporation of DNA, growth factors and enzymes, conjugated to fibers, preserves their bioactivity and functionality [87–90]. The modulation of drug release can also be obtained if surface modification is done on blended electrospun fibers. Im et al. fluorinated the electrospun fibers to obtain controlled release of the drug by introducing a hydrophobic group onto the surface [91]. In one modification, Yun et al. oxyfluorinated the multi-walled carbon nanotubes (MWCNTs) to introduce the functional groups and improve the compatibility with the PVA/polyacrylic acid (PAA) polymer solution before electrospinning the composite mixture [92]. Kim et al. surface modified the fiber and loaded it with small-interfering RNA (siRNA) to obtain better results in gene silencing and wound healing [93]. Co-axial electrospinning encapsulates biomolecules like DNA into the fiber, in contrast to surface localization of DNA fibers with the blending process. Luu et al. reported that the transfection efficiency of electrospun DNA was significantly lower than Fugene 6, a commercially available transfection mediation agent [94]. To overcome the drawback, the electrospinning method was changed to coaxial to get a polymer coating around the biomolecules, which not only modified the release, but also protected the core against the direct exposure to the environment [60,62,95]. For additional benefits, the shell polymer can also be loaded with other bioactive molecules, such as non-viral gene-delivery vectors, for delivering the released DNA [62].

4.3. Emulsion

Another approach is the process of forming an emulsion for electrospinning, where the drug or the protein solution is emulsified within a polymer solution. The latter acts as an oil phase, and spinning such an emulsion produces a well-distributed fiber for a low molecular weight drug [96] and a core-shell for a high molecular weight drug [97–99]. The success of this process is mainly dependent on the ratio of the aqueous solution to the polymer solution. This governs the distribution behavior of the molecule in fiber, which in turn determines the release profile, structural stability and bioactivity of the encapsulated biomolecules [97]. As the drug and the polymers are dissolved in appropriate solvents, avoiding the need of a common solvent, various combinations of hydrophilic drugs and lipophilic polymer can be used. Unlike coaxial spinning, emulsion spinning might damage macromolecules, such as pDNA, due to shearing force and interfacial tension between the two phases. Such instances can be avoided by preventing denaturation by the condensation of pDNA [98,99].

4.4. Multi-Drug Delivery

Multi-drug delivery is a recent approach in which multiple drugs with or without similar therapeutic effects are combined and electrospun with suitable polymer(s) [100,101]. Wang et al. have used drug-loaded polymeric nanoparticles for the core and drug-loaded polymer for the sheath to obtain a chain-like structure with a distinct release behavior, enabling a program or temporality release of multiple agents [100]. Xu et al. have developed a hydrophilic model of bovine serum albumin (BSA) drug-loaded chitosan microspheres and suspended them in poly(l-lactic acid) (PLLA) solution with a hydrophobic model drug (benzoin) and polyvinylpyrrolidone (PVP) as a release tuner [101]. It is difficult to achieve independent release of the drugs in a multidrug system, as both drugs are held by the carrier, which provides the same diffusion pathways and matrix-degradation rate [95]. Okuda et al. have developed a multilayered drug-loaded electrospun nanofiber mesh fabricated for time-programmed dual release by sequential electrospinning. The formulation has four layers: the drug-loaded mesh (the top layer), the barrier mesh (blank polymer), the second drug-loaded mesh and the last basement mesh. This system provided for the development of electrospun fibers with controlled drug release and time of release by optimizing the fiber size, thickness of each layer and relative position of the layer. Though the authors have used two dyes as model drugs, this approach is significant for the biochemical modulation in chemotherapy with multiple-anti tumor drugs [102]. A graphical presentation of the same is shown in Figure 5.

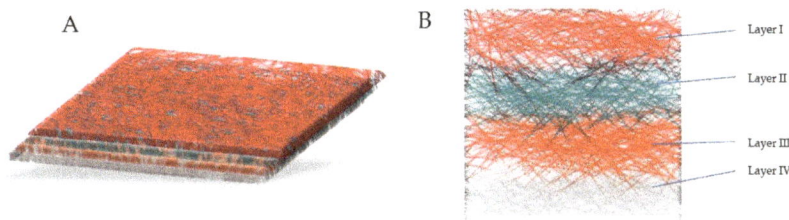

Figure 5. Graphical presentation of multi-drug delivery system: (**A**) overview; (**B**) cross sectional view of a tetra-layered sequential electrospun mesh. Cross-sectional view consists of drug loaded mesh (layer I), barrier mesh (layer II), second drug loaded mesh (layer III) and basement mesh (layer IV). Redrawn from [102].

4.5. Multilayer Coated

Yet another innovative method of incorporation and delivery of drug combines the large surface area of electrospun fibers with polyelectrolyte multilayer structures [95]. Such a multilayer uses either electrostatic or hydrogen bonding or acid-base pairing in layer-by-layer adsorption of polymers [103]. Chundar et al. have used two oppositely charged weak polyelectrolytes, polyacrylic acid (PAA) and poly allylamine hydrochloride (PAH), to produce nanofibers loaded with methylene blue as a model drug. In addition to polymers, a hydrophobic layer of perfluorosilane and PAA/poly(N-isopropylacrylamide) (PNIPAAM) was coated. The latter also provided temperature-controlled drug-release properties. Im et al. used alginate and chitosan to coat the lactobacillus-incorporated polyvinyl alcohol-based electrospun fibers. This formulation was designed to release lactobacillus in the large intestine after chitosan and alginate were dissolved in the acidic and then neutral environments of the GIT [104].

5. Electrospun Nanofibers in Drug Delivery

The electrospinning process has been used in drug delivery for treating various diseases. Electrospun fibers are administered mainly via oral and topical routes and as implantable systems.

5.1. Vitamins, NSAIDS and Natural Products

The transdermal drug delivery system (TDDS) delivers the drugs locally or systemically via the skin. This is mainly suitable for drugs that cannot be taken by the oral route, either because of extensive degradation in the GIT or because the drug undergoes extensive first pass metabolism [105]. Electrospun fibers of vitamins, anti-inflammatory and antioxidant drugs are mainly given by transdermal route [92,106–111]. Taepaiboon et al. have loaded vitamin A acid (all-*trans* retinoic acid) and vitamin E (α-tocopherol) in cellulose acetate polymer-based electrospun fibers and solvent cast films [110]. The results obtained revealed that the electrospun fiber mats showed a gradual and consistent increase in the cumulative vitamin release assayed using a total immersion technique over the test period of 24 h for vitamin E- and 6 h for vitamin A-loaded fiber. The corresponding solvent cast films showed a burst release of vitamins. A similar study performed by Nagwhirunpat et al. compared the electrospun and solvent cast film of polyvinyl alcohol loaded with meloxicam, an anti-arthritis drug [111]. They observed significantly higher skin permeation flux of the drug from electrospun fiber mats than with the solvent cast film, and the flux increased with an increase in drug concentration in both cases. Yun et al. developed an electro-responsive TDDS fiber by electrospinning poly(vinyl alcohol)/poly(acrylic acid)/multi-walled carbon nanotubes (PVA/PAA/MWCNT) with ketoprofen. The swelling, drug-release properties and conductivity of nanofibers were dependent upon the MWCNT, oxyfluorination and oxygen content during oxyfluorination [92]. The fibers were found to be non-toxic and biocompatible, with cell viability of more than 80%. In a similar study, Im et al. worked to understand the effect of MWCNT on ketoprofen delivery in an electro-sensitive

TDDS with polyethylene oxide and pentaerythritol triacrylate polymers [109]. This study supported the impact of MWCNT in influencing conductivity and drug-release behavior. Reda et al. formulated ketoprofen-loaded Eudragit® L and Eudragit® S electrospun nanofibers for treating oral mucositis. The rapid evaporation of solvent during electrospinning prevented the drug molecules from forming crystalline aggregates within the nanofibers. In addition, the amount of ketoprofen released from nanofibers was significantly higher than that released from corresponding solvent-casted films. Furthermore, a marked reduction in inflammatory infiltrate was seen in mucositis-induced rabbits with developed nanofibers [112]. Apart from the synthetic chemicals, a natural/herbal extract containing asiaticoside from *Centella asiatica* was incorporated into the electrospun fibers based on cellulose acetate polymer [106]. Suwantong et al. used two forms of the drug, pure asiaticoside and a crude extract from the plant. They observed a better release profile from the pure drug than from the extract assayed using the immersion method, while the release from both fiber mats was significantly low in the pigskin method. In addition, they checked the release profile of the solvent cast films, which were much lower. They further reported that the extract-loaded fibers and films were toxic to normal human dermal fibroblasts at the extraction concentrations of 5 and 10 mg/mL [106].

5.2. Antibiotics/Antibacterial Agents and Wound Dressing

In recent years, antibiotics and antibacterial agents have been the most common drug molecules that are encapsulated, using different polymers and their combinations as carriers. Different polymers, such as PLA, PLGA and PCL, are primarily used in the polymeric electrospun fibers for biodegradability, and other natural and synesthetic hydrophilic or hydrophobic polymers are used to control the release pattern of the drug. Kenaway et al. used tetracycline hydrochloride with poly(ethylene-co-vinyl acetate) (PEVA), PLA and their 50:50 blend to deliver the drug for treating periodontal disease [113]. They reported over five days of release with PEVA and the blend, suggesting their applicability in controlled-release technology. In another study by Alhusein et al., electrospun fibers of tetracycline HCl using PCL and PEVA were developed for potential application in wound healing and skin-structure infections. The developed three-layered electrospun matrix showed controlled release and also higher antibacterial efficacy when compared to the commercially available test disks of the drug [114]. The same group of researchers also reported high biological activity of the developed fiber matrices in complex models of biofilm formation. The fibers killed preformed biofilms and mature dense colonies of *Staphylococcus aureus* MRSA252 and also inhibited the formation of new biofilms [115]. Wang et al. have electrospun PVA nanofibers containing pleurocidin, a novel, broad-spectrum antimicrobial peptide, for food preservation applications [116]. Direct application of the active moiety is not possible because of the loss in its bioactivity. This study reported higher inhibition efficacy of the drug from nanofibers against *Escherichia coli* in apple cider.

Wound dressings protect the wound from external microorganisms and absorb/adsorb the exudate from the wound, providing an acceptable cosmetic appearance. The use of different components in the wound dressing prevents infection of the wound and accelerates the healing process [117]. The components added to the inert dressings are mainly bioactives in the form of films, hydrogels, foams and sponges [84]. With respect to wound healing, electrospun fiber mats have the advantage of high surface area for efficient absorption of exudates; in addition to adjusting the moisture of the wound and promoting scar-free regeneration of skin cells, these mats have porosity enough to supply oxygen for cell respiration, yet not enough for bacterial infections [58,117,118]. In one study by Jannesari et al., electrospun nanofibers of poly(vinyl alcohol) and poly(vinyl acetate) were prepared individually and in a 50:50 blend of the polymers. The nanofibers prepared using the polymer blend sustained the drug release and were found to be comfortable due to significant swelling [84]. In an in vitro microbial study, Said et al. have shown a faster bacterial colonization and biofilm formation in fusidic acid-loaded PLGA fibers, which in turn enhanced the release of the drug, eradicated planktonic bacteria and suppressed the biofilm [119]. Thakur et al. used the dual spinneret electrospinning apparatus to prepare a single scaffold of lidocaine and mupirocin [120]. Two drugs with varying lipophilicities were found to have different release profiles. Lidocaine showed a burst release, while mupirocin showed sustained release, providing action for over 72 h. Wang et al. have fabricated nanofibers of ethylene-co-vinyl alcohol (EVOH) with different antibacterial drugs and silver for wound dressings with superior germ killing capacity [121]. Silver nanoparticles have been used in many other studies for similar applications [66,122]. Recently, Chutipakdeevong et al. have utilized the hybridization method to combine the properties of *Bombyx mori* silk fibroin with poly(ε-caprolactone) (PCL) electrospun fibers [123]. The PCL fiber surfaces were coated with silk fibroin protein using the lyophilization technique and then surface modified with fibronectin to improve their biological function. The surface-modified hybrid showed significant proliferation of normal human dermal fibroblast (NHDF), followed by hybrid scaffold and then neat PCL fibers.

5.3. Delivery of Anticancer Agents

Anticancer agents, such as doxorubicin, paclitaxel, cisplatin and dichloroacetate, have been incorporated into electrospun fibers with polymers such as PLA, PLGA and PLLA for postoperative chemotherapy. A water-in-oil (w/o) emulsion, with water soluble drugs in aqueous phase and polymeric solutions of PEG-PLA in chloroform as oily phase, was prepared and electrospun to obtain fibers [124]. In a continuation study, hydrophobic paclitaxel and hydrophilic doxorubicin were simultaneously loaded in the emulsion based electrospinning process for multi-drug delivery [125]. The cytotoxicity study of rat Glioma C6 cells showed higher inhibition and apoptosis in combination therapy compared to the single-drug system. In another study, an in vitro cytotoxicity study of the same cells showed a sustained release of platinum-based cisplatin for more than 75 days without burst release and four times better cytotoxicity than the free drug [126]. Lee et al. have fabricated biodegradable PLGA fibers sheets for local delivery of epigallocatechin-3-O-gallate (EGCG) to reduce intimal hyperplasia in injured abdominal aorta [116]. The EGCG-loaded sheets exhibited initial burst release for 24 h, followed by sustained release for more than 30 days in phosphate buffer. In vivo studies showed promising results against intimal hyperplasia after application of the EGCG-loaded fibers, compared to PLGA control.

Recently, electrospun fibers have been used for local chemotherapy. Liu et al. encapsulated doxorubicin in PLLA polymer fiber and examined its efficacy for local chemotherapy against secondary hepatic carcinoma by wrapping the whole liver with carcinoma with the fiber-mat [127]. In the first 24 h, the drug was rapidly released from the fiber to localize in the liver tissue. It also significantly inhibited the tumor growth and increased the median survival time of the mice in the experiment. Luo et al. prepared fibers with core-loaded hydroxycamptothecin (HCPT) and 2-hydroxypropyl-β-cyclodextrin complexed HCPT, and observed that the inclusion complex showed superior antitumor activity and fewer side effects compared to the free drug [128]. Ma et al. loaded paclitaxel in the porous chitosan nanofiber and then encapsulated the fiber in polyanionic macromolecular hyaluronic acid (HA). The MTT assay in prostate cancer cells showed that the drug-loaded nanofiber mats were good at prohibiting cell attachment and proliferation [129]. The drawback of the fibers was an initial burst release of drug within the first 48 h. Chen et al. incorporated titanocene dichloride in PLLA polymer-based fibers [130]. The MTT assay in human lung tumor (SPCA-1) cells showed that drug contents of 40, 80, 160 and 240 mg/L had cell growth inhibition rates of 11.2%, 22.1%, 44.2% and 68.2%, respectively. Apart from the synthetic anticancer drug, natural products with anticancer properties and minimal side effects have been studied. Suwantong et al. electrospun curcumin in cellulose acetate solution and observed that curcumin is almost completely (~90 to ~95%) released in the total immersion method, while considerably low values were obtained for transdermal diffusion through pig skin [108]. In another study, Shao et al. fabricated green tea polyphenols (GTP) in poly(ε-caprolactone)/multi-walled carbon nanotube (PCL/MWCNTs) composite nanofibers by electrospinning. The cytotoxicity experiment showed a significant inhibitory effect in A549 and Hep G2 tumor cells [131]. Table 1 provides a compilation of studies involving the use of electrospun fibers in delivering antibiotics, anticancer agents and NSAIDS.

Table 1. Studies involving the use of electrospun fibers in drug delivery (partial listing).

Drug(s)	Polymer(s)	Solvent Composition	Spraying Type
		Antibacterial agents	
Tetracycline hydrochloride	PEUU and PLGA [71]; PLA, PEV, PLA/PEVA [113]; PLA/PCL [132]; PLLA [133,134]; PCL, PEVA [114]	1,1,3,3,3-Hexafluoro-2-propanol [71]; Chloroform [113]; Chloroform, dimethylformamide [132]; Chloroform: acetone (2:1) [133,134]; chloroform:methanol (9:1) [114]	Single nozzle; Coaxial [133,134]
Gentamycin sulfate and Resveratrol (antioxidant)	PCL [133]	Chloroform: ethanol (3:1)	Coaxial
Ciprofloxacin Hydrochloride	PVA, Poly(vinyl acetate) [84]	Diluted acetic acid solution	Single nozzle
Fusidic acid and rifampicin	PLGA [135]	Tetrahydro Furan/Dimethylformamide	Single nozzle
Mefoxin	PLGA [83]	DMF	Single nozzle
Metronidazole benzoate	PCL [136]	Dichloromethane (DCM:DMF)	Single nozzle
Ciprofloxacin hydrochloride, Levofloxacin hemihydrate, Moxifloxacin hydrochloride	coPLA, coPLA/PEG [137]	DCM:DMSO (3:1)	Single nozzle
Lidocaine and mupirocin	PLLA [120]	Hexafluoroisopropanol	Dual spinneret
Ornidazole (Biteral®)	PCL	Chloroform and DMF (3:7)	Single nozzle
Potassium 5-nitro-8-quinolinolate	Chitosan/PEO [138]	2% (w/v) acetic acid	Single nozzle
Itraconazole and ketanserin	PU [139]	DMF, DMAc	Single nozzle
Pleurocidin	PVA [116]	Distilled water	Single nozzle
		NSAIDS	
Ketoprofen	PVA/PAA/MWCNT [92]; PEO/PETA/MWCNT [109]; EC and PVP [140]; PVP/Zein [141]	Deionized water [92,109] Ethanol-water [140,141]	Single nozzle Coaxial [141]
Ibuprofen	PLGA PEG-g-CHN [142]	DMF	Side-by-side
Fenbufen	PLGA/Gelatin [82]	2,2,2-trifluoroethanol	Single nozzle
Rhodamine B/Naproxen	Chitosan nanoparticles/PCL composite [100]	Acetic acid/chloroform: methanol (3:1)	Single nozzle yet core/sheath fiber
Meloxicam	PVA [111]	Water	Single nozzle

Table 1. *Cont.*

Drug(s)	Polymer(s)	Solvent Composition	Spraying Type
Anticancer agents			
Doxorubicin [127]	PLLA [127]	Chloroform-methano-DMSO [127]	Single nozzle
Doxorubicin Hydrochloride	PEG-PLA [124,143]	Chloroform [143]	Emulsion [124]
		w/o emulsion [124]	
Hydroxycamptothecin	HPCD [128]	DMSO	Emulsion
Paclitaxel	Chitosan/PEO/HA [84]	Acetic acid/distilled water [84]	Single nozzle
	PLGA [144,145]	DCM and DMF	
Cisplatin	PLA/PLGA [126]	DCM	Single nozzle
Dichloroacetate	PLA [146]	Chloroform	Single nozzle
1,3-Bis(2-chloroethyl)-1-nitrosourea	PEO and PEG-PLLA [147]	Chloroform	Single nozzle/Emulsion
Curcumin	Cellulose acetate [108]	Acetone/dimethylacetamide (2:1)	Single nozzle
Green tea polyphenols (GTP)	PCL/MWCNT [131]	Dichloromethane	Single nozzle
Titanocene dichloride	PLLA [130]	Dichloromethane	Single nozzle

PLA: Polylactic acid); PEVA-Poly(ethylene-co-vinylacetate); PCL: poly(ε-caprolactone); PCL-co-PCLEEP: Copolymer of caprolactone and ethyl ethylene phosphate; PLGA: Poly(D,L-Lactic acid-co-glycolic acid); PEUU: poly(ester urethane) urea; EC: ethyl cellulose; PEO: Poly(ethylene oxide); PU: Polyurethane; DMAc: Dimethylacetamide; PETA: pentaerythritol triacrylate; PEI-HA: Poly(ethylenimine)-hyaluronic acid; PVP: polyvinylpyrrolidone; PEG-g-CHN: poly(ethylene glycol)-g-Chitosan; PEG-PLA: poly(ethylene glycol)-poly(lactic acid); PLLA: poly(L-lactic acid); HPCD: 2-hydroxypropyl-β-cyclodextrin; HA: Hyaluronic acid; MWCNT: multi-walled carbon nanotubes, PAA–Poly(acrylic acid); PECCL: poly(ethylene carbonate-ε-caprolactone); PDLLA: poly(D,L-lactic acid).

5.4. DNA, RNA, Protein and Growth Factor Delivery

The most commonly loaded bioactive materials in electrospun fibers include DNA, RNA, proteins and growth factors. The electrospinning process applied to the bioactive materials should be designed in such a way that the activity and functional efficacy of the material is preserved during and after electrospinning. Before coaxial electrospinning, few studies on bioactive materials had been done with the blending process. The stability of the growth factors is the limiting aspect in formulating them in tissue-engineered scaffolds. Human nerve growth factor (hNGF) was encapsulated with BSA as a carrier protein into the nanofibers of PCL and poly(ethyl ethylene phosphate) (PCLEEP). The protein released in a sustained manner for more than three months from the electrospun fibers and showed partial retention of bioactivity [148]. The same group also co-encapsulated small-interfering RNA (siRNA) and transfection reagent (TKO) complexes within a nanofiber of caprolactone and ethyl ethylene phosphate (PCLEEP, diameter ~400 nm) to obtain a sustained release of siRNA for up to 28 days [149]. The release of siRNA was enhanced and more significant gene knockdown was obtained when compared with electrospun fibers of PCL containing siRNA [150]. Schneider et al. demonstrated that biofunctionalized silk mats containing epidermal growth factor (EGF) are extremely promising in achieving bioactive wound dressings for the wound healing process [151]. Similarly, Zhang et al. showed that the poly(ethylene carbonate-ε-caprolactone) scaffolds with VEGF maintained good growth and spread morphology in human umbilical vein endothelial cells [152]. After the introduction of the coaxial electrospinning method, most biomolecules are preferentially encapsulated using this method, forming a core of biomolecule and shell of polymer in a core-shell structure. The polymeric shell protected and released biomolecules in a sustained manner. Saraf et al. prepared fiber scaffolds with plasmid DNA (pDNA) within the core of poly(ethylene glycol) and non-viral gene delivery vector poly(ethylenimine)-hyaluronic acid (PEI-HA) within the sheath polymer poly(ε-caprolactone) (PCL) by coaxial electrospinning [62]. They achieved variable transfection activity over extended periods of time upon the release of pDNA and non-viral gene delivery vectors from electrospun fiber scaffolds. Mickova et al. have proposed the use of liposomes in the core of polyvinyl alcohol (PVA) and shell of PCL for protecting the enzymatic activity of horseradish peroxidase [86]. The encapsulated enzyme retained its activity because of the shielding effect of the lipid sphere of liposome. Chen et al. encapsulated chitosan/siRNA nanoparticles in PLGA by electrospinning to control the release behavior at different pH conditions. In addition, the encapsulated siRNA showed up to 50% enhanced green fluorescent protein (EGFP) gene silencing activity after 48 h of transfection in H1299 cells [143]. Surface functionalization of nanofibers was performed for MMP-2-siRNA (Matrix metalloproteinase) in linear polyethyleneimine (LPEI) coated nanofibers with various nitrogen/phosphate (N/P) ratios [93]. In an animal study for seven days, it was observed that the siRNA in these fibers increased the MMP-2 gene silencing effect and neo-collagen accumulation at the wound site. Fabrication of surface modified electrospun fibers containing growth factors conjugated with heparin or polysaccharides is becoming common [87,89,153]. A burst release of nerve growth factor was observed from electrospun scaffolds conjugated with chitosan/poly(vinyl alcohol) [89]. Basic fibroblast growth factor was incorporated in heparin containing a polyelectrolyte nanoparticle, and that was electrostatically adsorbed on the chitosan matrix to overcome the problem of burst release [87]. Han et al. fabricated a composite design containing poly(ethylene glycol)-poly-(ε-caprolactone) diacrylate (PEGPCL) hydrogels coupled with electrospun mats of poly(ε-caprolactone) to control the burst release and to extend the release duration of nerve growth factor [154]. The bioactivity of the growth factor was demonstrated by PC-12 cells' neurite extension. Further, immobilization and delivery of the growth factor for the bone tissue engineering is discussed in the review by Chen and Lv [155]. In addition, electrospinning has extensively been used and reviewed for tissue scaffold engineering with or without any active moiety incorporated in the polymeric matrix. Table 2 provides a list of studies involving the use of electrospun fibers in delivering proteins, DNA, RNA and human factors.

5.5. Nanoparticle Impregnated Nanofibers

Electrospun nanofibers containing nanoparticles is another area of research that has been widely investigated for various applications, including surface-enhanced Raman scattering [156], antimicrobial packaging [157], dye-sensitized solar cells [158], food preservation [159], biowarfare decontamination [160], water treatment [161], high-performance gas sensing [162], and environmental remediation [163]. In drug delivery, these novel impregnated nanofibers are being explored in the areas of wound care, regenerative medicine, dental engineering, and for cancer treatment. In this section, we briefly summarized biomedical applications of nanoparticle impregnated nanofibers.

A study conducted by Lee et al. investigated the efficacy of chitosan (CTS) nanofibers containing silver nanoparticles for topical wound care. Silver nanoparticles were generated directly in the chitosan solution by chemical reduction using sodium borohydride. The nanoparticle solution obtained was then poured into sodium hydroxide resulting in the formation of CTS/AgNPs composite, which was further subjected to electrospinning to form nanofibers. The prepared fibers showed excellent antibacterial activity against *P. aeruginosa* and methicillin-resistant *S. aureus* when compared to the pure CTS nanofibers [164]. Similarly, Shi et al. prepared Ag/polyacrylonitrile (Ag/PAN) anti-bacterial nanofibers for use in implant scaffolds and biotextiles. Initially, PAN was dissolved in DMF and a known amount of $AgNO_3$ was added to form the pre-electrospinning solution. The solution was then treated using helium atmospheric plasma to reduce $AgNO_3$ into metallic silver nanoparticles. Finally, the solution obtained was electrospun to form nanofibers containing embedded Ag nanoparticles. SEM images revealed the smooth and continuous nature of the nanofibers. The nanofibers demonstrated a sustained release of silver ions and also showed higher antibacterial activity against Gram positive (*B. cereus*) and Gram negative bacteria (*E. coli*) when compared to the untreated nanofibers [165]. Another study conducted by Castro-Mayorga et al., investigated the antiviral properties of Ag nanoparticles in coated polyhydroxyalkonates. The films of poly(3-hydroxybutyrate-co-3-hydroxyvalerate) (PHBV) were developed by depositing a coat of electrospun fiber mat containing post-processed PHBV18/Ag nanoparticles over PHBV3 films formed by compression molding. Energy dispersive X-ray (EDX) analysis showed that Ag nanoparticles were homogeneously distributed into the coating and on the PHBV3/PHBV18 film. Moreover, cell culture analysis revealed no infectious feline calicivirus (FCV) recovery when treated with the prepared films, while murine norovirus (MNV) was decreased by 0.86 log [166].

Nie and Wang studied the complex of DNA and poly lactide-co-glycolide (PLGA)/hydroxyapatite (HAp) composite scaffolds fabricated by electrospinning for their use in bone tissue engineering. DNA was incorporated into the scaffolds in the form of naked DNA or DNA/chitosan nanoparticles before/after fiber fabrication. The results revealed that the scaffolds were non-woven and predominantly composed of PLGA with a dispersion of HAp nanoparticles. The addition of HAp nanoparticles showed an increase in the release rate of DNA from the scaffolds containing both naked and encapsulated DNA. Moreover, the scaffolds with encapsulated DNA/chitosan nanoparticles also showed a higher cell attachment, greater cell viability and desired transfection efficiency in human marrow stem cells (hMSCs) [167]. A similar study conducted by Tanaka and co-workers fabricated hydroxyapatite/PLA composite electrospun nanofibers for bone tissue engineering. The surface-modified HAp nanoparticles of stearic acid were dispersed uniformly in the PLA nanofibers and were evaluated for their mechanical strength. The authors concluded that the electrospun fibers showed higher strength when compared to the unmodified ones [168]. Table 3 provides a partial listing of studies involving the use of electrospun fibers in tissue engineering.

Table 2. Studies involving the use of electrospun fibers in delivery of proteins, DNA, RNA and human factors (partial listing).

Drug(s)	Polymer(s)	Solvent Composition	Spraying Type
plasmid DNA (pDNA)	PEI-HA [62]		Coaxial
siRNA	PCL [150]; PCLEEP [149] Chitosan/PLGA [169]	2,2,2-Trifluoroethanol (TFE) [150]; RNase-free water [149]; Hexafluoro-2-isopropanol/water [169]	Single nozzle
Human glial cell-derived neurotrophic factor	PCL-co-PCLEEP [170]	Dichloromethane	Single nozzle
Human β-nerve growth factor	PCL-co-PCLEEP [148]	Dichloromethane	Single nozzle
Endothelial growth factor VEGF	PECCL [152]	-	Single nozzle
Bovine Serum Albumin (BSA)	PEO [171]	Deionized water	Single nozzle
Lysozyme	PLA [97]	Chloroform	Emulsion
Human-nerve growth factor (NGF)	Poly(L-lactide-co-caprolactone) [172]	Chloroform	Emulsion
DNA	PLA-PEG and PLGA [94]	DMF	Single nozzle
Growth factors (VEGF, PDGF)	Poly(urethane) [63]	Chloroform: ethanol (75:25)	Coaxial
Horseradish peroxidase	PVA/PCL [86]	-	Coaxial

Table 3. Studies involving the use of electrospun fibers in tissue engineering (partial listing).

Drug(s)	Polymer(s)	Solvent Composition	Spraying Type
Wound healing, tissue engineering, hemostatic agent	Collagen-PEO [173,174]	Hydrochloric acid	Single nozzle
Adenovirus with gene for green fluorescent protein	Poly(ε-caprolactone) [60]	Chloroform: ethanol (75:25)	Coaxial
Guided tissue regeneration	PDLLA/PLGA [175]	Chloroform:DMF (9:1) and THF/DMF (3:1)	Single nozzle

Liposome-enriched nanofibers were investigated for delivering and preserving horseradish peroxidase (HRP) enzymatic activity. Liposomes were prepared using soybean derived L-α-phosphatidylcholine encapsulating horseradish peroxidase (HRP) by the extrusion technique. This study compared the activity of HRP in nanofibers developed by coaxial or blend electrospinning with and without liposomes. Blend nanofibers were prepared by electrospinning unilamellar liposomes dispersed in an aqueous solution of PVA and nanofibers, while the coaxial nanofibers were developed using PVA-core/PCL-shell with embedded liposomes. The results indicate that the blending of liposomes could not conserve the intact liposomes, while the nanofibers obtained by coaxial electrospinning retained liposomes. In addition, the core/shell nanofibers not only preserved the activity of encapsulated HRP enzyme but also enhanced the proliferation of mesenchymal stem cells (MSC) [86].

Poly (L-lactic acid-co-ε-caprolactone) (PLACL) nanofibers containing magnesium oxide (MgO) nanoparticles in synergy with aloe vera (AV), curcumin (CUR) and β-cyclodextrin (β-CD) were prepared and evaluated for treating breast cancer. In vitro toxicity of electrospun nanofibers composed of PLACL; PLACL with AV; PLACL with AV and MgO; PLACL with AV, MgO and CUR; and PLACL with AV, MgO, and β-CD was assessed in MCF-7 cells using the MTT assay. The results showed that PLACL nanofibers containing CUR showed the greatest cell death among all other nanofibrous scaffolds. However, PLACL nanofibers without MgO nanoparticles exhibited greatest tensile strength [176]. Sperm-shaped microrobots were studied for targeting breast cancer cells in vitro using fabricated nanoparticles. The microrobots were fabricated using electrospinning by a solution composed of polystyrene, dimethylformamide and nanoparticles of iron oxide. Under the influence of an oscillating magnetic field, the robotic sperm could controllably take S-shaped, U-shaped, square paths and selectively target the MCF-7 cells. Moreover, the cell membrane was not damaged after penetration of the robotic sperm into the cancerous cells [177].

Electrospun nanofibers composed of poly (ε-caprolactone) (PCL) and zero valent zinc nanoparticles were investigated by Sezer et al. to promote neuroglial cell proliferation. Chemical characterization studies indicated that the nanoparticles did not interact chemically with the PCL matrix. In addition, the nanofibers enhanced the tensile strength of the PCL matrix and promoted cell proliferation depending on the amount of zinc nanoparticles embedded inside the PCL matrix [178]. Another study investigated the efficiency of electrospun hybrid scaffolds composed of cyclosporine-loaded PLGA nanoparticles embedded in PCL scaffolds for promoting innervation of bioengineered teeth. The results from histological studies showed that the implantation of designed scaffolds in adult ICR mice did not alter the development of teeth. In addition, the transmission electron microscopy (TEM) and indirect immunofluorescence studies showed that 88% of the teeth were innervated upon treating with designed hybrid scaffolds [179].

6. Commercialization Challenges of Electrospinning

Although the benefits of electrospinning have been largely demonstrated in various fields of science, there is still a great need to implement the production in an efficient way. Several challenges relating to the electrospinning process are yet to be addressed. These include: (a) large-scale manufacturing; (b) accuracy and reproducibility during all the fabrication steps; and, (c) safety and environmental aspects of electrospinning [45]. The major challenges involved in mass production of electrospun fibers include low output per spinneret, clogging of the spinneret tip, inter-jet interference, recovery of vaporized solvents involved in the process, and fiber alignment over a large area of substantial thickness. To produce electrospun nanofibers without any morphology defects, the solution concentration is kept to a minimum, with solvent making up more than 70% of the solution mass. Therefore, only a fraction of the solution passing through the spinneret actually contributes to the mass of the nanofiber produced [180]. Also, there is a limit on the feed-rate per nozzle and higher rates might result in dripping of the solution from the nozzle, especially if the nozzle is placed in the middle. This is due to the insufficient electric field experienced by the nozzles, which results in inadequate drawing of the solution.

Clogging of the spinneret due to the solution gelation is highly disruptive and causes production losses. This problem is more apparent with solutions of higher concentration, as they are more viscous [181] and with polymers of high degree of crystallinity [182]. In addition, a solvent with low boiling point also causes clogging of the spinneret tip [183]. While the productivity of the microfiber spinning process can be increased by placing many spinnerets per spinning head, this is not feasible in the case of electrospinning. In electrospinning, the ejected solution spreads out to form an expanding cone and it interferes with the neighboring jets if the spinnerets are packed too close to each other [68]. Uniformity in the fiber layer thickness deposited onto substrate material is also comprised by the inter-jet interference [180].

Another important concern is regarding the solvent used in the electrospinning process. This particular issue is highly important not only for safety reasons during fabrication, but also for the final products, as solvent residues might be trapped inside the electrospun nanofibers. Accurate control over solvent residues becomes crucial in the case of large-volume, solvent-based electrospinning for biomedical and pharmaceutical applications [45]. However, the use of solvent-free spinning should eliminate the risk of solvent residues and recovery of solvents [184]. Due to the lack of reliable and affordable electrospinning technologies, the use of many different active polymeric materials for the fabrication of nanofibers is still limited [45]. In tissue engineering, the other main challenges that impede the progress of electrospinning applications are increasing scaffold thickness and pore size. Moreover, it is highly difficult to produce identical scaffolds, especially between research groups, which narrows the use of electrospun fiber mats for tissue engineering applications. Also, with tailored electrospun fibers, it is challenging to ensure uniformity of the fibers with specific morphologies and properties [185].

The recent development of needleless electrospinning offers the possibility for fabricating electrospun nanofibers on a large scale and addresses the issue of clogging at the spinnerets [186]. Needleless electrospinning systems using rotating disks [187], rollers [188], balls [189], and bubbles [190] that produce huge amounts of nanofibers have been reported by a few researchers. This method involves the formation of numerous small droplets on the drum surface or disk/coil. Moreover, this method does not require the maintenance of Taylor cones throughout the process making it highly advantageous over conventional needle-based method. Nonetheless, this process consumes a lot of energy in order to maintain the high voltage required and thus increases the chance of spark generation in the system. Therefore, solvents with low flash points, such as chloroform, tetrahydrofuran (THF), and toluene cannot be used for needless electrospinning [182]. Another area where considerable progress has been made in recent years is the development of smart electrospun nanofibers. These nanofibers respond to various kinds of stimuli, including pH, ionic strength, temperature, light, electricity, and magnetic field, and undergo physical and/or chemical changes. Studies involving smart electrospun nanofibers, their advantages and shortcomings are detailed in recent review by Weng and Xie [191].

7. Conclusions

The electrospinning process has generated a lot of interest in various medical applications due to its ease of use, adaptability and flexibility in controlling the fiber diameter from the micrometer down to the nanometer range. Though this method has been in use for a few decades now, the techniques and the equipment used in the electrospinning process are ever-evolving. Electrospinning began with a single nozzle configuration and evolved into multi-nozzle configurations through coaxial and emulsion spinning configurations. Further studies are being carried out to modify the nozzle configuration and collector design in order to significantly improve fiber properties and simplify the manufacturing process. This review summarizes several key aspects of electrospinning in the use of electrospun fibers in drug delivery with a special emphasis on electrospun nanofibers impregnated with nanoparticles. Studies involving biomedical applications of electrospun nanofibers are also discussed. By careful selection of polymers, it is now possible to deliver various antibacterial agents and anticancer drugs in a required manner using electrospun nanofibers. In order to make further progress, particularly in the field of drug delivery, it is necessary to identify ways that allow large-scale fabrication of nanofibers with desired morphological and mechanical properties in a reproducible manner. Despite the relentless efforts being made by academic and industrial scientists, much of the research conducted with electrospun fibers is in vitro. Further progress in the field of electrospun nanofibers will require continued assessment in vivo. Scientists working in this field have to identify ways to use nanofibers for immunotherapy, gene therapy and regenerative medicine in order to meet the current, as well as any future, demands in drug delivery.

Funding: This work was partially supported by the grant from the deArce Memorial Endowment Fund from The University of Toledo.

Conflicts of Interest: The authors declare no conflict of interest. The funders had no role in the writing of the manuscript.

References

1. Nayak, R.; Padhye, R.; Kyratzis, I.L.; Truong, Y.; Arnold, L. Recent advances in nanofibre fabrication techniques. *Text. Res. J.* **2011**. [CrossRef]
2. Greiner, A.; Wendorff, J.H. Electrospinning: A fascinating method for the preparation of ultrathin fibers. *Angew. Chem. Int. Ed.* **2007**, *46*, 5670–5703. [CrossRef] [PubMed]
3. Reneker, D.H.; Yarin, A.L. Electrospinning jets and polymer nanofibers. *Polymer* **2008**, *49*, 2387–2425. [CrossRef]
4. Kiyohiko, H. Process for Manufacturing Artificial Silk and Other Filaments by Applying Electric Current. U.S. Patents No. US1699615A, 22 January 1929.
5. Huang, Z.-M.; Zhang, Y.-Z.; Kotaki, M.; Ramakrishna, S. A review on polymer nanofibers by electrospinning and their applications in nanocomposites. *Compos. Sci. Technol.* **2003**, *63*, 2223–2253. [CrossRef]
6. Sill, T.J.; von Recum, H.A. Electrospinning: Applications in drug delivery and tissue engineering. *Biomaterials* **2008**, *29*, 1989–2006. [CrossRef] [PubMed]
7. Taylor, G. Electrically driven jets. *Proc. R. Soc. Lond. A Math. Phys. Eng. Sci.* **1969**, *313*, 453–475. [CrossRef]
8. Yarin, A.; Koombhongse, S.; Reneker, D.H. Bending instability in electrospinning of nanofibers. *J. Appl. Phys.* **2001**, *89*, 3018–3026. [CrossRef]
9. Doshi, J.; Reneker, D.H. Electrospinning process and applications of electrospun fibers. *J. Electrost.* **1995**, *35*, 154–160. [CrossRef]
10. Yang, Q.; Li, Z.; Hong, Y.; Zhao, Y.; Qiu, S.; Wang, C.; Wei, Y. Influence of solvents on the formation of ultrathin uniform poly(vinyl pyrrolidone) nanofibers with electrospinning. *J. Polym. Sci. Part B Polym. Phys.* **2004**, *42*, 3721–3726. [CrossRef]
11. Shin, Y.; Hohman, M.; Brenner, M.; Rutledge, G. Electrospinning: A whipping fluid jet generates submicron polymer fibers. *Appl. Phys. Lett.* **2001**, *78*, 1149–1151. [CrossRef]
12. Jaeger, R.; Bergshoef, M.M.; Batlle, C.M.I.; Schönherr, H.; Julius Vancso, G. Electrospinning of ultra-thin polymer fibers. *Macromol. Symp.* **1998**, *127*, 141–150. [CrossRef]
13. Carson, R.; Hendricks, C.; Hogan, J.; Schneider, J. Factors influencing electrically sprayed liquids. *AIAA J.* **1964**, *2*, 1460–1461. [CrossRef]
14. Buchko, C.J.; Chen, L.C.; Shen, Y.; Martin, D.C. Processing and microstructural characterization of porous biocompatible protein polymer thin films. *Polymer* **1999**, *40*, 7397–7407. [CrossRef]
15. Deitzel, J.; Kleinmeyer, J.; Harris, D.; Tan, N.B. The effect of processing variables on the morphology of electrospun nanofibers and textiles. *Polymer* **2001**, *42*, 261–272. [CrossRef]
16. Reneker, D.H.; Chun, I. Nanometre diameter fibres of polymer, produced by electrospinning. *Nanotechnology* **1996**, *7*, 216. [CrossRef]
17. Zhang, C.; Yuan, X.; Wu, L.; Han, Y.; Sheng, J. Study on morphology of electrospun poly(vinyl alcohol) mats. *Eur. Polym. J.* **2005**, *41*, 423–432. [CrossRef]
18. Li, Z.; Wang, C. Effects of working parameters on electrospinning. In *One-Dimensional Nanostructures*; Springer: Berlin, Germany, 2013; pp. 15–28.
19. Megelski, S.; Stephens, J.S.; Chase, D.B.; Rabolt, J.F. Micro-and nanostructured surface morphology on electrospun polymer fibers. *Macromolecules* **2002**, *35*, 8456–8466. [CrossRef]

20. Kilic, A.; Oruc, F.; Demir, A. Effects of polarity on electrospinning process. *Text. Res. J.* **2008**, *78*, 532–539. [CrossRef]
21. Varesano, A.; Carletto, R.A.; Mazzuchetti, G. Experimental investigations on the multi-jet electrospinning process. *J. Mater. Process. Technol.* **2009**, *209*, 5178–5185. [CrossRef]
22. Zargham, S.; Bazgir, S.; Tavakoli, A.; Rashidi, A.S.; Damerchely, R. The effect of flow rate on morphology and deposition area of electrospun nylon 6 nanofiber. *J. Eng. Fibers Fabr.* **2012**, *7*, 42–49.
23. Bhardwaj, N.; Kundu, S.C. Electrospinning: A fascinating fiber fabrication technique. *Biotechnol. Adv.* **2010**, *28*, 325–347. [CrossRef] [PubMed]
24. Nurwaha, D.; Han, W.; Wang, X. Investigation of a new needleless electrospinning method for the production of nanofibers. *J. Eng. Fibers Fabr.* **2013**, *8*, 42–49.
25. Sukigara, S.; Gandhi, M.; Ayutsede, J.; Micklus, M.; Ko, F. Regeneration of Bombyx mori silk by electrospinning—Part 1: Processing parameters and geometric properties. *Polymer* **2003**, *44*, 5721–5727. [CrossRef]
26. Fong, H.; Chun, I.; Reneker, D. Beaded nanofibers formed during electrospinning. *Polymer* **1999**, *40*, 4585–4592. [CrossRef]
27. Baumgarten, P.K. Electrostatic spinning of acrylic microfibers. *J. Colloid Interface Sci.* **1971**, *36*, 71–79. [CrossRef]
28. Meechaisue, C.; Dubin, R.; Supaphol, P.; Hoven, V.P.; Kohn, J. Electrospun mat of tyrosine-derived polycarbonate fibers for potential use as tissue scaffolding material. *J. Biomater. Sci. Polym. Ed.* **2006**, *17*, 1039–1056. [CrossRef] [PubMed]
29. Koski, A.; Yim, K.; Shivkumar, S. Effect of molecular weight on fibrous PVA produced by electrospinning. *Mater. Lett.* **2004**, *58*, 493–497. [CrossRef]
30. Zhao, Y.; Yang, Q.; Lu, X.-F.; Wang, C.; Wei, Y. Study on correlation of morphology of electrospun products of polyacrylamide with ultrahigh molecular weight. *J. Polym. Sci. Part B Polym. Phys.* **2005**, *43*, 2190–2195. [CrossRef]
31. Lyons, J.; Li, C.; Ko, F. Melt-electrospinning part I: Processing parameters and geometric properties. *Polymer* **2004**, *45*, 7597–7603. [CrossRef]
32. Larrondo, L.; St John Manley, R. Electrostatic fiber spinning from polymer melts. I. Experimental observations on fiber formation and properties. *J. Polym. Sci. Polym. Phys. Ed.* **1981**, *19*, 909–920. [CrossRef]
33. Ding, B.; Kim, H.Y.; Lee, S.C.; Shao, C.L.; Lee, D.R.; Park, S.J.; Kwag, G.B.; Choi, K.J. Preparation and characterization of a nanoscale poly(vinyl alcohol) fiber aggregate produced by an electrospinning method. *J. Polym. Sci. Part B Polym. Phys.* **2002**, *40*, 1261–1268. [CrossRef]
34. Inai, R.; Kotaki, M.; Ramakrishna, S. Structure and properties of electrospun PLLA single nanofibres. *Nanotechnology* **2005**, *16*, 208. [CrossRef] [PubMed]
35. Kim, K.-H.; Jeong, L.; Park, H.-N.; Shin, S.-Y.; Park, W.-H.; Lee, S.-C.; Kim, T.-I.; Park, Y.-J.; Seol, Y.-J.; Lee, Y.-M. Biological efficacy of silk fibroin nanofiber membranes for guided bone regeneration. *J. Biotechnol.* **2005**, *120*, 327–339. [CrossRef] [PubMed]
36. Lee, J.S.; Choi, K.H.; Ghim, H.D.; Kim, S.S.; Chun, D.H.; Kim, H.Y.; Lyoo, W.S. Role of molecular weight of atactic poly(vinyl alcohol)(PVA) in the structure and properties of PVA nanofabric prepared by electrospinning. *J. Appl. Polym. Sci.* **2004**, *93*, 1638–1646. [CrossRef]
37. Pillay, V.; Dott, C.; Choonara, Y.E.; Tyagi, C.; Tomar, L.; Kumar, P.; du Toit, L.C.; Ndesendo, V.M. A review of the effect of processing variables on the fabrication of electrospun nanofibers for drug delivery applications. *J. Nanomater.* **2013**, *2013*. [CrossRef]
38. Zong, X.; Kim, K.; Fang, D.; Ran, S.; Hsiao, B.S.; Chu, B. Structure and process relationship of electrospun bioabsorbable nanofiber membranes. *Polymer* **2002**, *43*, 4403–4412. [CrossRef]
39. Hayati, I.; Bailey, A.; Tadros, T.F. Investigations into the mechanisms of electrohydrodynamic spraying of liquids: I. Effect of electric field and the environment on pendant drops and factors affecting the formation of stable jets and atomization. *J. Colloid Interface Sci.* **1987**, *117*, 205–221. [CrossRef]
40. Huang, C.; Chen, S.; Lai, C.; Reneker, D.H.; Qiu, H.; Ye, Y.; Hou, H. Electrospun polymer nanofibres with small diameters. *Nanotechnology* **2006**, *17*, 1558. [CrossRef] [PubMed]
41. Gupta, B.; Revagade, N.; Hilborn, J. Poly(lactic acid) fiber: An overview. *Prog. Polym. Sci.* **2007**, *32*, 455–482. [CrossRef]

42. Cicero, J.A.; Dorgan, J.R.; Garrett, J.; Runt, J.; Lin, J. Effects of molecular architecture on two-step, melt-spun poly (lactic acid) fibers. *J. Appl. Polym. Sci.* **2002**, *86*, 2839–2846. [CrossRef]

43. Kim, M.S.; Kim, J.C.; Kim, Y.H. Effects of take-up speed on the structure and properties of melt-spun poly(L-lactic acid) fibers. *Polym. Adv. Technol.* **2008**, *19*, 748–755. [CrossRef]

44. Postema, A.; Luiten, A.; Pennings, A. High-strength poly(L-lactide) fibers by a dry-spinning/hot-drawing process. I. Influence of the ambient temperature on the dry-spinning process. *J. Appl. Polym. Sci.* **1990**, *39*, 1265–1274. [CrossRef]

45. Persano, L.; Camposeo, A.; Tekmen, C.; Pisignano, D. Industrial upscaling of electrospinning and applications of polymer nanofibers: A review. *Macromol. Mater. Eng.* **2013**, *298*, 504–520. [CrossRef]

46. Tan, E.; Ng, S.; Lim, C. Tensile testing of a single ultrafine polymeric fiber. *Biomaterials* **2005**, *26*, 1453–1456. [CrossRef] [PubMed]

47. Liu, J.; Shen, Z.; Lee, S.-H.; Marquez, M.; McHugh, M.A. Electrospinning in compressed carbon dioxide: Hollow or open-cell fiber formation with a single nozzle configuration. *J. Supercrit. Fluids* **2010**, *53*, 142–150. [CrossRef]

48. Stitzel, J.; Liu, J.; Lee, S.J.; Komura, M.; Berry, J.; Soker, S.; Lim, G.; Van Dyke, M.; Czerw, R.; Yoo, J.J. Controlled fabrication of a biological vascular substitute. *Biomaterials* **2006**, *27*, 1088–1094. [CrossRef] [PubMed]

49. Zhou, Y.; Freitag, M.; Hone, J.; Staii, C.; Johnson, A., Jr.; Pinto, N.J.; MacDiarmid, A. Fabrication and electrical characterization of polyaniline-based nanofibers with diameter below 30 nm. *Appl. Phys. Lett.* **2003**, *83*, 3800–3802. [CrossRef]

50. Agarwal, S.; Burgard, M.; Greiner, A.; Wendorff, J. *Electrospinning: A Practical Guide to Nanofibers*; Walter de Gruyter GmbH & Co KG: Berlin, Germany, 2016.

51. Gupta, P.; Wilkes, G.L. Some investigations on the fiber formation by utilizing a side-by-side bicomponent electrospinning approach. *Polymer* **2003**, *44*, 6353–6359. [CrossRef]

52. Townsend-Nicholson, A.; Jayasinghe, S.N. Cell electrospinning: A unique biotechnique for encapsulating living organisms for generating active biological microthreads/scaffolds. *Biomacromolecules* **2006**, *7*, 3364–3369. [CrossRef] [PubMed]

53. Ravichandran, R.; Venugopal, J.R.; Sundarrajan, S.; Mukherjee, S.; Sridhar, R.; Ramakrishna, S. Expression of cardiac proteins in neonatal cardiomyocytes on PGS/fibrinogen core/shell substrate for Cardiac tissue engineering. *Int. J. Cardiol.* **2013**, *167*, 1461–1468. [CrossRef] [PubMed]

54. Wang, X.; Yuan, Y.; Huang, X.; Yue, T. Controlled release of protein from core–shell nanofibers prepared by emulsion electrospinning based on green chemical. *J. Appl. Polym. Sci.* **2015**, *132*. [CrossRef]

55. Su, Y.; Su, Q.; Liu, W.; Lim, M.; Venugopal, J.R.; Mo, X.; Ramakrishna, S.; Al-Deyab, S.S.; El-Newehy, M. Controlled release of bone morphogenetic protein 2 and dexamethasone loaded in core–shell PLLACL–collagen fibers for use in bone tissue engineering. *Acta Biomater.* **2012**, *8*, 763–771. [CrossRef] [PubMed]

56. Rubert, M.; Dehli, J.; Li, Y.-F.; Taskin, M.B.; Xu, R.; Besenbacher, F.; Chen, M. Electrospun PCL/PEO coaxial fibers for basic fibroblast growth factor delivery. *J. Mater. Chem. B* **2014**, *2*, 8538–8546. [CrossRef]

57. Liao, I.; Chew, S.; Leong, K. Aligned core–shell nanofibers delivering bioactive proteins. *Nanomedicine* **2006**, *1*, 465–471. [CrossRef] [PubMed]

58. Tian, L.; Prabhakaran, M.P.; Ding, X.; Kai, D.; Ramakrishna, S. Emulsion electrospun vascular endothelial growth factor encapsulated poly(L-lactic acid-*co*-ε-caprolactone) nanofibers for sustained release in cardiac tissue engineering. *J. Mater. Sci.* **2012**, *47*, 3272–3281. [CrossRef]

59. Choi, J.S.; Choi, S.H.; Yoo, H.S. Coaxial electrospun nanofibers for treatment of diabetic ulcers with binary release of multiple growth factors. *J. Mater. Chem.* **2011**, *21*, 5258–5267. [CrossRef]

60. Liao, I.-C.; Chen, S.; Liu, J.B.; Leong, K.W. Sustained viral gene delivery through core-shell fibers. *J. Control. Release* **2009**, *139*, 48–55. [CrossRef] [PubMed]

61. Wang, C.; Yan, K.-W.; Lin, Y.-D.; Hsieh, P.C. Biodegradable core/shell fibers by coaxial electrospinning: Processing, fiber characterization, and its application in sustained drug release. *Macromolecules* **2010**, *43*, 6389–6397. [CrossRef]

62. Saraf, A.; Baggett, L.S.; Raphael, R.M.; Kasper, F.K.; Mikos, A.G. Regulated non-viral gene delivery from coaxial electrospun fiber mesh scaffolds. *J. Control. Release* **2010**, *143*, 95–103. [CrossRef] [PubMed]

63. Liao, I.-C.; Leong, K.W. Efficacy of engineered FVIII-producing skeletal muscle enhanced by growth factor-releasing co-axial electrospun fibers. *Biomaterials* **2011**, *32*, 1669–1677. [CrossRef] [PubMed]

64. Huang, W.; Zou, T.; Li, S.; Jing, J.; Xia, X.; Liu, X. Drug-loaded zein nanofibers prepared using a modified coaxial electrospinning process. *AAPS PharmSciTech* **2013**, *14*, 675–681. [CrossRef] [PubMed]

65. Zhu, T.; Chen, S.; Li, W.; Lou, J.; Wang, J. Flurbiprofen axetil loaded coaxial electrospun poly (vinyl pyrrolidone)–nanopoly(lactic-*co*-glycolic acid) core–shell composite nanofibers: Preparation, characterization, and anti-adhesion activity. *J. Appl. Polym. Sci.* **2015**, *132*. [CrossRef]

66. Ignatova, M.; Rashkov, I.; Manolova, N. Drug-loaded electrospun materials in wound-dressing applications and in local cancer treatment. *Expert Opin. Drug Deliv.* **2013**, *10*, 469–483. [CrossRef] [PubMed]

67. Ding, B.; Kimura, E.; Sato, T.; Fujita, S.; Shiratori, S. Fabrication of blend biodegradable nanofibrous nonwoven mats via multi-jet electrospinning. *Polymer* **2004**, *45*, 1895–1902. [CrossRef]

68. Theron, S.; Yarin, A.; Zussman, E.; Kroll, E. Multiple jets in electrospinning: Experiment and modeling. *Polymer* **2005**, *46*, 2889–2899. [CrossRef]

69. Teo, W.; Ramakrishna, S. Electrospun fibre bundle made of aligned nanofibres over two fixed points. *Nanotechnology* **2005**, *16*, 1878. [CrossRef]

70. Kim, G.; Cho, Y.-S.; Kim, W.D. Stability analysis for multi-jets electrospinning process modified with a cylindrical electrode. *Eur. Polym. J.* **2006**, *42*, 2031–2038. [CrossRef]

71. Hong, Y.; Fujimoto, K.; Hashizume, R.; Guan, J.; Stankus, J.J.; Tobita, K.; Wagner, W.R. Generating elastic, biodegradable polyurethane/poly(lactide-*co*-glycolide) fibrous sheets with controlled antibiotic release via two-stream electrospinning. *Biomacromolecules* **2008**, *9*, 1200–1207. [CrossRef] [PubMed]

72. Wang, X.; Um, I.C.; Fang, D.; Okamoto, A.; Hsiao, B.S.; Chu, B. Formation of water-resistant hyaluronic acid nanofibers by blowing-assisted electro-spinning and non-toxic post treatments. *Polymer* **2005**, *46*, 4853–4867. [CrossRef]

73. Sundaray, B.; Subramanian, V.; Natarajan, T.; Xiang, R.-Z.; Chang, C.-C.; Fann, W.-S. Electrospinning of continuous aligned polymer fibers. *Appl. Phys. Lett.* **2004**, *84*, 1222–1224. [CrossRef]

74. Li, D.; Wang, Y.; Xia, Y. Electrospinning nanofibers as uniaxially aligned arrays and layer-by-layer stacked films. *Adv. Mater.* **2004**, *16*, 361–366. [CrossRef]

75. Ki, C.S.; Kim, J.W.; Hyun, J.H.; Lee, K.H.; Hattori, M.; Rah, D.K.; Park, Y.H. Electrospun three-dimensional silk fibroin nanofibrous scaffold. *J. Appl. Polym. Sci.* **2007**, *106*, 3922–3928. [CrossRef]

76. Smit, E.; Büttner, U.; Sanderson, R.D. Continuous yarns from electrospun fibers. *Polymer* **2005**, *46*, 2419–2423. [CrossRef]

77. Xu, C.; Inai, R.; Kotaki, M.; Ramakrishna, S. Aligned biodegradable nanofibrous structure: A potential scaffold for blood vessel engineering. *Biomaterials* **2004**, *25*, 877–886. [CrossRef]

78. Bazilevsky, A.V.; Yarin, A.L.; Megaridis, C.M. Co-electrospinning of core-shell fibers using a single-nozzle technique. *Langmuir* **2007**, *23*, 2311–2314. [CrossRef] [PubMed]

79. Bhattarai, N.; Edmondson, D.; Veiseh, O.; Matsen, F.A.; Zhang, M. Electrospun chitosan-based nanofibers and their cellular compatibility. *Biomaterials* **2005**, *26*, 6176–6184. [CrossRef] [PubMed]

80. Theron, A.; Zussman, E.; Yarin, A. Electrostatic field-assisted alignment of electrospun nanofibres. *Nanotechnology* **2001**, *12*, 384. [CrossRef]

81. Zeng, J.; Yang, L.; Liang, Q.; Zhang, X.; Guan, H.; Xu, X.; Chen, X.; Jing, X. Influence of the drug compatibility with polymer solution on the release kinetics of electrospun fiber formulation. *J. Control. Release* **2005**, *105*, 43–51. [CrossRef] [PubMed]

82. Meng, Z.; Xu, X.; Zheng, W.; Zhou, H.; Li, L.; Zheng, Y.; Lou, X. Preparation and characterization of electrospun PLGA/gelatin nanofibers as a potential drug delivery system. *Colloids Surf. B Biointerfaces* **2011**, *84*, 97–102. [CrossRef] [PubMed]

83. Kim, K.; Luu, Y.K.; Chang, C.; Fang, D.; Hsiao, B.S.; Chu, B.; Hadjiargyrou, M. Incorporation and controlled release of a hydrophilic antibiotic using poly(lactide-*co*-glycolide)-based electrospun nanofibrous scaffolds. *J. Control. Release* **2004**, *98*, 47–56. [CrossRef] [PubMed]

84. Jannesari, M.; Varshosaz, J.; Morshed, M.; Zamani, M. Composite poly (vinyl alcohol)/poly (vinyl acetate) electrospun nanofibrous mats as a novel wound dressing matrix for controlled release of drugs. *Int. J. Nanomed.* **2011**, *6*, 993–1003.

85. Nair, R.; Arunkumar, K.; Vishnu Priya, K.; Sevukarajan, M. Recent advances in solid lipid nanoparticle based drug delivery systems. *J. Biomed. Sci. Res.* **2011**, *3*, 368–384.

86. Mickova, A.; Buzgo, M.; Benada, O.; Rampichova, M.; Fisar, Z.; Filova, E.; Tesarova, M.; Lukas, D.; Amler, E. Core/shell nanofibers with embedded liposomes as a drug delivery system. *Biomacromolecules* **2012**, *13*, 952–962. [CrossRef] [PubMed]

87. Volpato, F.Z.; Almodóvar, J.; Erickson, K.; Popat, K.C.; Migliaresi, C.; Kipper, M.J. Preservation of FGF-2 bioactivity using heparin-based nanoparticles, and their delivery from electrospun chitosan fibers. *Acta Biomater.* **2012**, *8*, 1551–1559. [CrossRef] [PubMed]

88. Kim, H.S.; Yoo, H.S. MMPs-responsive release of DNA from electrospun nanofibrous matrix for local gene therapy: In vitro and in vivo evaluation. *J. Control. Release* **2010**, *145*, 264–271. [CrossRef] [PubMed]

89. Mottaghitalab, F.; Farokhi, M.; Mottaghitalab, V.; Ziabari, M.; Divsalar, A.; Shokrgozar, M.A. Enhancement of neural cell lines proliferation using nano-structured chitosan/poly(vinyl alcohol) scaffolds conjugated with nerve growth factor. *Carbohydr. Polym.* **2011**, *86*, 526–535. [CrossRef]

90. Choi, J.S.; Leong, K.W.; Yoo, H.S. In vivo wound healing of diabetic ulcers using electrospun nanofibers immobilized with human epidermal growth factor (EGF). *Biomaterials* **2008**, *29*, 587–596. [CrossRef] [PubMed]

91. Im, J.S.; Yun, J.; Lim, Y.-M.; Kim, H.-I.; Lee, Y.-S. Fluorination of electrospun hydrogel fibers for a controlled release drug delivery system. *Acta Biomater.* **2010**, *6*, 102–109. [CrossRef] [PubMed]

92. Yun, J.; Im, J.S.; Lee, Y.-S.; Kim, H.-I. Electro-responsive transdermal drug delivery behavior of PVA/PAA/MWCNT nanofibers. *Eur. Polym. J.* **2011**, *47*, 1893–1902. [CrossRef]

93. Kim, H.; Yoo, H. Matrix metalloproteinase-inspired suicidal treatments of diabetic ulcers with siRNA-decorated nanofibrous meshes. *Gene Ther.* **2013**, *20*, 378–385. [CrossRef] [PubMed]

94. Luu, Y.; Kim, K.; Hsiao, B.; Chu, B.; Hadjiargyrou, M. Development of a nanostructured DNA delivery scaffold via electrospinning of PLGA and PLA–PEG block copolymers. *J. Control. Release* **2003**, *89*, 341–353. [CrossRef]

95. Zamani, M.; Prabhakaran, M.P.; Ramakrishna, S. Advances in drug delivery via electrospun and electrosprayed nanomaterials. *Int. J. Nanomed.* **2013**, *8*, 2997–3017.

96. Xu, X.; Yang, L.; Xu, X.; Wang, X.; Chen, X.; Liang, Q.; Zeng, J.; Jing, X. Ultrafine medicated fibers electrospun from W/O emulsions. *J. Control. Release* **2005**, *108*, 33–42. [CrossRef] [PubMed]

97. Yang, Y.; Li, X.; Qi, M.; Zhou, S.; Weng, J. Release pattern and structural integrity of lysozyme encapsulated in core–sheath structured poly(DL-lactide) ultrafine fibers prepared by emulsion electrospinning. *Eur. J. Pharm. Biopharm.* **2008**, *69*, 106–116. [CrossRef] [PubMed]

98. He, S.; Xia, T.; Wang, H.; Wei, L.; Luo, X.; Li, X. Multiple release of polyplexes of plasmids VEGF and bFGF from electrospun fibrous scaffolds towards regeneration of mature blood vessels. *Acta Biomater.* **2012**, *8*, 2659–2669. [CrossRef] [PubMed]

99. Yang, Y.; Li, X.; Cheng, L.; He, S.; Zou, J.; Chen, F.; Zhang, Z. Core–sheath structured fibers with pDNA polyplex loadings for the optimal release profile and transfection efficiency as potential tissue engineering scaffolds. *Acta Biomater.* **2011**, *7*, 2533–2543. [CrossRef] [PubMed]

100. Wang, Y.; Qiao, W.; Yin, T. A novel controlled release drug delivery system for multiple drugs based on electrospun nanofibers containing nanoparticles. *J. Pharm. Sci.* **2010**, *99*, 4805–4811. [CrossRef] [PubMed]

101. Xu, J.; Jiao, Y.; Shao, X.; Zhou, C. Controlled dual release of hydrophobic and hydrophilic drugs from electrospun poly(L-lactic acid) fiber mats loaded with chitosan microspheres. *Mater. Lett.* **2011**, *65*, 2800–2803. [CrossRef]

102. Okuda, T.; Tominaga, K.; Kidoaki, S. Time-programmed dual release formulation by multilayered drug-loaded nanofiber meshes. *J. Control. Release* **2010**, *143*, 258–264. [CrossRef] [PubMed]

103. Chunder, A.; Sarkar, S.; Yu, Y.; Zhai, L. Fabrication of ultrathin polyelectrolyte fibers and their controlled release properties. *Colloids Surf. B Biointerfaces* **2007**, *58*, 172–179. [CrossRef] [PubMed]

104. Im, J.S.; Lee, S.K.; Bai, B.C.; Lee, Y.-S. Prediction and characterization of drug release in a multi-drug release system. *J. Ind. Eng. Chem.* **2012**, *18*, 325–330. [CrossRef]

105. Prausnitz, M.R.; Langer, R. Transdermal drug delivery. *Nat. Biotechnol.* **2008**, *26*, 1261–1268. [CrossRef] [PubMed]

106. Suwantong, O.; Ruktanonchai, U.; Supaphol, P. Electrospun cellulose acetate fiber mats containing asiaticoside or Centella asiatica crude extract and the release characteristics of asiaticoside. *Polymer* **2008**, *49*, 4239–4247. [CrossRef]

107. Taepaiboon, P.; Rungsardthong, U.; Supaphol, P. Drug-loaded electrospun mats of poly (vinyl alcohol) fibres and their release characteristics of four model drugs. *Nanotechnology* **2006**, *17*, 2317. [CrossRef]

108. Suwantong, O.; Opanasopit, P.; Ruktanonchai, U.; Supaphol, P. Electrospun cellulose acetate fiber mats containing curcumin and release characteristic of the herbal substance. *Polymer* **2007**, *48*, 7546–7557. [CrossRef]

109. Im, J.S.; Bai, B.C.; Lee, Y.-S. The effect of carbon nanotubes on drug delivery in an electro-sensitive transdermal drug delivery system. *Biomaterials* **2010**, *31*, 1414–1419. [CrossRef] [PubMed]

110. Taepaiboon, P.; Rungsardthong, U.; Supaphol, P. Vitamin-loaded electrospun cellulose acetate nanofiber mats as transdermal and dermal therapeutic agents of vitamin A acid and vitamin E. *Eur. J. Pharm. Biopharm.* **2007**, *67*, 387–397. [CrossRef] [PubMed]

111. Ngawhirunpat, T.; Opanasopit, P.; Rojanarata, T.; Akkaramongkolporn, P.; Ruktanonchai, U.; Supaphol, P. Development of meloxicam-loaded electrospun polyvinyl alcohol mats as a transdermal therapeutic agent. *Pharm. Dev. Technol.* **2009**, *14*, 73–82. [CrossRef] [PubMed]

112. Reda, R.I.; Wen, M.M.; El-Kamel, A.H. Ketoprofen-loaded eudragit electrospun nanofibers for the treatment of oral mucositis. *Int. J. Nanomed.* **2017**, *12*, 2335. [CrossRef] [PubMed]

113. Kenawy, E.-R.; Bowlin, G.L.; Mansfield, K.; Layman, J.; Simpson, D.G.; Sanders, E.H.; Wnek, G.E. Release of tetracycline hydrochloride from electrospun poly(ethylene-*co*-vinylacetate), poly (lactic acid), and a blend. *J. Control. Release* **2002**, *81*, 57–64. [CrossRef]

114. Alhusein, N.; Blagbrough, I.S.; De Bank, P.A. Electrospun matrices for localised controlled drug delivery: Release of tetracycline hydrochloride from layers of polycaprolactone and poly(ethylene-*co*-vinyl acetate). *Drug Deliv. Transl. Res.* **2012**, *2*, 477–488. [CrossRef] [PubMed]

115. Alhusein, N.; De Bank, P.A.; Blagbrough, I.S.; Bolhuis, A. Killing bacteria within biofilms by sustained release of tetracycline from triple-layered electrospun micro/nanofibre matrices of polycaprolactone and poly (ethylene-*co*-vinyl acetate). *Drug Deliv. Transl. Res.* **2013**, *3*, 531–541. [CrossRef] [PubMed]

116. Wang, X.; Yue, T.; Lee, T.-C. Development of Pleurocidin-poly(vinyl alcohol) electrospun antimicrobial nanofibers to retain antimicrobial activity in food system application. *Food Control* **2015**, *54*, 150–157. [CrossRef]

117. Zhang, Y.; Lim, C.T.; Ramakrishna, S.; Huang, Z.-M. Recent development of polymer nanofibers for biomedical and biotechnological applications. *J. Mater. Sci. Mater. Med.* **2005**, *16*, 933–946. [CrossRef] [PubMed]

118. Boateng, J.S.; Matthews, K.H.; Stevens, H.N.; Eccleston, G.M. Wound healing dressings and drug delivery systems: A review. *J. Pharm. Sci.* **2008**, *97*, 2892–2923. [CrossRef] [PubMed]

119. Said, S.S.; Aloufy, A.K.; El-Halfawy, O.M.; Boraei, N.A.; El-Khordagui, L.K. Antimicrobial PLGA ultrafine fibers: Interaction with wound bacteria. *Eur. J. Pharm. Biopharm.* **2011**, *79*, 108–118. [CrossRef] [PubMed]

120. Thakur, R.; Florek, C.; Kohn, J.; Michniak, B. Electrospun nanofibrous polymeric scaffold with targeted drug release profiles for potential application as wound dressing. *Int. J. Pharm.* **2008**, *364*, 87–93. [CrossRef] [PubMed]

121. Wang, A.; Xu, C.; Zhang, C.; Gan, Y.; Wang, B. Experimental investigation of the properties of electrospun nanofibers for potential medical application. *J. Nanomater.* **2015**, *2015*, 5. [CrossRef]

122. GhavamiNejad, A.; Rajan Unnithan, A.; Ramachandra Kurup Sasikala, A.; Samarikhalaj, M.; Thomas, R.G.; Jeong, Y.Y.; Nasseri, S.; Murugesan, P.; Wu, D.; Hee Park, C. Mussel-inspired electrospun nanofibers functionalized with size-controlled silver nanoparticles for wound dressing application. *ACS Appl. Mater. Interfaces* **2015**, *7*, 12176–12183. [CrossRef] [PubMed]

123. Chutipakdeevong, J.; Ruktanonchai, U.; Supaphol, P. Hybrid biomimetic electrospun fibrous mats derived from poly(ε-caprolactone) and silk fibroin protein for wound dressing application. *J. Appl. Polym. Sci.* **2015**, *132*, 41653. [CrossRef]

124. Xu, X.; Chen, X.; Ma, P.; Wang, X.; Jing, X. The release behavior of doxorubicin hydrochloride from medicated fibers prepared by emulsion-electrospinning. *Eur. J. Pharm. Biopharm.* **2008**, *70*, 165–170. [CrossRef] [PubMed]

125. Xu, X.; Chen, X.; Wang, Z.; Jing, X. Ultrafine PEG–PLA fibers loaded with both paclitaxel and doxorubicin hydrochloride and their in vitro cytotoxicity. *Eur. J. Pharm. Biopharm.* **2009**, *72*, 18–25. [CrossRef] [PubMed]

126. Xie, J.; Tan, R.S.; Wang, C.H. Biodegradable microparticles and fiber fabrics for sustained delivery of cisplatin to treat C6 glioma in vitro. *J. Biomed. Mater. Res. Part A* **2008**, *85*, 897–908. [CrossRef] [PubMed]

127. Liu, S.; Zhou, G.; Liu, D.; Xie, Z.; Huang, Y.; Wang, X.; Wu, W.; Jing, X. Inhibition of orthotopic secondary hepatic carcinoma in mice by doxorubicin-loaded electrospun polylactide nanofibers. *J. Mater. Chem. B* **2013**, *1*, 101–109. [CrossRef]

128. Luo, X.; Xie, C.; Wang, H.; Liu, C.; Yan, S.; Li, X. Antitumor activities of emulsion electrospun fibers with core loading of hydroxycamptothecin via intratumoral implantation. *Int. J. Pharm.* **2012**, *425*, 19–28. [CrossRef] [PubMed]

129. Gupta, S. Biocompatible microemulsion systems for drug encapsulation and delivery. *Curr Sci* **2011**, *101*, 174–188.

130. Chen, P.; Wu, Q.-S.; Ding, Y.-P.; Chu, M.; Huang, Z.-M.; Hu, W. A controlled release system of titanocene dichloride by electrospun fiber and its antitumor activity in vitro. *Eur. J. Pharm. Biopharm.* **2010**, *76*, 413–420. [CrossRef] [PubMed]

131. Shao, S.; Li, L.; Yang, G.; Li, J.; Luo, C.; Gong, T.; Zhou, S. Controlled green tea polyphenols release from electrospun PCL/MWCNTs composite nanofibers. *Int. J. Pharm.* **2011**, *421*, 310–320. [CrossRef] [PubMed]

132. Zahedi, P.; Karami, Z.; Rezaeian, I.; Jafari, S.H.; Mahdaviani, P.; Abdolghaffari, A.H.; Abdollahi, M. Preparation and performance evaluation of tetracycline hydrochloride loaded wound dressing mats based on electrospun nanofibrous poly(lactic acid)/poly(ε-caprolactone) blends. *J. Appl. Polym. Sci.* **2012**, *124*, 4174–4183. [CrossRef]

133. He, C.L.; Huang, Z.M.; Han, X.J.; Liu, L.; Zhang, H.S.; Chen, L.S. Coaxial electrospun poly(L-lactic acid) ultrafine fibers for sustained drug delivery. *J. Macromol. Sci. Part B* **2006**, *45*, 515–524. [CrossRef]

134. He, C.L.; Huang, Z.M.; Han, X.J. Fabrication of drug-loaded electrospun aligned fibrous threads for suture applications. *J. Biomed. Mater. Res. Part A* **2009**, *89*, 80–95. [CrossRef] [PubMed]

135. Gilchrist, S.E.; Lange, D.; Letchford, K.; Bach, H.; Fazli, L.; Burt, H.M. Fusidic acid and rifampicin *co*-loaded PLGA nanofibers for the prevention of orthopedic implant associated infections. *J. Control. Release* **2013**, *170*, 64–73. [CrossRef] [PubMed]

136. Zamani, M.; Morshed, M.; Varshosaz, J.; Jannesari, M. Controlled release of metronidazole benzoate from poly ε-caprolactone electrospun nanofibers for periodontal diseases. *Eur. J. Pharm. Biopharm.* **2010**, *75*, 179–185. [CrossRef] [PubMed]

137. Toncheva, A.; Paneva, D.; Maximova, V.; Manolova, N.; Rashkov, I. Antibacterial fluoroquinolone antibiotic-containing fibrous materials from poly (L-lactide-*co*-D, L-lactide) prepared by electrospinning. *Eur. J. Pharm. Sci.* **2012**, *47*, 642–651. [CrossRef] [PubMed]

138. Spasova, M.; Manolova, N.; Paneva, D.; Rashkov, I. Preparation of chitosan-containing nanofibres by electrospinning of chitosan/poly(ethylene oxide) blend solutions. *e-Polymers* **2004**, *4*, 624–635. [CrossRef]

139. Verreck, G.; Chun, I.; Rosenblatt, J.; Peeters, J.; Van Dijck, A.; Mensch, J.; Noppe, M.; Brewster, M.E. Incorporation of drugs in an amorphous state into electrospun nanofibers composed of a water-insoluble, nonbiodegradable polymer. *J. Control. Release* **2003**, *92*, 349–360. [CrossRef]

140. Huang, L.-Y.; Branford-White, C.; Shen, X.-X.; Yu, D.-G.; Zhu, L.-M. Time-engineeringed biphasic drug release by electrospun nanofiber meshes. *Int. J. Pharm.* **2012**, *436*, 88–96. [CrossRef] [PubMed]

141. Jiang, Y.-N.; Mo, H.-Y.; Yu, D.-G. Electrospun drug-loaded core–sheath PVP/zein nanofibers for biphasic drug release. *Int. J. Pharm.* **2012**, *438*, 232–239. [CrossRef] [PubMed]

142. Jiang, H.; Fang, D.; Hsiao, B.; Chu, B.; Chen, W. Preparation and characterization of ibuprofen-loaded poly(lactide-*co*-glycolide)/poly(ethylene glycol)-*g*-chitosan electrospun membranes. *J. Biomater. Sci. Polym. Ed.* **2004**, *15*, 279–296. [CrossRef] [PubMed]

143. Lu, T.; Jing, X.; Song, X.; Wang, X. Doxorubicin-loaded ultrafine PEG-PLA fiber mats against hepatocarcinoma. *J. Appl. Polym. Sci.* **2012**, *123*, 209–217. [CrossRef]

144. Ranganath, S.H.; Wang, C.-H. Biodegradable microfiber implants delivering paclitaxel for post-surgical chemotherapy against malignant glioma. *Biomaterials* **2008**, *29*, 2996–3003. [CrossRef] [PubMed]

145. Xie, J.; Wang, C.-H. Electrospun micro-and nanofibers for sustained delivery of paclitaxel to treat C6 glioma in vitro. *Pharm. Res.* **2006**, *23*, 1817–1826. [CrossRef] [PubMed]

146. Liu, D.; Liu, S.; Jing, X.; Li, X.; Li, W.; Huang, Y. Necrosis of cervical carcinoma by dichloroacetate released from electrospun polylactide mats. *Biomaterials* **2012**, *33*, 4362–4369. [CrossRef] [PubMed]

147. Xu, X.; Zhuang, X.; Chen, X.; Wang, X.; Yang, L.; Jing, X. Preparation of core-sheath composite nanofibers by emulsion electrospinning. *Macromol. Rapid Commun.* **2006**, *27*, 1637–1642. [CrossRef]

148. Chew, S.Y.; Wen, J.; Yim, E.K.; Leong, K.W. Sustained release of proteins from electrospun biodegradable fibers. *Biomacromolecules* **2005**, *6*, 2017–2024. [CrossRef] [PubMed]

149. Rujitanaroj, P.-o.; Wang, Y.-C.; Wang, J.; Chew, S.Y. Nanofiber-mediated controlled release of siRNA complexes for long term gene-silencing applications. *Biomaterials* **2011**, *32*, 5915–5923. [CrossRef] [PubMed]

150. Cao, H.; Jiang, X.; Chai, C.; Chew, S.Y. RNA interference by nanofiber-based siRNA delivery system. *J. Control. Release* **2010**, *144*, 203–212. [CrossRef] [PubMed]

151. Schneider, A.; Wang, X.; Kaplan, D.; Garlick, J.; Egles, C. Biofunctionalized electrospun silk mats as a topical bioactive dressing for accelerated wound healing. *Acta Biomater.* **2009**, *5*, 2570–2578. [CrossRef] [PubMed]

152. Zhang, X.; Shi, Z.; Fu, W.; Liu, Z.; Fang, Z.; Lu, W.; Wang, Y.; Chen, F. In vitro biocompatibility study of electrospun copolymer ethylene carbonate-ε-caprolactone and vascular endothelial growth factor blended nanofibrous scaffolds. *Appl. Surf. Sci.* **2012**, *258*, 2301–2306. [CrossRef]

153. Cho, Y.I.; Choi, J.S.; Jeong, S.Y.; Yoo, H.S. Nerve growth factor (NGF)-conjugated electrospun nanostructures with topographical cues for neuronal differentiation of mesenchymal stem cells. *Acta Biomater.* **2010**, *6*, 4725–4733. [CrossRef] [PubMed]

154. Han, N.; Johnson, J.; Lannutti, J.J.; Winter, J.O. Hydrogel–electrospun fiber composite materials for hydrophilic protein release. *J. Control. Release* **2012**, *158*, 165–170. [CrossRef] [PubMed]

155. Chen, G.; Lv, Y. Immobilization and application of electrospun nanofiber scaffold-based growth factor in bone tissue engineering. *Curr. Pharm. Des.* **2015**, *21*, 1967–1978. [CrossRef] [PubMed]

156. Ren, S.; Dong, L.; Zhang, X.; Lei, T.; Ehrenhauser, F.; Song, K.; Li, M.; Sun, X.; Wu, Q. Electrospun Nanofibers Made of Silver Nanoparticles, Cellulose Nanocrystals, and Polyacrylonitrile as Substrates for Surface-Enhanced Raman Scattering. *Materials* **2017**, *10*, 68. [CrossRef] [PubMed]

157. Segala, K.; Nista, S.V.G.; Cordi, L.; Bizarria, M.T.M.; Ávila Júnior, J.D.; Kleinubing, S.A.; Cruz, D.C.; Brocchi, M.; Lona, L.M.F.; Caballero, N.E.D. Silver nanoparticles incorporated into nanostructured biopolymer membranes produced by electrospinning: A study of antimicrobial activity. *Braz. J. Pharm. Sci.* **2015**, *51*, 911–921. [CrossRef]

158. Li, J.; Chen, X.; Ai, N.; Hao, J.; Chen, Q.; Strauf, S.; Shi, Y. Silver nanoparticle doped TiO_2 nanofiber dye sensitized solar cells. *Chem. Phys. Lett.* **2011**, *514*, 141–145. [CrossRef]

159. Cui, H.; Yuan, L.; Li, W.; Lin, L. Antioxidant property of SiO_2-eugenol liposome loaded nanofibrous membranes on beef. *Food Packag. Shelf Life* **2017**, *11*, 49–57. [CrossRef]

160. Yarin, A.L.; Pourdeyhimi, B.; Ramakrishna, S. *Fundamentals and Applications of Micro-and Nanofibers*; Cambridge University Press: Cambridge, UK, 2014.

161. Zou, H.; Lv, P.F.; Wang, X.; Wu, D.; Yu, D.G. Electrospun poly(2-aminothiazole)/cellulose acetate fiber membrane for removing Hg (II) from water. *J. Appl. Polym. Sci.* **2017**, *134*. [CrossRef]

162. Zhou, J.; Zhang, J.; Rehman, A.U.; Kan, K.; Li, L.; Shi, K. Synthesis, characterization, and ammonia gas sensing properties of Co_3O_4@ CuO nanochains. *J. Mater Sci.* **2016**, *52*, 1–14. [CrossRef]

163. Homaeigohar, S.; Elbahri, M. Nanocomposite electrospun nanofiber membranes for environmental remediation. *Materials* **2014**, *7*, 1017–1045. [CrossRef] [PubMed]

164. Lee, S.J.; Heo, D.N.; Moon, J.-H.; Ko, W.-K.; Lee, J.B.; Bae, M.S.; Park, S.W.; Kim, J.E.; Lee, D.H.; Kim, E.-C. Electrospun chitosan nanofibers with controlled levels of silver nanoparticles. Preparation, characterization and antibacterial activity. *Carbohydr. Polym.* **2014**, *111*, 530–537. [CrossRef] [PubMed]

165. Shi, Q.; Vitchuli, N.; Nowak, J.; Caldwell, J.M.; Breidt, F.; Bourham, M.; Zhang, X.; McCord, M. Durable antibacterial Ag/polyacrylonitrile (Ag/PAN) hybrid nanofibers prepared by atmospheric plasma treatment and electrospinning. *Eur. Polym. J.* **2011**, *47*, 1402–1409. [CrossRef]

166. Castro-Mayorga, J.; Randazzo, W.; Fabra, M.; Lagaron, J.; Aznar, R.; Sánchez, G. Antiviral properties of silver nanoparticles against norovirus surrogates and their efficacy in coated polyhydroxyalkanoates systems. *LWT Food Sci. Technol.* **2017**, *79*, 503–510. [CrossRef]

167. Nie, H.; Wang, C.-H. Fabrication and characterization of PLGA/HAp composite scaffolds for delivery of BMP-2 plasmid DNA. *J. Control. Release* **2007**, *120*, 111–121. [CrossRef] [PubMed]

168. Tanaka, K.; Shiga, T.; Katayama, T. Fabrication of Hydroxyapatite/PLA Composite Nanofiber by Electrospinning. *WIT Trans. Built Environ.* **2016**, *166*, 371–379.

169. Chen, M.; Gao, S.; Dong, M.; Song, J.; Yang, C.; Howard, K.A.; Kjems, J.; Besenbacher, F. Chitosan/siRNA nanoparticles encapsulated in PLGA nanofibers for siRNA delivery. *ACS Nano* **2012**, *6*, 4835–4844. [CrossRef] [PubMed]

170. Chew, S.Y.; Mi, R.; Hoke, A.; Leong, K.W. Aligned Protein–Polymer Composite Fibers Enhance Nerve Regeneration: A Potential Tissue-Engineering Platform. *Adv. Funct. Mater.* **2007**, *17*, 1288–1296. [CrossRef] [PubMed]

171. Kowalczyk, T.; Nowicka, A.; Elbaum, D.; Kowalewski, T.A. Electrospinning of bovine serum albumin. Optimization and the use for production of biosensors. *Biomacromolecules* **2008**, *9*, 2087–2090. [CrossRef] [PubMed]

172. Li, X.; Su, Y.; Liu, S.; Tan, L.; Mo, X.; Ramakrishna, S. Encapsulation of proteins in poly (L-lactide-*co*-caprolactone) fibers by emulsion electrospinning. *Colloids Surf. B Biointerfaces* **2010**, *75*, 418–424. [CrossRef] [PubMed]

173. Huang, L.; Apkarian, R.P.; Chaikof, E.L. High-resolution analysis of engineered type I collagen nanofibers by electron microscopy. *Scanning* **2001**, *23*, 372–375. [CrossRef] [PubMed]

174. Huang, L.; Nagapudi, K.; Apkarian, R.P.; Chaikof, E.L. Engineered collagen–PEO nanofibers and fabrics. *J. Biomater. Sci. Polym. Ed.* **2001**, *12*, 979–993. [CrossRef] [PubMed]

175. Zhang, E.; Zhu, C.; Yang, J.; Sun, H.; Zhang, X.; Li, S.; Wang, Y.; Sun, L.; Yao, F. Electrospun PDLLA/PLGA composite membranes for potential application in guided tissue regeneration. *Mater. Sci. Eng. C* **2016**, *58*, 278–285. [CrossRef] [PubMed]

176. Sudakaran, S.V.; Venugopal, J.R.; Vijayakumar, G.P.; Abisegapriyan, S.; Grace, A.N.; Ramakrishna, S. Sequel of MgO nanoparticles in PLACL nanofibers for anti-cancer therapy in synergy with curcumin/β-cyclodextrin. *Mater. Sci. Eng. C* **2017**, *71*, 620–628. [CrossRef] [PubMed]

177. Khalil, I.S.; Abdel-Kader, R.M.; Gomaa, I.E.; Serag, N.; Klingner, A.; Elwi, M. Targeting of Cancer Cells using Controlled Nanoparticles and Robotics Sperms. *Int. J. Adv. Robot. Syst.* **2016**, *13*, 123. [CrossRef]

178. Sezer, U.A.; Ozturk, K.; Aru, B.; Demirel, G.Y.; Sezer, S.; Bozkurt, M.R. Zero valent zinc nanoparticles promote neuroglial cell proliferation: A biodegradable and conductive filler candidate for nerve regeneration. *J. Mater. Sci. Mater. Med.* **2017**, *28*, 19. [CrossRef] [PubMed]

179. Kuchler-Bopp, S.; Larrea, A.; Petry, L.; Idoux-Gillet, Y.; Sebastian, V.; Ferrandon, A.; Schwinté, P.; Arruebo, M.; Benkirane-Jessel, N. Promoting Bioengineered Tooth Innervation Using Nanostructured and Hybrid Scaffolds. *Acta Biomater.* **2017**, *50*, 493–501. [CrossRef] [PubMed]

180. Teo, W.-E. Addressing the Needs of Nanofiber Mass Production (Limitation of Nozzle System). Available online: http://electrospintech.com/mpchallenge.html#.WK2nq28rLIX (accessed on 27 October 2018).

181. Li, L.; Frey, M.W.; Green, T.B. Modification of air filter media with nylon-6 nanofibers. *J. Eng. Fibers Fabr.* **2006**, *1*, 1–22.

182. Moon, S.; Gil, M.; Lee, K.J. Syringeless Electrospinning toward Versatile Fabrication of Nanofiber Web. *Sci. Rep.* **2017**, *7*, 41424. [CrossRef] [PubMed]

183. Liu, W.; Huang, C.; Jin, X. Electrospinning of grooved polystyrene fibers: Effect of solvent systems. *Nanoscale Res. Lett.* **2015**, *10*, 237. [CrossRef] [PubMed]

184. Zhang, B.; Yan, X.; He, H.-W.; Yu, M.; Ning, X.; Long, Y.-Z. Solvent-free electrospinning: Opportunities and challenges. *Polym. Chem.* **2017**, *8*, 333–352. [CrossRef]

185. Fakirov, S. *Nano-Size Polymers: Preparation, Properties, Applications*; Springer: Berlin, Germany, 2016.

186. Niu, H.; Lin, T. Fiber generators in needleless electrospinning. *J. Nanomater.* **2012**, 12. [CrossRef]

187. Niu, H.; Lin, T.; Wang, X. Needleless electrospinning. I. A comparison of cylinder and disk nozzles. *J. Appl. Polym. Sci.* **2009**, *114*, 3524–3530. [CrossRef]

188. Cengiz, F.; Dao, T.A.; Jirsak, O. Influence of solution properties on the roller electrospinning of poly(vinyl alcohol). *Polym. Eng. Sci.* **2010**, *50*, 936–943. [CrossRef]

189. Niu, H.; Wang, X.; Lin, T. Needleless electrospinning: Influences of fibre generator geometry. *J. Text. Inst.* **2012**, *103*, 787–794. [CrossRef]

190. Liu, Y.; He, J. Bubble electrospinning for mass production of nanofibers. *Int. J. Nonlinear Sci. Numer. Simul.* **2007**, *8*, 393. [CrossRef]

191. Weng, L.; Xie, J. Smart electrospun nanofibers for controlled drug release: Recent advances and new perspectives. *Curr. Pharm. Des.* **2015**, *21*, 1944–1959. [CrossRef] [PubMed]

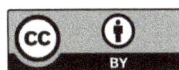

pharmaceutics

MDPI

Review

Engineering of Nanofibrous Amorphous and Crystalline Solid Dispersions for Oral Drug Delivery

Laura Modica de Mohac [1,2], Alison Veronica Keating [2], Maria de Fátima Pina [3] and Bahijja Tolulope Raimi-Abraham [2,*]

1   DIBIMIS Department, University of Study of Palermo, 90128 Palermo, Italy; laura.modicademohac@unipa.it
2   Drug Delivery Group, Institute of Pharmaceutical Science Faculty of Life Sciences and Medicine,
     King's College London, London SE1 9NH, UK; Alison.Keating@kcl.ac.uk
3   Department of Pharmaceutics, University College London School of Pharmacy, London WC1N 1AX, UK;
     mariafatima.gpina@gmail.com
*   Correspondence: bahijja.raimi-abraham@kcl.ac.uk; Tel.: +44-207-836-5454

Received: 22 June 2018; Accepted: 19 October 2018; Published: 24 December 2018

Abstract: Poor aqueous solubility (<0.1 mg/mL) affects a significant number of drugs currently on the market or under development. Several formulation strategies including salt formation, particle size reduction, and solid dispersion approaches have been employed with varied success. In this review, we focus primarily on the emerging trends in the generation of amorphous and micro/nano-crystalline solid dispersions using electrospinning to improve the dissolution rate and in turn the bioavailability of poorly water-soluble drugs. Electrospinning is a simple but versatile process that utilizes electrostatic forces to generate polymeric fibers and has been used for over 100 years to generate synthetic fibers. We discuss the various electrospinning studies and spinneret types that have been used to generate amorphous and crystalline solid dispersions.

Keywords: solid dispersion; aqueous solubility enhancement; amorphous; crystalline; oral drug delivery

1. Introduction

Approximately 40% of marketed oral drugs are categorized as having poor aqueous solubility (i.e., <0.1 mg/mL) [1] resulting in a significant challenge in drug development. Several formulation strategies such as co-crystals [2], salt formation [3], particle size reduction [4], and more commonly, solid dispersion (SD) approaches [5–7] have been employed to increase aqueous solubility (and in turn enhance the oral bioavailability) of Biopharmaceutics Classification System (BCS) II (i.e., low solubility and high permeability) and IV (i.e., low solubility and permeability) drugs.

SDs have been redefined several times over time. For example, in 1961, Sekiguchi and Obi suggested that when the drug was formulated as a SD, it was present in a microcrystalline state as a eutectic mixture i.e., a combination of crystalline components (drug and a carrier) that are miscible in the molten liquid state, but show little to no miscibility in the solid state and on cooling would crystallize as two components [8]. Later, Chiou and Riegelman (1971) referred to SDs as a dispersion of one or more active ingredients present within an inert carrier or matrix in the solid state prepared by the melting (fusion), solvent-based, or melting-solvent method [9]. This was further defined by Lerner et al. (2000) as a dispersion in which the drug is only partially molecularly dispersed and is generated from physical mixtures of the carrier and drug [10]. In 2002, Craig described SDs as a delivery system whereby the drug is dispersed in a biologically inert matrix, to enhance oral bioavailability [11]. A range of materials are used as the inert matrix or carrier in a SD ranging from sugars [12,13], wax based systems [14] and, more commonly, polymers.

There are several hypotheses regarding the mechanism of drug release from SD systems amorphous and crystalline alike. The most agreed hypothesis is the existence of two different mechanisms of drug release, carrier-controlled or drug-controlled (Figure 1). This hypothesis is based on key findings by Corrigan et al. [15] in their drug release study of a phenobarbitone-(poly)ethylene glycol (PEG) SD where the rate of phenobarbitone release from the SD was the same as that of PEG on its own. Craig [11] further suggested that, if a system underwentcarrier-controlled dissolution then the physical properties such as initial particle size of the drug or crystallinity should be largely irrelevant. In comparison with drug-controlled dissolution, the physical property of the drug as well as its solubility is of greater relevance [11], highlighting the potential of SDs to enhance drug dissolution rate through a preferential selection of the appropriate carrier (in this case polymer) or a combination of carrier and carrier types (e.g., wax and polymers polymer blends [14]).

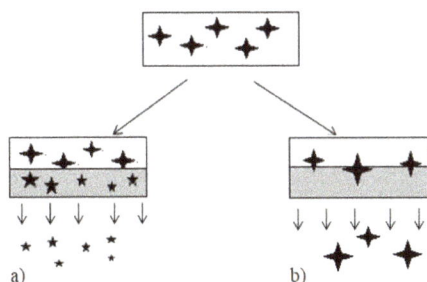

Figure 1. Schematic diagram shows (**a**) Carrier-controlled dissolution and (**b**) drug-controlled dissolution (Adapted with permission from [11], copyright Elsevier, 2002). *The larger* ✦ *represents dissolved drug, the smaller* ✦ *represent the partially dissolved drug. Grey box represents an aqueous environment.*

In most cases where SDs are generated, a comparison is made with the physical mixture (PM). The PM is essentially where the drug and carrier are not chemically combined through a process but prepared through gentle or mild mixing. To ensure drug release compared to SD is not influenced by additional factors such as particle size, it is good practice for both drug and carrier to be passed through a dry sieve of known aperture so any effects observed are due entirely to the properties of the PM. Examples in the literature exist that demonstrate enhanced drug release of a PM compared to its SD counterpart. For example Leonardi and Salomon (2013) PM of benznidazole and PEG 6000 offered greater dissolution compared to it a SD prepared by a solvent method [16].

SDs have been characterized into two main classifications, firstly in accordance to carrier type and secondly taking into account the correlation to stability and solubility, preparation, and characterization techniques [17].

When classifying SDs by carrier type, there are four generations that have been discussed and explored in the literature. The first generation SDs were introduced by Sekiguchi and Obi as eutectic mixtures where both drug and carrier were present in the crystalline state [18]. Second generation SDs were carriers are generally polymeric and present in the amorphous state with the drug dispersed molecularly within the inert matrix. The drug is generally supersaturated to ensure its solubilization in the carriers in second generation SDs [19]. Third generation SDs were the carriers can be a co-polymer system or a mixture of surfactants and polymers and improvement of the drug release profile is due to the carrier's surface activity or self-emulsifying properties which in addition could reduce drug re-crystallization and improve SD stability [20]. Finally, fourth generation SDs are the carriers are bifunctional in nature and have solubilizing as well as surfactant properties [21]. The carriers are non-ionic and so the solubility is independent of pH changes making these carriers more suited for SD development. Soluplus®, a polyvinyl caprolactam-polyvinyl acetate-polyethylene glycol graft co-polymer solubilizer with an amphiphilic chemical structure has been highlighted as a fourth generation SD carrier [22].

When classifying SDs in accordance to their correlation to stability and solubility, preparation and characterization techniques, six classes have been identified [23]. Class C–C and Class C–A where the Active Pharmaceutical Ingredient (API) is present in the crystalline state are dispersed in either a crystalline or amorphous carrier respectively. Class C–C and C–A SDs are deemed stable, however, less soluble due to the crystalline nature of the API. Class A–C and Class A-A were the API is present in the amorphous state dispersed in either a crystalline or amorphous carrier. Class A–C and CC SDs are considered to increase API solubility enhancement, however, low miscibility is observed between the API and carrier has been highlighted as an issue. Class M–C and Class M–A are where the drug is molecularly dispersed within either a crystalline or amorphous carrier. These systems have been shown to greatly improve drug dissolution behavior with great physical stability due to the high miscibility and strong molecular interaction between the two components with the API being molecularly dispersed [23].

In this review, we discuss amorphous and crystalline SDs which we define as a system where the drug is molecularly dispersed with an amorphous polymer matrix and as a system where the micronized or nanosized crystalline drug is dispersed within an amorphous polymer matrix with or without the use of stabilizing agents respectively.

SD stability has been studied at length over the years and factors influencing can be summarized as follows: physical stability, crystallization tendency, amorphization, drug-polymer miscibility, dissolution enhancement, and method of preparation. Electrospinning is a rapid solvent evaporation method and is well suited for drugs with thermal instability and can avoid drug re-crystallization or amorphization during processing [24]. Many polymers have been used to prepare SDs such as poly(*N*-vinvylpyrrolidone) (PVP) [25], polyethylene glycol (PEG) [26], zein [27], hydroxypropyl methylcellulose (HPMC) [28,29], polycaprolactone [30], and polyacrylic acid [31], expanding the potential of processes used to make SDs from the traditional solvent-based methods [32,33], hot melt extrusion (HME) [34–36], spray-drying [22,37], to polymer-based nanofabrication methods such as electrospinning [38–40] and other centrifugal spinning based methods [12,13,41,42].

In this review, we focus primarily on the emerging trends in the generation of amorphous and crystalline SDs using nanofabrication techniques namely electrospinning to improve the dissolution rate and in turn bioavailability of poorly water-soluble drugs. It is important to note that there are more studies investigating the generation of electrospun nanofibrous amorphous solid dispersions than crystalline SDs suggesting that electrospun nanofibrous crystalline SDs are still a relatively under-investigated formulation strategy.

2. Nanofibrous Amorphous Solid Dispersions

Amorphous materials have higher enthalpy, entropy, and free energy compared to their crystalline counterparts, leading to higher apparent solubility. The weaker attractive intermolecular forces of amorphous materials are more easily broken, allowing molecules to move from the material's surface into the medium greater ease compared to crystalline counterparts. As a result, amorphous materials are more soluble and have a faster dissolution rate. Unfortunately, even with such advantages the success and usefulness of amorphous materials in drug development is greatly dependent on their long stability within a dosage form [3,43,44]. Given the high solubility of amorphous compounds (compared to their crystalline counterparts), amorphous solid dispersions (ASDs) are an important strategy to improve the apparent solubility, dissolution rate, and in turn bioavailability of poorly water-soluble drugs [45].

Nanofibers possess a high surface area to volume ratio and have gained increased interest in drug delivery beyond their known application in areas such as tissue engineering scaffolds [46] or wound dressing for example [47]. Due to their high drug-loading capacity, internal architecture, porosity, and malleability the addition of therapeutically relevant molecules has several benefits. For further information on recent developments in the application of micro and nanofabrication techniques in drug delivery and on nanofibres in drug delivery, the reader is directed to a recent review by Qi and Craig [26].

2.1. Electrospinning

Electrospinning is a simple but versatile process that utilizes electrostatic forces to generate polymeric fibers and has been used for over 100 years to generate synthetic fibers [48–50]. Typically, electrospinning involves pushing a viscous polymer or polymer/drug solution through a spinneret (narrow gauge syringe needle) at a constant flow rate. A voltage is applied to the polymer solution, creating repulsive forces between the like charges in the solution and attractive forces between the charged solution and the grounded collector. When the electrostatic forces equal the surface tension of the liquid, a Taylor cone is formed. If the electric field is increased beyond this point, the electrostatic repulsion will exceed the surface tension and result in the ejection of a fiber jet from the apex of the cone which accelerates towards the grounded collector [51,52]. As the fiber jet accelerates towards the collector it undergoes chaotic whipping instability which increases the transit time and path length to the collector, allowing the solvent to evaporate leaving solid, thin fibers. Cheng et al. presented electrospinning as a novel processing method to generate functional nanomaterials with many applications ranging from wound healing and medical textiles, to production of oral-dispersible film SD and controlled delivery systems [27,53–55]. Electrospinning is a rapid solvent evaporation process well suited to amorphous materials as by this process the drug does not have time to form a crystal lattice within the nanofiber and remains distributed in its amorphous form at a molecular scale [56]. Additionally, the internal structure of the fibers themselves can be altered to be hollow or biphasic by using specific electrospinning approaches [57].

2.1.1. Mono-Axial Electrospinning

Mono-axial electrospinning is the simplest and as a result of this the most common electrospinning experiment. The polymer (and API) in solution or suspension is dispensed through a single-bore blunt-end needle resulting in a monolithic product, with the API and polymer typically evenly and homogeneously blended throughout the fibers [58].

In Verreck et al.'s study, Itraconazole-HPMC SDs were generated by electrospinning and properties of the resultant nanofibres were compared relative to other SD techniques namely HME and solvent casting with regards their dissolution behavior [59]. Though the dissolution methods varied for the different presentations, several apparent trends were observed. PMs of itraconazole and HPMC generated little (<1–3%) drug release in any of the dissolution approaches assessed. Interestingly, electrospun ASDs samples resulted in complete in vitroitraconazole release over but however, the dissolution rate was slower compared to the cast thin films, melt extruded and milled powders [59]. The authors concluded that for this drug-polymer system, there could be potential as a controlled drug delivery system. Nagy et al. compared the drug dissolution behavior of spironolactone-soluplus SDs generated by electrospinning to those prepared by HME with key findings confirming the generation of ASDs with the electrospun nanofibers showing enhanced drug dissolution behavior compared to the HME SDs [60,61].

PVP-acetaminophen SDs prepared by electrospinning generating non-woven nanofibrous meshes were compared to traditional SD preparation processes namely freeze drying, vacuum drying, and heat drying with an advantage of the electrospinning process over the traditional processes being the unique microstructural characteristics of the electrospun nanofibres generated. Freeze dried samples and electrospun fibers did not show any evidence of phase separation phenomenon which was evident in heat-dried and vacuum-dried samples which led to visible (in scanning electron microscopy studies) microparticles on the sample surfaces. The in vitro dissolution tests illustrated that the electrospun SDs nanofibers released 93.8% acetaminophen in the first 2 min and the dissolution rates of acetaminophen from the different SDs had the following order: electrospun > vacuum-dried ≈ freeze-dried > heating-dried [62]. They also highlighted [62] the advantage of third generation SDs (where the state the carrier has surface activity or self-emulsifying properties) and the potential for these to be generated using mono-axial electrospinning. Third generation SDs of ferulic acid in composite nanofibers with three-dimensional continuous web structure were generated by electrospinning co-dissolving solutions of ferulic acid, PVP with the surfactant sodium dodecyl sulfate (SDS) and sucralose. In vitro dissolution and permeation tests showed that the nanofiber-based SDs rapidly released all of the ferulic acid within in 1 min and had a 13-fold greater permeation rate across sublingual mucosa compared to crude ferulic acid particles [63,64].

2.1.2. Coaxial and Multi-Axial Electrospinning

Coaxial electrospinning (also known as co-electrospinning) involves the use of a two-needle spinneret, with one needle nested inside another in a concentric fashion. Fires generated tend to have greater versatility in terms of the range of materials used, therapeutic agents incorporated (ranging from small molecules to biological molecules), size (e.g., from 100 nm to 300 μm), and can offer complete drug encapsulation and higher drug stability compared to mono-axial fibers [58]. The use of coaxial and multi-axial electrospinning approaches has been applied in drug delivery with great success to generate biphasic [65], targeted release [66,67] and multifunctional materials [68] as well as SDs. Yang et al. [69] explored three types of electrospinning namely coaxial, modified coaxial, and tri-axial (characterized by the use of un-spinnable liquids as the sheath working fluids) electrospinning to generate nanofibrous ferulic acid-cellulose acetate ASDs depot systems [69]. In vitro dissolution tests revealed that the fibers were able to provide close to zero-order release over 36 h, with no initial burst release and minimal tailing-off. The release properties of the depot systems generated showed improved properties over the monolithic fibers, which exhibited a significant burst release and also considerable tailing-off at the end of the drug release studies [69]. Tri-axial electrospinning has also been successfully used to fabricate nanofibres of lecithin (known to be un-spinnable), diclofenac sodium with Eudragit S100 a methacrylic acid/methyl methacrylate copolymer (which only dissolves at pH > 7.0) as the carrier matrix for oral colon targeting [70].

2.1.3. Others

Several other electrospinning systems exist which have been used to generate ASDs. The core-cut nozzle system where the exit pipe of the core nozzle is removed so that the core fluid can form an envelope inside the shell solution [71] has been shown to improve spinnability of two fluids by reducing jet instability. This system is also suitable for the production of multi-layered nanofibers where the drug is in the internal layer. Due to this, drug release is shown to start from the core then moving through to the external environment with applications as a controlled drug delivery system as the thickness of each layer can be tailored to vary the drug release [71]. Side-by-side electrospinning is a two-liquid process and the structure of the spinneret is propagated into the solid products creating Janus fibers with two different sides [72]. The different sides could hold two different polymers with two different drugs loaded resulting in concomitant drug release [73].

Unfortunately, in spite of the enormous research efforts both in academia and in industry very few ASDs products let alone nanofibrous ASDs have reached the market so far [74]. Works by Démuth et al. have successfully turned ASDs nanofibers into a viable nanofibrous ASDs solid dosage forms by compressing them into tablets with enhanced drug dissolution rates [75,76]. With promising work on-going in the field, there is the potential to have a commercially available nanofibrous ASD based dosage form.

3. Nanofibrous Micro/Nano-Crystalline Solid Dispersions

Due to the challenges associated with the stability of ASDs, there is a push to reconsider the crystalline state in the micron or nanoscale as an alternative method for SD production. It is well-known that the dissolution rate of smaller particles is greater due to the increased surface area in accordance with Noyes–Whitney equation and Nernst–Brunner theory [66–68]. Several investigations into drug particle size reduction [77–79] have shown that particle size reduction leads to increased drug solubility. It has also been demonstrated that a further increase in drug bioavailability is observed when the particle size of a drug is reduced from micrometer to nanometer [80].

Nanosuspensions are sub-micron colloidal dispersions of the drug, which are stabilized by surfactants [81]. This technology has shown great promise as a strategy to improve the dissolution rate of poorly soluble drugs by maintaining the drug in its preferred crystalline state of a size sufficiently small for pharmaceutical acceptability [82,83]. Major advantages of this technology are its general applicability to most drugs and its simplicity [80]. Solid micro/nano-crystalline dispersions have been generated using techniques such as film making [82,84], solvent casting method [32], spray drying [84,85], hot melt extrusion [25], and electrospinning [86].

4. Conclusions

In this review, we focused on the emerging trends in the generation of amorphous and micro/nano-crystalline solid dispersions using electrospinning to improve the dissolution rate and in turn the bioavailability of poorly water-soluble drugs. With electrospinning being a simple but versatile process, various studies have successfully generated mainly amorphous solid dispersions with few studies exploring the generation of crystalline solid dispersions. The scalability of electrospinning and its products for commercial drug delivery applications is a topic of great discussion and debate. The industrial upscaling of electrospinning and application of resultant fibers is discussed by Taylor et al. [86]. The electrospinning equipment market for laboratory research and industrial production is expected to grow significantly in the future due to the continuous development of new electrospinning technologies influenced by demand.

Funding: This research is funded by Universita degli Studi di Palermo DIBIMIS Department.

Conflicts of Interest: The authors declare no conflicts of interest.

References

1. Vo, C.L.N.; Park, C.; Lee, B.J. Current trends and future perspectives of solid dispersions containing poorly water-soluble drugs. *Eur. J. Pharm. Biopharm.* **2013**, *85*, 799–813. [CrossRef] [PubMed]
2. Demetzos, C. *Pharmaceutical Nanotechnology*; Springer Singapore: Singapore, 2016; ISBN 978-981-10-0790-3.
3. Serajuddln, A.T.M. Solid dispersion of poorly water-soluble drugs: Early promises, subsequent problems, and recent breakthroughs. *J. Pharm. Sci.* **1999**, *88*, 1058–1066. [CrossRef]
4. Loh, Z.H.; Samanta, A.K.; Sia Heng, P.W. Overview of milling techniques for improving the solubility of poorly water-soluble drugs. *Asian J. Pharm. Sci.* **2015**, *10*, 255–274. [CrossRef]
5. Paudel, A.; Worku, Z.A.; Meeus, J.; Guns, S.; Van den Mooter, G. Manufacturing of solid dispersions of poorly water soluble drugs by spray drying: Formulation and process considerations. *Int. J. Pharm.* **2013**, *453*, 253–284. [CrossRef] [PubMed]
6. Shah, N.; Iyer, R.M.; Mair, H.-J.; Choi, D.; Tian, H.; Diodone, R.; Fahnrich, K.; Pabst-Ravot, A.; Tang, K.; Scheubel, E.; et al. Improved human bioavailability of vemurafenib, a practically insoluble drug, using an amorphous polymer-stabilized solid dispersion prepared by a solvent-controlled coprecipitation process. *J. Pharm. Sci.* **2013**, *102*, 967–981. [CrossRef] [PubMed]
7. Huang, Y.; Dai, W.-G. Fundamental aspects of solid dispersion technology for poorly soluble drugs. *Acta Pharm. Sin. B.* **2014**, *4*, 18–25. [CrossRef]
8. Sekiguchi, K.; Obi, N. Studies on absorption of eutectic mixture I. A comparison of the behaviour of eutectic mixture of sulfathiazole and that of ordinary sulfathiazole in man. *Chem. Pharm. Bull.* **1961**, *9*, 866–872. [CrossRef]
9. Chiou, W.L.; Riegelman, S. Pharmaceutical applications of solid dispersion systems. *J. Pharm. Sci.* **1971**, *60*, 1281–1302. [CrossRef]

10. Leuner, C.; Dressman, J. Improving drug solubility for oral delivery using solid dispersions. *Eur. J. Pharm. Biopharm.* **2000**, *50*, 47–60. [CrossRef]

11. Craig, D.Q.M. The mechanisms of drug release from solid dispersions in water-soluble polymers. *Int. J. Pharm.* **2002**, *231*, 131–144. [CrossRef]

12. Marano, S.; Barker, S.A.; Raimi-Abraham, B.T.; Missaghi, S.; Rajabi-Siahboomi, A.; Aliev, A.E.; Craig, D.Q.M. Microfibrous solid dispersions of poorly water-soluble drugs produced via centrifugal spinning: unexpected dissolution behavior on recrystallization. *Mol. Pharm.* **2017**, *14*, 1666–1680. [CrossRef] [PubMed]

13. Marano, S.; Barker, S.A.; Raimi-Abraham, B.T.; Missaghi, S.; Rajabi-Siahboomi, A.; Craig, D.Q.M. Development of micro-fibrous solid dispersions of poorly water-soluble drugs in sucrose using temperature-controlled centrifugal spinning. *Eur. J. Pharm. Biopharm.* **2016**, *103*, 84–94. [CrossRef]

14. Yan, H.-X.; Zhang, S.-S.; He, J.-H.; Liu, J.-P. Application of ethyl cellulose, microcrystalline cellulose and octadecanol for wax based floating solid dispersion pellets. *Carbohydr. Polym.* **2016**, *148*, 143–152. [CrossRef] [PubMed]

15. Corrigan, O.I. Retardation of polymeric carrier dissolution by dispersed drugs: factors influencing the dissolution of solid dispersions containing polyethlene glycols. *Drug Dev. Ind. Pharm.* **1986**, *12*, 1777–1793. [CrossRef]

16. Leonardi, D.; Salomon, C.J. Unexpected performance of physical mixtures over solid dispersions on the dissolution behavior of benznidazole from tablets. *J. Pharm. Sci.* **2013**, *102*, 1016–1023. [CrossRef] [PubMed]

17. Sharma, P.K.; Panda, A.; Pradhan, A.; Zhang, J.; Thakkar, R.; Whang, C.-H.; Repka, M.A.; Murthy, S.N. Solid-state stability issues of drugs in transdermal patch formulations. *AAPS PharmSciTech* **2017**, *19*. [CrossRef] [PubMed]

18. Vasconcelos, T.; Sarmento, B.; Costa, P. Solid dispersions as strategy to improve oral bioavailability of poor water soluble drugs. *Drug Discov. Today* **2007**, *12*, 1068–1075. [CrossRef]

19. van Drooge, D.J.; Braeckmans, K.; Hinrichs, W.L.J.; Remaut, K.; De Smedt, S.C.; Frijlink, H.W. Characterization of the mode of incorporation of lipophilic compounds in solid dispersions at the nanoscale using fluorescence resonance energy transfer (FRET). *Macromol. Rapid Commun.* **2006**, *27*, 1149–1155. [CrossRef]

20. Pouton, C.W. Formulation of poorly water-soluble drugs for oral administration: Physicochemical and physiological issues and the lipid formulation classification system. *Eur. J. Pharm. Sci.* **2006**, *29*, 278–287. [CrossRef] [PubMed]

21. Khan, A.W.; Kotta, S.; Ansari, S.H.; Sharma, R.K.; Ali, J. Enhanced dissolution and bioavailability of grapefruit flavonoid Naringenin by solid dispersion utilizing fourth generation carrier. *Drug Dev. Ind. Pharm.* **2015**, *41*, 772–779. [CrossRef]

22. Shamma, R.N.; Basha, M. Soluplus: A novel polymeric solubilizer for optimization of Carvedilol solid dispersions: Formulation design and effect of method of preparation. *Powder Technol.* **2013**, *237*, 406–414. [CrossRef]

23. Meng, F.; Gala, U.; Chauhan, H. Classification of solid dispersions: correlation to (i) stability and solubility (ii) preparation and characterization techniques. *Drug Dev. Ind. Pharm.* **2015**, *41*, 1401–1415. [CrossRef] [PubMed]

24. Kumar, B. Solid Dispersion—A Review. *PharmaTutor* **2017**, *5*, 24–29.

25. Pina, M.F.; Zhao, M.; Pinto, J.F.; Sousa, J.J.; Craig, D.Q.M. The influence of drug physical state on the dissolution enhancement of solid dispersions prepared via hot-melt extrusion: A case study using olanzapine. *J. Pharm. Sci.* **2014**, *103*, 1214–1223. [CrossRef] [PubMed]

26. Qi, S.; Craig, D. Recent developments in micro- and nanofabrication techniques for the preparation of amorphous pharmaceutical dosage forms. *Adv. Drug Deliv. Rev.* **2016**, *100*, 67–84. [CrossRef] [PubMed]

27. Alhusein, N.; Blagbrough, I.S.; Beeton, M.L.; Bolhuis, A.; De Bank, P.A. Electrospun Zein/PCL fibrous matrices release tetracycline in a controlled manner, killing *Staphylococcus aureus* both in biofilms and *ex vivo* on pig skin, and are compatible with human skin cells. *Pharm. Res.* **2016**, *33*, 237–246. [CrossRef] [PubMed]

28. Li, B.; Konecke, S.; Harich, K.; Wegiel, L.; Taylor, L.S.; Edgar, K.J. Solid dispersion of quercetin in cellulose derivative matrices influences both solubility and stability. *Carbohydr. Polym.* **2013**, *92*, 2033–2040. [CrossRef]

29. Zidan, A.S.; Rahman, Z.; Sayeed, V.; Raw, A.; Yu, L.; Khan, M.A. Crystallinity evaluation of tacrolimus solid dispersions by chemometric analysis. *Int. J. Pharm.* **2012**, *423*, 341–350. [CrossRef]

30. Alhusein, N.; De Bank, P.A.; Blagbrough, I.S.; Bolhuis, A. Killing bacteria within biofilms by sustained release of tetracycline from triple-layered electrospun micro/nanofibre matrices of polycaprolactone and poly (ethylene-co-vinyl acetate). *Drug Deliv. Transl Res.* **2013**, *3*, 531–541. [CrossRef]

31. Alshahrani, S.M.; Lu, W.; Park, J.-B.; Morott, J.T.; Alsulays, B.B.; Majumdar, S.; Langley, N.; Kolter, K.; Gryczke, A.; Repka, M.A. Stability-enhanced hot-melt extruded amorphous solid dispersions via combinations of soluplus®and hpmcas-hf. *AAPS PharmSciTech* **2015**, *16*, 824–834. [CrossRef]

32. Modica de Mohac, L.; de Fátima Pina, M.; Raimi-Abraham, B.T. Solid microcrystalline dispersion films as a new strategy to improve the dissolution rate of poorly water soluble drugs: A case study using olanzapine. *Int. J. Pharm.* **2016**, *508*, 42–50. [CrossRef] [PubMed]

33. De Caro, V.; Ajovalasit, A.; Sutera, F.M.; Murgia, D.; Sabatino, M.A.; Dispenza, C. Development and characterization of an amorphous solid dispersion of furosemide in the form of a sublingual bioadhesive film to enhance bioavailability. *Pharmaceutics* **2017**, *9*, 22. [CrossRef] [PubMed]

34. Li, Y.; Pang, H.; Guo, Z.; Lin, L.; Dong, Y.; Li, G.; Lu, M.; Wu, C. Interactions between drugs and polymers influencing hot melt extrusion. *J. Pharm. Pharmacol.* **2014**, *66*, 148–166. [CrossRef] [PubMed]

35. Zhang, K.; Yu, H.; Luo, Q.; Yang, S.; Lin, X.; Zhang, Y.; Tian, B.; Tang, X. Increased dissolution and oral absorption of itraconazole/Soluplus extrudate compared with itraconazole nanosuspension. *Eur. J. Pharm. Biopharm.* **2013**, *85*, 1285–1292. [CrossRef] [PubMed]

36. Keating, A.V.; Soto, J.; Tuleu, C.; Forbes, C.; Zhao, M.; Craig, D.Q.M. Solid state characterisation and taste masking efficiency evaluation of polymer based extrudates of isoniazid for paediatric administration. *Int. J. Pharm.* **2018**, *536*, 536–546. [CrossRef] [PubMed]

37. Davis, M.T.; Potter, C.B.; Mohammadpour, M.; Albadarin, A.B.; Walker, G.M. Design of spray dried ternary solid dispersions comprising itraconazole, soluplus and HPMCP: Effect of constituent compositions. *Int. J. Pharm.* **2017**, *519*, 365–372. [CrossRef] [PubMed]

38. Qi, S.; Moffat, J.G.; Yang, Z. Early stage phase separation in pharmaceutical solid dispersion thin films under high humidity: improved spatial understanding using probe based thermal and spectroscopic nano-characterisation methods. *Mol. Pharm.* **2013**, *10*, 918–930. [CrossRef]

39. Ng, Y.C.; Yang, Z.; McAuley, W.J.; Qi, S. Stabilisation of amorphous drugs under high humidity using pharmaceutical thin films. *Eur. J. Pharm. Biopharm.* **2013**, *84*, 555–565. [CrossRef]

40. Luo, C.J.; Stoyanov, S.D.; Stride, E.; Pelan, E.; Edirisinghe, M. Electrospinning versus fibre production methods: from specifics to technological convergence. *Chem. Soc. Rev.* **2012**, *41*, 4708–4735. [CrossRef]

41. Illangakoon, U.E.; Nazir, T.; Williams, G.R.; Chatterton, N.P. Mebeverine-loaded electrospun nanofibers: physicochemical characterization and dissolution studies. *J. Pharm. Sci.* **2014**, *103*, 283–292. [CrossRef]

42. Raimi-Abraham, B.T.; Mahalingam, S.; Davies, P.J.; Edirisinghe, M.; Craig, D.Q.M. Development and characterization of amorphous nanofiber drug dispersions prepared using pressurized gyration. *Mol. Pharm.* **2015**, *12*, 3851–3861. [CrossRef] [PubMed]

43. Bhut, V.Z.; Prajapati, A.B.; Patel, K.N.; Patel, B.A.; Patel, P.A. Solid dispersion as a strategy to enhance solubility: A review article. *IJPRS* **2012**, *5*, 490–498.

44. Thakral, S.; Thakral, N.K. Prediction of drug–polymer miscibility through the use of solubility parameter based flory–huggins interaction parameter and the experimental validation: PEG as model polymer. *J. Pharm. Sci.* **2013**, *102*, 2254–2263. [CrossRef] [PubMed]

45. Son, Y.J.; Kim, W.J.; Yoo, H.S. Therapeutic applications of electrospun nanofibers for drug delivery systems. *Arch. Pharm. Res.* **2013**, *37*, 69–78. [CrossRef]

46. Liu, M.; Duan, X.-P.; Li, Y.-M.; Yang, D.-P.; Long, Y.-Z. Electrospun nanofibers for wound healing. *Mater. Sci. Eng. C* **2017**, *76*, 1413–1423. [CrossRef] [PubMed]

47. Jun, I.; Han, H.S.; Edwards, J.R.; Jeon, H. Electrospun Fibrous Scaffolds for Tissue Engineering: Viewpoints on Architecture and Fabrication. *Int. J. Mol. Sci.* **2018**, *19*, 745. [CrossRef] [PubMed]

48. Cooley, J.F. Improved methods of and apparatus for electrically separating the relatively volatile liquid component from the component of relatively fixed substances of composite fluids. *United Kingdom Patent* **1900**, *6385*, 19.

49. Cooley, J.F. Apparatus for Electrically Dispersing Fluids. U.S. Patent Application No. 692,631, 4 February 1902.

50. Morton, W.J. Method of Dispersing Fluids. U.S. Patent US705691A, 29 July 1902.

51. Sill, T.J.; von Recum, H.A. Electrospinning: applications in drug delivery and tissue engineering. *Biomaterials* **2008**, *29*, 1989–2006. [CrossRef] [PubMed]

52. Williams, G.R.; Chatterton, N.P.; Nazir, T.; Yu, D.G.; Zhu, L.M.; Branford-White, C.J. Electrospun nanofibers in drug delivery: recent developments and perspectives. *Ther. Deliv.* **2012**, *3*, 515–533. [CrossRef]
53. Cheng, H.; Yang, X.; Che, X.; Yang, M.; Zhai, G. Biomedical application and controlled drug release of electrospun fibrous materials. *Mater. Sci. Eng. C* **2018**, *90*, 750–763. [CrossRef]
54. Vogt, L.; Liverani, L.; Roether, J.; Boccaccini, A. Electrospun Zein Fibers Incorporating Poly(glycerol sebacate) for Soft Tissue Engineering. *Nanomaterials* **2018**, *8*, 150. [CrossRef]
55. Alhusein, N.; Blagbrough, I.S.; De Bank, P.A. Zein/polycaprolactone electrospun matrices for localised controlled delivery of tetracycline. *Drug Deliv. Transl. Res.* **2013**, *3*, 542–550. [CrossRef] [PubMed]
56. Zhang, H.; Lou, S.; Williams, G.R.; Branford-White, C.; Nie, H.; Quan, J.; Zhu, L.-M. A systematic study of captopril-loaded polyester fiber mats prepared by electrospinning. *Int. J. Pharm.* **2012**, *439*, 100–108. [CrossRef] [PubMed]
57. Qu, H.; Wei, S.; Guo, Z. Coaxial electrospun nanostructures and their applications. *J. Mater. Chem. A* **2013**, *1*, 11513–11518. [CrossRef]
58. Williams, G.R.; Raimi-Abraham, B.T.; Luo, C.J. *Nanofibres in Drug Delivery*; UCL Press: London, UK, 2018; ISBN 9781787350182.
59. Verreck, G.; Chun, I.; Peeters, J.; Rosenblatt, J.; Brewster, M.E. Preparation and characterization of nanofibers containing amorphous drug dispersions generated by electrostatic spinning. *Pharm. Res.* **2003**, *20*, 810–817. [CrossRef] [PubMed]
60. Nagy, Z.K.; Balogh, A.; Vajna, B.; Farkas, A.; Patyi, G.; Kramarics, Á.; Marosi, G. Comparison of electrospun and extruded soluplus®-based solid dosage forms of improved dissolution. *J. Pharm. Sci.* **2012**, *101*, 322–332. [CrossRef] [PubMed]
61. Nagy, Z.K.; Balogh, A.; Démuth, B.; Pataki, H.; Vigh, T.; Szabó, B.; Molnár, K.; Schmidt, B.T.; Horák, P.; Marosi, G.; et al. High speed electrospinning for scaled-up production of amorphous solid dispersion of itraconazole. *Int. J. Pharm.* **2015**, *480*, 137–142. [CrossRef] [PubMed]
62. Yu, D.-G.; Branford-White, C.; White, K.; Li, X.-L.; Zhu, L.-M. dissolution improvement of electrospun nanofiber-based solid dispersions for acetaminophen. *AAPS PharmSciTech* **2010**, *11*, 809–817. [CrossRef]
63. Huang, Z.-M.; Zhang, Y.-Z.; Kotaki, M.; Ramakrishna, S. A review on polymer nanofibers by electrospinning and their applications in nanocomposites. *Compos. Sci. Technol.* **2003**, *63*, 2223–2253. [CrossRef]
64. Li, D.; Xia, Y. Electrospinning of nanofibers: reinventing the wheel? *Adv. Mater.* **2004**, *16*, 1151–1170. [CrossRef]
65. Yu, D.G.; Wang, X.; Li, X.Y.; Chian, W.; Li, Y.; Liao, Y.Z. Electrospun biphasic drug release polyvinylpyrrolidone/ethyl cellulose core/sheath nanofibers. *Acta Biomater.* **2013**, *9*, 5665–5672. [CrossRef]
66. Maincent, J.; Williams, R.O. Sustained-release amorphous solid dispersions. *Drug Deliv. Transl. Res.* **2018**, *8*, 1–12. [CrossRef] [PubMed]
67. Lin, W.C.; Yeh, I.T.; Niyama, E.; Huang, W.R.; Ebara, M.; Wu, C.S. Electrospun poly(ε-caprolactone) nanofibrous mesh for imiquimod delivery in melanoma therapy. *Polymers* **2018**, *10*, 231. [CrossRef]
68. Wei, Q.; Xu, F.; Xu, X.; Geng, X.; Ye, L.; Zhang, A.; Feng, Z. The multifunctional wound dressing with core–shell structured fibers prepared by coaxial electrospinning. *Front. Mater. Sci.* **2016**, *10*, 113–121. [CrossRef]
69. Yang, G.; Li, J.; Yu, D.; He, M.; Yang, J.; Williams, G.R. Nanosized sustained-release drug depots fabricated using modified tri-axial electrospinning. *Acta Biomater.* **2017**, *53*, 233–241. [CrossRef] [PubMed]
70. Yang, C.; Yu, D.-G.; Pan, D.; Liu, X.-K.; Wang, X.; Bligh, S.W.A.; Williams, G.R. Electrospun pH-sensitive core–shell polymer nanocomposites fabricated using a tri-axial process. *Acta Biomater.* **2016**, *35*, 77–86. [CrossRef]
71. Lee, B.S.; Jeon, S.Y.; Park, H.; Lee, G.; Yang, H.S.; Yu, W.R. New electrospinning nozzle to reduce jet instability and its application to manufacture of multi-layered nanofibers. *Sci. Rep.* **2014**, *4*, 6758. [CrossRef] [PubMed]
72. Yu, D.-G.; Yang, C.; Jin, M.; Williams, G.R.; Zou, H.; Wang, X.; Bligh, S.W.A. Medicated Janus fibers fabricated using a Teflon-coated side-by-side spinneret. *Colloids Surf B Biointerfaces* **2016**, *138*, 110–116. [CrossRef]
73. Geng, Y.; Zhang, P.; Wang, Q.; Liu, Y.; Pan, K. Novel PAN/PVP Janus ultrafine fiber membrane and its application for biphasic drug release. *J. Mater. Chem. B* **2017**, *5*, 5390–5396. [CrossRef]
74. Van Den Mooter, G. The use of amorphous solid dispersions: A formulation strategy to overcome poor solubility and dissolution rate. *Drug Discov. Today Technol.* **2012**, *9*, 79–86. [CrossRef]

75. Démuth, B.; Farkas, A.; Balogh, A.; Bartosiewicz, K.; Kállai-Szabó, B.; Bertels, J.; Vigh, T.; Mensch, J.; Verreck, G.; Van Assche, I.; et al. Lubricant-induced crystallization of itraconazole from tablets made of electrospun amorphous solid dispersion. *J. Pharm. Sci.* **2016**, *105*, 2982–2988. [CrossRef]

76. Démuth, B.; Farkas, A.; Szabó, B.; Balogh, A.; Nagy, B.; Vágó, E.; Vigh, T.; Tinke, A.P.; Kazsu, Z.; Demeter, Á.; et al. Development and tableting of directly compressible powder from electrospun nanofibrous amorphous solid dispersion. *Adv. Powder Technol.* **2017**, *28*, 1554–1563. [CrossRef]

77. Li, M.; Gogos, C.G.; Ioannidis, N. Improving the API dissolution rate during pharmaceutical hot-melt extrusion I: Effect of the API particle size, and the co-rotating, twin-screw extruder screw configuration on the API dissolution rate. *Int. J. Pharm.* **2015**, *478*, 103–112. [CrossRef] [PubMed]

78. Ige, P.P.; Baria, R.K.; Gattani, S.G. Fabrication of fenofibrate nanocrystals by probe sonication method for enhancement of dissolution rate and oral bioavailability. *Colloids Surf. B Biointerfaces* **2013**, *108*, 366–373. [CrossRef] [PubMed]

79. Frizon, F.; de Oliveira Eloy, J.; Donaduzzi, C.M.; Mitsui, M.L.; Marchetti, J.M. Dissolution rate enhancement of loratadine in polyvinylpyrrolidone K-30 solid dispersions by solvent methods. *Powder Technol.* **2013**, *235*, 532–539. [CrossRef]

80. Gao, L.; Liu, G.; Wang, X.; Liu, F.; Xu, Y.; Ma, J. Preparation of a chemically stable quercetin formulation using nanosuspension technology. *Int. J. Pharm.* **2011**, *404*, 231–237. [CrossRef] [PubMed]

81. Rabinow, B.E. Nanosuspensions in drug delivery. *Drug Deliv.* **2004**, *3*, 785–796. [CrossRef] [PubMed]

82. Bodmeier, R.; Oh, K.H.; Chen, H. The effect of the addition of low molecular weight poly(DL-lactide) on drug release from biodegradable poly(DL-lactide) drug delivery systems. *Int. J. Pharm.* **1989**, *51*, 1–8. [CrossRef]

83. Tinke, A.P.; Carnicer, A.; Govoreanu, R.; Scheltjens, G.; Lauwerysen, L.; Mertens, N.; Vanhoutte, K.; Brewster, M.E. Particle shape and orientation in laser diffraction and static image analysis size distribution analysis of micrometer sized rectangular particles. *Powder Technol.* **2008**, *186*, 154–167. [CrossRef]

84. Choi, H.J.; Kim, S.G.; Hyun, Y.H.; Jhon, M.S. Preparation and rheological characteristics of solvent-cast poly (ethylene oxide)/ montmorillonite nanocomposites. *Macromol. Rapid Commun.* **2001**, *22*, 320–325. [CrossRef]

85. Singh, A.; Van den Mooter, G. Spray drying formulation of amorphous solid dispersions. *Adv. Drug Deliv. Rev.* **2016**, *100*, 27–50. [CrossRef]

86. Taylor, M.J.; Tanna, S.; Sahota, T. In vivo study of a polymeric glucose-sensitive insulin delivery system using a rat model. *J. Pharm. Sci.* **2010**, *99*, 4215–4227. [CrossRef] [PubMed]

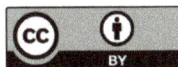

pharmaceutics

MDPI

Review

Electrospun Nanofibers for Tissue Engineering with Drug Loading and Release

Kaiqiang Ye [1], Haizhu Kuang [1], Zhengwei You [2], Yosry Morsi [3] and Xiumei Mo [1,*]

[1] State Key Laboratory for Modification of Chemical Fibers and Polymer Materials, College of Chemistry, Chemical Engineering and Biotechnology, Donghua University, Shanghai 201620, China; yekaiqiang91@gmail.com (K.Y.); kuanghaizhu@gmail.com (H.K.)

[2] State Key Laboratory for Modification of Chemical Fibers and Polymer Materials, College of Materials Science and Engineering, Donghua University, Shanghai 201620, China; zyou@dhu.edu.cn

[3] Faculty of Engineering and Industrial Sciences, Swinburne University of Technology, Boroondara, VIC 3122, Australia; ymorsi@swin.edu.au

* Correspondence: xmm@dhu.edu.cn; Tel.: +86-21-67792653

Received: 17 December 2018; Accepted: 29 March 2019; Published: 15 April 2019

Abstract: Electrospinning technologies have been applied in the field of tissue engineering as materials, with nanoscale-structures and high porosity, can be easily prepared via this method to bio-mimic the natural extracellular matrix (ECM). Tissue engineering aims to fabricate functional biomaterials for the repairment and regeneration of defective tissue. In addition to the structural simulation for accelerating the repair process and achieving a high-quality regeneration, the combination of biomaterials and bioactive molecules is required for an ideal tissue-engineering scaffold. Due to the diversity in materials and method selection for electrospinning, a great flexibility in drug delivery systems can be achieved. Various drugs including antibiotic agents, vitamins, peptides, and proteins can be incorporated into electrospun scaffolds using different electrospinning techniques and drug-loading methods. This is a review of recent research on electrospun nanofibrous scaffolds for tissue-engineering applications, the development of preparation methods, and the delivery of various bioactive molecules. These studies are based on the fabrication of electrospun biomaterials for the repair of blood vessels, nerve tissues, cartilage, bone defects, and the treatment of aneurysms and skin wounds, as well as their applications related to oral mucosa and dental fields. In these studies, due to the optimal selection of drugs and loading methods based on electrospinning, in vitro and in vivo experiments demonstrated that these scaffolds exhibited desirable effects for the repair and treatment of damaged tissue and, thus, have excellent potential for clinical application.

Keywords: electrospinning; tissue engineering; drug delivery

1. Introduction

Electrospinning technology has been widely utilized for the preparation of tissue-engineering scaffolds [1]. The set-up of a typical electrospinning apparatus mainly consists of a spinneret (e.g., a medical injector with a blunt tip), a boost pump for controlling the extrusion rate of a polymer solution, a direct-current electric field, and a grounded collector [2]. The electrospinning technique applies electrostatic principles to fabricate electrospun nanofibers [3]. Generally, in the electrospinning process, a polymer solution generates a cone-shaped drop beneath the needle under a strong electric field; then, the polymer drops overcome the surface tension to eject polymer nanofibers into the low electric field [4,5]. Using electrospinning, various polymers including synthetic and natural materials (as well as blends of the two in consideration of the mechanical properties) can be fabricated as diverse tissue-engineering scaffolds possessing nanofibrous structure. Scaffolds prepared by electrospinning have tremendous advantages for tissue engineering, such as a large specific surface area, high porosity, extracellular matrix (ECM)-biomimetic structures, and better biocompatibility [6–10]. Furthermore, the ECM can bind, release, and activate signaling molecules and can also modulate the cell's reaction to soluble factors [11]. In order to functionalize the scaffolds for the promotion of cell adhesion, proliferation, and differentiation, nanofibers of the scaffold can be loaded with many bioactive substances, such as proteins, peptides, and small-molecule drugs [12–18]. Therefore, electrospun scaffolds have remarkable advantages in both ECM-biomimetic structures and the loading of bioactive substances. Electrospun drug delivery scaffolds have emerged as essential applications in the biomedical field [19].

The diversity in material selection and preparation methods gives electrospun scaffolds great flexibility for the application of drug delivery [20]. By utilizing different kinds of electrospinning methods, drugs can be incorporated into electrospun scaffolds in many ways, such as coatings, embedded loading, and encapsulated loading (coaxial and emulsion electrospinning). Traditional electrospinning is the simplest method to prepare electrospun scaffolds. In this method, polymers are directly dissolved into solvent to obtain the electrospinning solution and fabricate the scaffolds. In traditional electrospinning, drugs can be incorporated into the scaffolds either by blending or surface modification. In blending electrospinning, drugs and polymers are simultaneously dissolved in the solvent. Later on, this blended solution is used to fabricate the scaffold [21]. In surface modification, electrospun scaffolds are prepared firstly, then drugs are loaded onto the scaffolds via physical adsorption, covalent binding, and other surface-treatment methods [22]. Accordingly, drugs incorporated into scaffolds via different methods exhibit diverse release characteristics. In blending, the release rate mainly depends on the properties of polymers and drugs in the physiological environment. In physical adsorption, the drug usually shows a faster release rate because of the weaker interaction between drugs and the surface of scaffolds, such as electrostatic adsorption, hydrogen bonding, and hydrophobic interactions [23]. However, drugs covalently bound to the scaffolds hardly release from the scaffolds unless the surface polymers are degraded [24].

Coaxial electrospinning is a special method to generate nanofibers with a core–shell structure. Using a coaxial configuration, two separate polymer solutions (core and shell solutions) flow through two different but coaxial aisles. Core and shell solutions are simultaneously pushed into the configuration. With the slow push of a syringe, the drops are jetted out to form nanofibers under a strong electric field. This technique attracted great attention due to its potential applications in controlled drug delivery [25–27]. In coaxial electrospinning, the shell solutions should have spinnability to form the main part of the nanofibers. However, the core solutions have no need for spinnability; thus, some substances without spinnability, such as drugs, proteins, and some bioactive substances, can be incorporated into the core structure of nanofibers by dissolving in the core solution. In this way, these drugs and bioactive substances can be released from the nanofibers in a sustained manner. Therefore, coaxial electrospinning can prepare electrospun scaffolds with bioactivity and functionality. This method is widely used for the preparation of functional nanofibrous scaffolds. A controlled release of functional molecules from the core layer of core–shell scaffolds loaded with drugs, bio-macromolecules, and growth factors could sustainably exert biological functions. For example, tetracycline hydrochloride encapsulated into electrospun core–shell nanofibers showed a sustained release, and exhibited great antibacterial capability, as shown in *Escherichia coli* growth-inhibiting tests [28]. ZnO and Zn acetate nanoparticles were embedded in polycaprolactone coaxial-fiber and uniaxial-fiber matrices to develop potential antibacterial nanocomposite wound dressings [29]. In order to guide tissue regeneration in an infectious environment, coaxial electrospinning was firstly conducted to fabricate dual drug-loaded fiber mats with a core/shell structure. Naringin-loaded polyvinylpyrrolidone was designed as a core fiber to enrich tissue regeneration, and metronidazole-loaded poly(lactic-*co*-glycolic acid) was designed as a shell fiber to inhibit bacterial growth [30].

In addition, nanofibers prepared via the emulsion electrospinning possess the analogous core–shell structure generated by coaxial electrospinning. Therefore, emulsion electrospinning can also be used to prepare core–shell nanofibers for loading and releasing drugs, proteins, and growth factors.

However, the process and needle used for emulsion electrospinning are different compared to coaxial electrospinning. Emulsion electrospinning has no need for a coaxial configuration, and the spinning solution is made into a uniform emulsifying solution by blending emulsifier into a polymer–drug mixed solution. However, the polymers and drugs are dissolved in different solvents before blending. Then, the solution is used for the electrospinning process via a single syringe needle as in traditional electrospinning. Finally, nanofibers with multicore or core–shell structures can be obtained. In order to verify the controlled delivery of drugs from this novel type of tissue-engineering scaffold, rhodamine B and bovine serum albumin (BSA) were incorporated into nanofibers via emulsion electrospinning [31]. In vitro dual drug-release studies of different types of electrospun mats indicated that the emulsion electrospun mats had the most desirable controllable release behaviors.

Therefore, electrospun scaffolds, due to their ECM-biomimetic structure and diversity of drug delivery applications, are widely applied in the field of tissue engineering [32]. In the upcoming section, we further introduce their specific applications, such as aneurysm treatment, nerve tissue engineering, vascular tissue engineering, wound dressing, and bone tissue engineering.

2. Electrospun Scaffolds for Aneurysm Treatment

Intracranial aneurysms represent one of the most common cerebrovascular diseases, and they cause serious healthcare problems, such as brain damage, hemorrhagic stroke, and even death [33,34]. Many studies demonstrated that a covered stent is a desirable solution to treat aneurysms [35,36]. However, the common problem is that the stent-graft easily causes platelet aggregation when implanted into the blood vessel, leading to thrombosis and intimal hyperplasia. Rapid endothelialization, antithrombotic coatings, and anti-clotting drugs are favorable methods to avoid thrombosis. A covered stent is formed by a covered sheet wrapping a metallic stent, where the anticoagulation properties of the covered sheet play a crucial role in avoiding thrombosis of the covered stent. The emulsion electrospinning technique was used to fabricate heparin-loaded poly(L-lactide-co-caprolactone) (PLCL) core–shell nanofibers as an anticoagulant cover sheet. Heparin aqueous solution and emulsifier Span-80 were added dropwise into dichloromethane while stirring until a uniform water-in-oil emulsion formed. PLCL was then added into the emulsion for electrospinning to fabricate PLCL/heparin core–shell nanofibers. The covered stent effectively separated the aneurysm dome in the bloodstream of the rabbit model [37]. In addition, vascular endothelial growth factor (VEGF) was mixed with heparin and loaded into the core of a PLCL nanofiber via emulsion electrospinning to promote rapid endothelialization [38]. An aqueous solution of VEGF, heparin, and Span-80 was mixed in dichloromethane to form a uniform water-in-oil emulsion via consistent stirring. PLCL was then dissolved in the emulsion to obtain a uniform electrospinning solution. Finally, the solution was electrospun to obtain PLCL–Hep–VEGF scaffolds. The release of heparin and VEGF lasted for more than 30 days. That sustained release of heparin and VEGF enhanced cell proliferation and the spread of pig iliac endothelial cells onto the stent. Rosuvastatin calcium can facilitate endothelialization with the ability to enhance the adhesion and proliferation of vascular endothelial cells (VECs). A novel type of covered stent was prepared via coaxial electrospinning to cover the stent with heparin and rosuvastatin calcium-loaded PLCL nanofibers [39]. The fabrication process of the covered stent is shown in Figure 1, showing heparin and rosuvastatin calcium as the core solution and PLCL as the shell solution. The release curves of heparin and rosuvastatin calcium have two stages, including an initial release that occurred during the first 48 h and a slow release that lasted more than 45 days. The covered stent showed remarkable anticoagulation ability, and the HUVECs proliferated well on the covered stent, due to the sustained release of rosuvastatin calcium and heparin from the PLCL coaxial nanofibers.

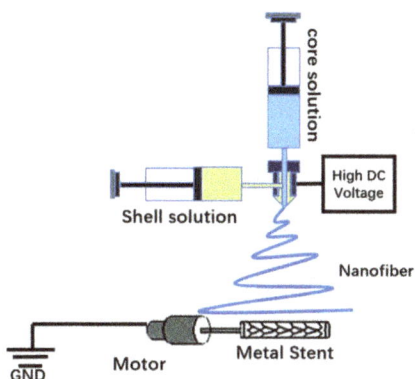

Figure 1. Schematic diagram of the set-up for coaxial electrospinning [39]. Reproduced by permission of The Royal Society of Chemistry (RSC) on behalf of the Centre National de la Recherche Scientifique (CNRS) and the RSC, 2017.

3. Electrospun Scaffolds for Nerve Tissue Engineering

Peripheral nerve defects represent a serious clinical issue which results in high morbidity among trauma patients [40]. To address the limited regenerative ability of the human nervous system and the shortage of therapeutic options, nerve tissue engineered graft transplantation is a potential treatment for peripheral nerve injury [41,42]. Conduit scaffolds, cells, and growth factors are the three elements for nerve tissue engineering [43]. Core–shell poly(D,L-lactide-*co*-glycolide) (PLGA) nanofibrous nerve guidance conduits loaded with nerve growth factor (NGF) were fabricated via coaxial electrospinning and were used to construct nerve guidance conduits for a 13-mm rat sciatic nerve defect. [44]. The shell solution was PLGA, and the core solution was β-NGF with 400 mg of PEG dissolved in distilled water. A rotating wheel drum with a speed of 4000 rpm was used to received nanofibers to form an aligned construct. The release of NGF from nanofibers lasted 30 days. After 12-weeks implantation, the regeneration of nerve cells in the PLGA/NGF conduit was superior to other groups. Another type of nerve guidance conduit (NGC) was fabricated via coaxial electrospinning. NGF in silk solution as a core layer was encapsulated in PLCL via coaxial electrospinning. NGF presented a sustained release and remained biologically active over 60 days because NGF was stabilized by silk fibroin (SF) in the core [45]. The graft was implanted across a 15-mm defect in the sciatic nerve of rats to evaluate nerve regeneration. Results of electrophysiological assessment, histochemistry, and electron microscopy at 12 weeks suggested that the released NGF from nanofibers could effectively promote the regeneration of the peripheral nerve. In order to further promote cell differentiation, the nanofibers with PLCL as the shell and BSA/NGF as the core were fabricated via coaxial electrospinning [46]. Sustained release of BSA/NGF from nanofibers was verified, and it promoted the differentiation of rat pheochromocytoma cells (PC12). Monosialoganglioside (GM1) can promote neuronal development, cell growth, and differentiation, and it plays an essential role in neuronal excitability of myelinated and nonmyelinated fibers. It was reported that the combination of GM1 with NGF can enhance the effects of protecting nerve cells. NGF and GM1 were loaded into the PLCL/silk fibroin (PLCL/SF) nanofibers via a coaxial electrospinning technique [47]. NGF reached $55.8 \pm 1.6\%$ release at 71 days. Schwann cell (SC) proliferation and pheochromocytoma (PC12) differentiation were enhanced by the synergistic effect of GM1 and NGF. The graft loading with GM1 and NGF performed good nerve function recovery in a rabbit sciatic nerve defect model. Vitamins play an important role in tissue growth and differentiation. The water-soluble vitamin B5 was blended with PLCL/silk solutions to form an electrospinning solution. Then, the electrospinning solution was aligned with nanofiber meshes via electrospinning technique [48]. Vitamin B5 was added to a PLCL/silk solution and constantly stirred overnight to form the electrospinning solution. Nanofibers with aligned structure were collected by a rotating drum collector with a speed of 3000 rpm. Vitamin B5 was released up to 80% in 24 h. This nanofibrous material might have potential applications in nerve repair or regeneration. A laminin-coated and yarn-encapsulated PLGA nerve guidance conduit (LC-YE-PLGA NGC) was fabricated to perform the cooperative effects of a topological structure promoting Schwann cell (SC) proliferation and migration [49]. The PLGA fiber yarns were fabricated through a double-nozzle electrospinning system; then, the PLGA fibrous outer layer was collected using a general electrospinning method. Subsequently, laminin was coated on the yarn-encapsulated PLGA NGC through covalent bonding (Figure 2). The cell growth test showed that SC growth and SC migration were much better in the LC-YE-PLGA NGCs than in those without yarn encapsulation or laminin coating. Polycaprolactone (PCL) and chitosan were blended and fabricated to form nanofibrous scaffolds via electrospinning. Taking advantage of the amine groups on the chitosan, the surface of the scaffolds was functionalized with laminin via carbodiimide-based cross-linking. Schwann cells grew well on PCL–chitosan scaffolds with excellent mechanical and surface properties [50]. NGF and GDNF were encapsulated in poly(D,L-lactic acid) (PDLLA) and poly(lactic-*co*-glycolic acid) (PLGA) nanofibers, respectively, via a dual-source dual-power (DS-DP) emulsion electrospinning technique. Scaffolds were developed providing dual GF delivery, and sustained release of both types of GFs was also achieved [51].

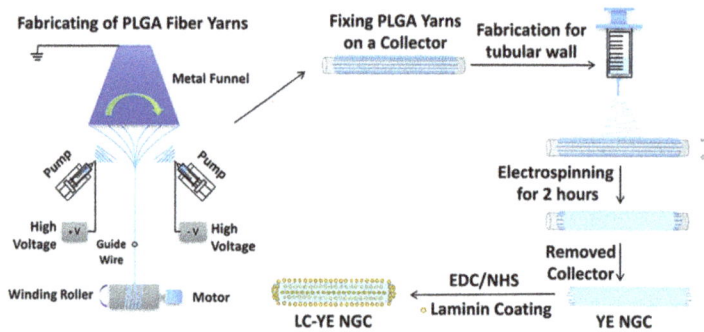

Figure 2. A schematic diagram of the fabrication of the laminin-coated and yarn-encapsulated PLGA (LC-YE-PLGA) nerve guidance conduit (YE NGC: yarn-encapsulated nerve guidance conduit; LC-YE NGC: laminin-coated and yarn-encapsulated nerve guidance conduit) [49]. Reproduced by permission of The Royal Society of Chemistry, 2017.

4. Electrospun Scaffolds for Vascular Tissue Engineering

Coronary heart and peripheral vascular diseases are now the leading cause of death worldwide [52]. Autologous and allogeneic vascular transplantation has limitations caused by many factors such as donor-site morbidity and the shortage of donors in clinic treatment. Developing artificial blood vessels shows increasing significance [53]. Electrospinning is an ideal technique to prepare grafts for small-diameter blood vessels. Heparin-loaded PLCL nanofibers were prepared via a coaxial electrospinning technique, fabricating tubular grafts with an inner diameter of 4 mm [54]. The release of heparin experienced two stages: an initial burst release of 50% followed by continuous release up to 72% from day 2 to 14. Evaluation with a canine artery model demonstrated that heparin loading could greatly enhance the patency rate of small-diameter grafts. To promote endothelial progenitor cell proliferation, vascular endothelial growth factors (VEGFs) are often loaded into scaffolds. Heparin and VEGF were encapsulated into a PLCL nanofiber via emulsion electrospinning to construct vascular grafts for anticoagulation and rapid endothelization [55]. Heparin/VEGF aqueous solution and Span-80 were added dropwise into methylene dichloride and stirred magnetically to form a uniform water-in-oil emulsion. Then, PLCL was dissolved in the emulsion and stirred overnight to obtain the electrospinning solution. Finally, electrospun vascular grafts were prepared using the electrospinning solution. Heparin and VEGF exhibited sustained release for 29 days. The controlled release of heparin and VEGF from the grafts showed good capability for anticoagulation and promoted EPC growth. Platelet-rich growth factor (PRGF) was added into PLCL/SF solutions at a concentration of 20 mg/mL to obtain the electrospinning solution; then, a tubular graft 4 nm in diameter was prepared via an electrospinning process. The graft promoted fast SMC growth and cell penetration into grafts [56]. Salvianolic acid B (SAB), a traditional Chinese plant medicine, can promote the proliferation and migration of endothelial cells. Heparin was dissolved in reverse osmosis (RO) water as a core solution. PLCL and collagen were dissolved in a solution of 1,1,1,3,3,3-hexafluoro-2-propanol (HFIP) with SAB-MSN as a shell solution. Heparin and SAB-MSN were separately encapsulated into the core and the shell of nanofibers via coaxial electrospinning to construct an inner layer of a small-diameter blood vessel graft. The electrospinning process is shown in Figure 3 [57]. SAB was gently released, and no burst release was observed; this is because SAB was adsorbed onto the MSN and blended into the coaxial fiber shell. The total release of 56% was attained within 30 days. The release of heparin was observed, with an initial burst followed by a steady increase up to 30 days. At the end of the test, the cumulative amount of heparin released was 68%. Assessment of the graft in a rat subcutaneous embedding model demonstrated that it possessed good biocompatibility and did not cause significant immune responses, suggesting that the graft is promising for preventing acute thrombosis and for promoting rapid endothelialization. Some findings provide evidence that surface-immobilized growth factors display enhanced stability and induce prolonged function. PCL nano- or microfibers were produced via electrospinning, and they were coated in a radio frequency (RF) plasma process to induce an oxygen functional hydrocarbon layer. Implemented carboxylic acid groups were converted into amine-reactive esters and covalently coupled to VEGF by forming stable amide bonds. Endothelial cell number was significantly enhanced on VEGF-functionalized scaffolds compared to native PCL scaffolds [58].

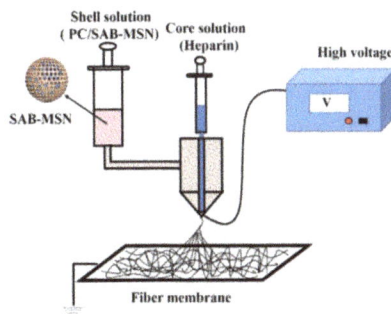

Figure 3. Process of fabricating the core (heparin)–shell (PC/SAB-MSN) fiber. Reprinted with permission from [57] Copyright (2018) American Chemical Society.

5. Electrospun Scaffolds for Wound Dressing Application

Skin wounds are a common issue for surgeons. Clinically, the injured skin should be disposed of and carefully protected with wound dressing immediately. Figure 4 exhibits the classic stages of wound repair. There are three classic stages of wound repair: inflammation (a), new tissue formation (b), and remodeling (c) [59]. The effective promotion of the healing of wounds and the prevention of any infection are the functions of wound dressing. Traditional wound dressings are no longer applicable for the required high-quality healing of heavy and chronic skin wounds [60]. In recent years, wound dressings fabricated via electrospinning methods have received a lot of attention in tissue engineering. Electrospinning is a simple and effective technology for preparing materials with a nanofibrous structure which is similar to the ECM. Wound dressing with this structure was proven to promote the repair of injured skin [61–63]. This is because the electrospun mats possess nanofibrous porous webs, which are not only suitable for the volatilization of tissue fluid, but also for the permeation of oxygen from the external environment. In addition, many growth factors and antibacterial substances can be loaded onto the electrospun wound dressings in various ways during the fabrication process.

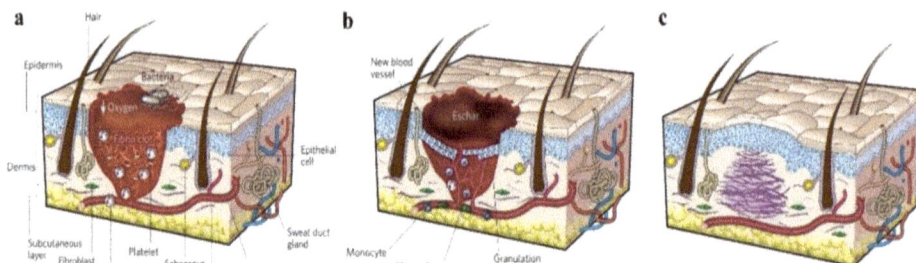

Figure 4. Classic stages of wound repair. There are three classic stages of wound repair: inflammation (a), new tissue formation (b), and remodeling (c) [59]. Reproduced with permission from Springer Nature, 2008.

Generally, electrospun wound dressings are fabricated through a typical electrospinning process to obtain membrane materials. Electrospinning solutions were prepared by dissolving single polymers or by blending natural and synthetic polymers; in some cases, the antibacterial substances could be directly mixed into the solutions [64,65]. Moreover, the healing of skin wounds is a complex biological process. In this process, many cellular pathways are activated to regulate cell behaviors to promote the repair of the wound and reduce the probability of infection [66,67]. Furthermore, different growth factors and important active substances in the wound healing process attracted attention in wound dressing applications, such as epidermal growth factor (EGF), platelet-derived growth factor (PDGF), fibroblast growth factor (FGF), transforming growth factor (TGF), insulin-like growth factor (IGF), and human growth hormone and granulocyte-macrophage colony-stimulating factor (GM-CSF) [60]. Other important active compounds in the healing of a wound are vitamins A, C, and E, zinc, iodine, silver nanoparticles, and copper minerals. Therefore, in many studies, there was a growing tendency to incorporate growth factors or antibacterial molecules into the electrospun materials for enhancing the healing quality of wounds [68–72].

Specifically, Sheng et al. [73] prepared a novel vitamin E (VE)-loaded silk fibroin (SF) nanofiber mat for skin care application. Studies suggested that VE possesses antioxidant and skin barrier stabilizing properties, which make VE a suitable agent for skin protection. In this study, water-soluble VE, RRR-α-tocopherol polyethylene glycol 1000 succinate (VE TPGS), was incorporated into SF nanofibers to investigate its potential application in skin care and tissue regeneration. An in vitro study showed that VE TPGS exhibited sustained-release behavior from the nanofiber mats in a physiological environment. In addition, cell experiments demonstrated that nanofibers containing VE TPGS promoted the proliferation of mouse skin fibroblasts (L929 cells) and protected the cell from oxidation.

El-Aassar et al. [74] developed electrospun polyvinyl alcohol (PVA)/pluronic F127 (Plur)/polyethyleneimine (PEI) composite mats containing titanium dioxide nanoparticles (TiO$_2$ NPs) for wound dressing application. Titanium ions having wound-healing and antimicrobial properties could be released from TiO$_2$ nanoparticles in a slow way, so as to accelerate the wound healing. In this study, TiO$_2$ nanoparticles were used as an antimicrobial agent by directly blending them into the electrospinning solution, and antibacterial tests demonstrated that the fabricated PVA-Plur-PEI/TiO$_2$ nanofibers exhibited better bactericidal activity than PVA-Plur-PEI nanofibers.

Lv et al. [75] reported an electrospun poly(caprolactone) (PCL)/gelatin scaffold containing silicate-based bioceramic particles (Nagelschmidtite, NAGEL, Ca$_7$P$_2$Si$_2$O$_{16}$) for wound healing. In this study, via a co-electrospinning process, the NAGEL bioceramic particles could be uniformly incorporated into PCL/gelatin fibers, and, with the degradation of the scaffold, the Si ions could be released from the fibers in a sustained way. Figure 5 shows the SEM and TEM images of electrospun fibers containing different amounts of NAGEL bioceramic particles which were well embedded inside polymer fibers [75]. Human umbilical vein endothelial cells (HUVECs) and human keratinocytes (HaCaTs) were cultured into the scaffolds, and cell tests indicated that the scaffolds could significantly promote cell adhesion, proliferation, and migration. Wound healing assessment also displayed that wound sites repaired by these scaffolds exhibited desirable healing results in the aspects of angiogenesis, collagen deposition, re-epithelialization, and inhibiting an inflammation reaction. Furthermore, the mechanism of the high-quality healing of the bioceramic/polymer composite biomaterial was identified as being related to the activation of the epithelial-to-mesenchymal transition (EMT) and endothelial-to-mesenchymal transition (EndMT) pathway.

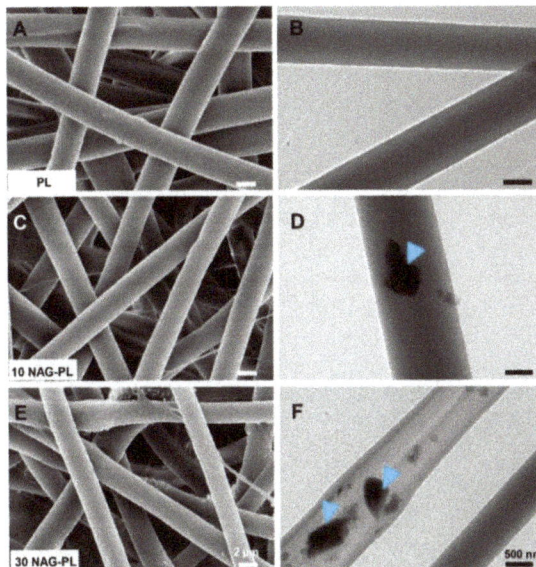

Figure 5. SEM (**A,C,E**) and TEM (**B,D,F**) images of the composite electrospun scaffolds with different contents of NAG bioceramic particles: (**A,B**) pure polymer (PL); (**C,D**) polymer with 10% NAG bioceramic particles (10 NAG-PL); (**E,F**) polymer with 30% NAG bioceramic particles (30 NAG-PL). Blue arrows identify the NAG bioceramic particles which were well embedded inside polymer fibers [75]. Reproduced with permission from Elsevier, 2017.

As a result of incorporating various bioactive molecules into the nanofibers, these novel electrospun biomaterials provided strategies to design functional dressings for the rapid and high-quality healing of skin wounds.

6. Electrospun Scaffolds for Tendon Tissue Engineering

Surgical repair utilizing autografts, allografts, xenografts, tendon prostheses, and suture techniques are the main therapies in the current approach to the treatment of tendon injuries [76]. However, tendon grafts clinically used in surgical treatments fail to meet the demands of adaptability, flexibility, and perpetual remodeling. To address these problems, tissue-engineering scaffolds based on electrospun fibers provide potential alternatives for the treatment and regeneration of damaged tendon tissue. The combination of synthetic polymers and natural materials was an easy method to obtain electrospun scaffolds with both biocompatibility and excellent mechanical strength. Electrospun fibers materials have been investigated in tissue engineering for the potential application of tendon treatment [77–79];

these studies revealed that electrospun composite scaffolds for tendon tissue engineering performed much better than conventional tendon materials in the aspects of biocompatibility, cell adhesion, proliferation, and mechanical properties.

A desirable scaffold that possesses both suitable mechanical properties and biological signals is required for tendon tissue engineering [80]. In recent years, novel spinning approaches were used to fabricate scaffolds mimicking the hierarchical structures of natural tendon tissue [81,82], and to accelerate the healing of tendon defects and further induce tendon regeneration. In addition to varying the preparation method, tendon scaffolds containing various bioactive molecules were also fabricated [83,84].

Sahoo et al. [85]. developed a hybrid scaffold containing both microfibers and nanofibers. Specifically speaking, the knitted silk scaffolds were firstly prefabricated and coated with an aqueous silk solution; then, the knitted scaffolds were installed onto a rotating collector during electrospinning, and the solution for electrospinning was prepared by dissolving PLGA and basic fibroblast growth factor (bFGF) into HFIP. As a result, the knitted scaffolds were wrapped around the electrospun PLGA ultrafine fibers. In this biohybrid scaffold system, silk microfibers were responsible for enhancing mechanical properties, while PLGA nanofibers, coated on the silk scaffolds, could release bFGF in a sustained manner, which was incorporated into PLGA nanofibers via blending electrospinning. As shown in Figure 6A,B, the bFGF was randomly distributed in the PLGA fibers; Figure 6C shows the biohybrid scaffold developed by coating protein-containing (FGF+ group) electrospun fibers (eF) onto microfibrous knitted silk scaffolds (μF). In cell evaluation, mesenchymal progenitor cell (MPC) was seeded into the biohybrid scaffold. Results showed that the biohybrid scaffold system not only promoted MPC attachment and cell proliferation, but also stimulated the tenogeneic differentiation of seeded MPCs. Figure 6D,E exhibits the BMSC-seeded ligament/tendon analogs after seven days of culture. Moreover, following a three-week co-culture of MPCs and scaffold, the generated tendon analog indicated that the scaffold has potential for repairing tendon defects.

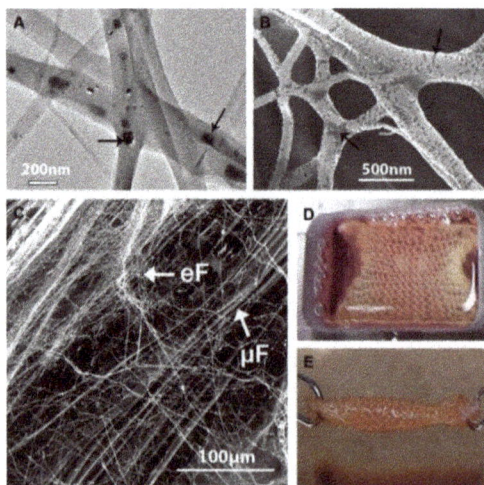

Figure 6. (**A**) TEM and (**B**) back-scattered SEM images of electrospun bFGF-containing PLGA fibers showing the random distribution of proteins (indicated by black arrows) in the fibers; (**C**) SEM image of biohybrid scaffold developed by coating FGF(+) electrospun fibers (eF) on microfibrous knitted silk scaffolds (mF); (**D,E**) BMSC-seeded biohybrid scaffold cultured in a custom-made chamber before being rolled up into cylindrical ligament/tendon analogs after seven days of culture [85]. Reproduced with permission from Elsevier, 2010.

Manning et al. [86] reported a scaffold with the capacity for controlled delivery of growth factors and cells for tendon tissue engineering. Platelet-derived growth factor BB (PDGF-BB), together with adipose-derived mesenchymal stem cells (ASCs), was firstly incorporated into a heparin/fibrin-based delivery system (HBDS). Then, the hydrogel was layered with electrospun nanofibers to obtain the resulting composite scaffold. In vitro and in vivo studies verified that this fabricating strategy allowed the novel layered scaffold to simultaneously and effectively deliver growth factors and fulfill cell migration in a controlled manner in the tendon repair environment so as to promote the tendon healing. Figure 7 shows the fluorescence dyed cells on the scaffold and the schematic of the scaffold structure and ingredients.

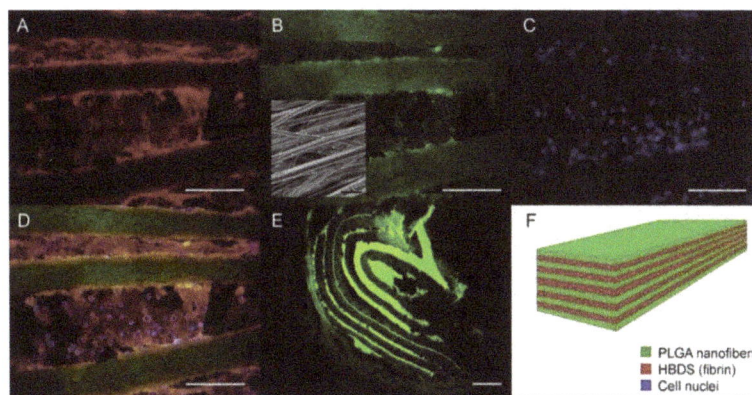

Figure 7. A representative HBDS/nanofiber scaffold with 11 alternating layers of aligned electrospun PLGA nanofiber mats separated by HBDS containing 1×10^6 ASCs is shown. (**A–D**) Micrograph showing the HBDS/nanofiber scaffold in vitro; the PLGA is labeled with FITC (green), the HBDS is labeled with Alexa Fluor 546 (red), and the ASC nuclei are labeled with Hoescht 33258 (blue) (scale bar = 200 μm). (**B**, inset) SEM image of the scaffold showing PLGA nanofiber alignment. (**E**) Micrograph showing the HBDS/nanofiber scaffold in vivo nine days after implantation in tendon repair. Eleven alternating layers of PLGA and HBDS can be seen (i.e., six layers of PLGA and five layers of fibrin); the PLGA is labeled with FITC (green) (scale bar = 100 μm). (**F**) A schematic of the layered scaffold is shown [86]. Reproduced with permission from Elsevier, 2013.

7. Electrospun Scaffolds for Bone Tissue Engineering

Bone tissue-engineering scaffolds are applied to repair bone defects mainly caused by tumors, trauma, osteoporosis, and infection. Due to a limited donor site in autografting treatment, bone tissue engineering aims to produce functional bone scaffolds as alternatives for clinical treatments [87]. An ideal bone scaffold should mimic the architecture of the native ECM to provide a three-dimensional (3D) environment for cell adhesion, proliferation, and differentiation [88]. However, nanofiber materials prepared via traditional electrospinning only possess nanofibrous structure on a two-dimensional level, lacking a 3D porous structure essential for nutrient transport and tissue regeneration; it is estimated that the interconnected spaces >100 μm are required for vascularized bone tissue growth [89]. Recently, emerging strategies were applied to prepare 3D nanofibrous scaffolds based on electrospun nanofibers, which have attracted attention in tissue engineering, especially bone tissue engineering [90–92]. Figure 8 shows the typical strategy of the preparation of electrospun 3D nanofibrous scaffolds; this method mainly consists of nanofiber preparation, homogenization, freeze-drying, and cross-linking processes. These scaffolds possess nanofibrous morphologies and interconnected pores. In addition, a prevailing strategy in bone engineering is the combination of growth factors and scaffolds to facilitate the osteogenic differentiation of stem cells in vitro, and bone regeneration in vivo.

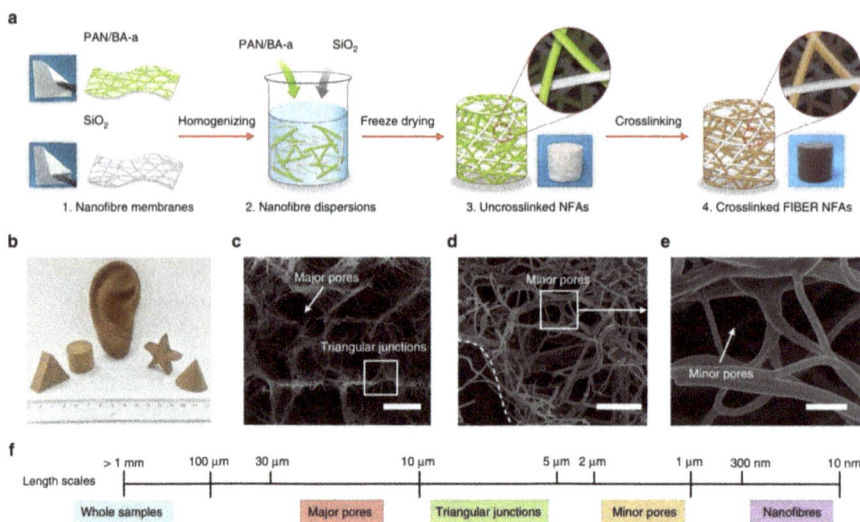

Figure 8. (**a**) Schematic of the synthetic steps. (**b**) The pictures of fabricated scaffolds. (**c–e**) SEM images of the electrospun nanofibrous scaffolds. (**f**) Length scales: 20 μm (**c**), 5 μm (**d**), 1 μm (**e**) [92]. Reproduced with permission from Springer Nature, 2014.

Several studies verified the crucial role of growth factors in regulating cell behaviors, such as recruitment, proliferation, and differentiation [93,94]. Currently, bone morphogenetic proteins (BMPs) are the most effective osteoinductive growth factors investigated in bone tissue engineering [24]. In particular, BMP-2 was approved for clinical application by the FDA. Su et al. [95] developed a BMP-2-and dexamethasone (DEX)-loaded core–shell electrospun mat for use in bone tissue engineering. BMP-2 and DEX were successfully incorporated into nanofibers via blending or coaxial electrospinning, and evaluation of release in vitro indicated that coaxial electrospinning nanofibers exhibited better controlled release of the two substances than blending electrospinning nanofibers. Moreover, the BMP-2 and DEX released from nanofibers induced human mesenchymal stromal cells (hMSC) to differentiate into osteogenic cells.

However, BMP-2 has the disadvantages of rapid enzymatic hydrolysis, ectopic bone formation, immune reactions, and high cost [96,97]. Recently, BMP-2-derived peptides gained much attention as alternative bioactive molecules. The sequences of the peptides were synthesized based on the "wrist" epitope and "knuckle" epitope, which are supposed to bind to BMP receptors [98]. Studies based on BMP-2-derived peptides indicated that these peptides had positive impacts on osteogenic differentiation of stem-cell and bone formation in defects [99,100]. For example, Ye et al. [23] developed a scaffold with a 3D nanofibrous porous structure for bone tissue engineering. In this study, by combining homogenization, freeze-drying, and thermal treatment, nano-hydroxyapatite/PLLA/gelatin (nHA/PLA/GEL) 3D nanofibrous scaffolds were fabricated using pre-prepared electrospun nanofibers. Then, utilizing a polydopamine (pDA)-assisted coating strategy, BMP-2-derived peptides (PEP, sequence: $S_{[PO4]}$KIPKASSVPTELSAISTLYLDDD) were immobilized onto the 3D scaffolds to obtain the resulting nHA/PLA/GEL-PEP 3D nanofibrous scaffolds capable of sustained release of BMP-2 peptides. Figure 9 illustrates the highlights of the study from fabrication to animal experiment. In vitro studies demonstrated that nHA/PLA/GEL-PEP scaffolds promoted the activity of alkaline phosphatase of bone mesenchymal stem cells (BMSCs) and gene expression related to osteogenic differentiation. Moreover, in vivo evaluation was performed using a rat cranial bone defect model, and the results of radiology and histology analysis indicated that this scaffold facilitated bone formation in the defects. Therefore, the scaffold has excellent potential in bone defect repair [23].

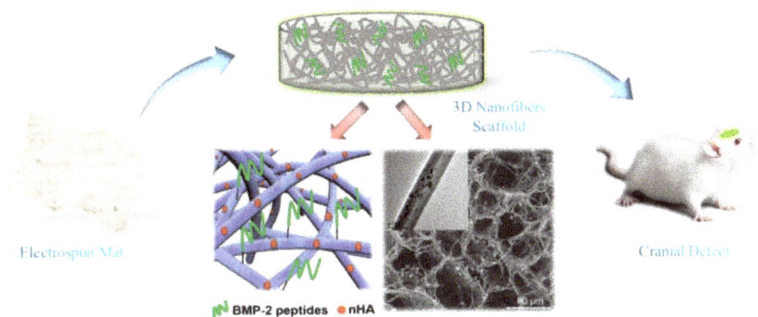

Figure 9. Three-dimensional (3D) electrospun nanofibrous scaffold for rat cranial bone regeneration [23]. Reproduced with permission from Elsevier, 2019.

8. Conclusions

In this review, various scaffolds based on electrospinning for tissue engineering have been discussed, and various strategies for designing novel scaffolds explained. Preparation and delivery methods highlighted indicate that electrospinning technology is a useful tool to fabricate scaffolds with nanofibrous structure. Moreover, bioactive molecules can also be incorporated into the scaffolds via method selection or surface modification for controlling the drug delivery. The ECM-mimicking structure, along with the delivery system based on electrospinning, makes electrospun scaffolds ideal biomaterials for tissue-engineering applications. Key aims going forward should be to address the relationship between mass production and material stability, and the deeper impacts on cells generated by these drug-loaded scaffolds should be illustrated.

Funding: This research was supported by National Major Research Program of China (2016YFC1100202), National Natural Science Foundation of China (31771023).

Conflicts of Interest: The authors declare no conflicts of interest.

References

1. Qasim, S.B.; Zafar, M.S.; Najeeb, S.; Khurshid, Z.; Shah, A.H.; Husain, S.; Rehman, I.U. Electrospinning of chitosan-based solutions for tissue engineering and regenerative medicine. *Int. J. Mol. Sci.* **2018**, *19*, 407.
2. Liu, W.; Thomopoulos, S.; Xia, Y. Electrospun nanofibers for regenerative medicine. *Adv. Healthc. Mater.* **2012**, *1*, 10–25. [PubMed]
3. Zamani, R.; Aval, S.F.; Pilehvar-Soltanahmadi, Y.; Nejati-Koshki, K.; Zarghami, N. Recent advances in cell electrospining of natural and synthetic nanofibers for regenerative medicine. *Drug Res.* **2018**, *68*, 425–435.
4. Greiner, A.; Wendorff, J.H. Electrospinning: A fascinating method for the preparation of ultrathin fibers. *Angew. Chem. Int. Ed.* **2007**, *46*, 5670–5703.
5. Zafar, M.; Najeeb, S.; Khurshid, Z.; Vazirzadeh, M.; Zohaib, S.; Najeeb, B.; Sefat, F. Potential of electrospun nanofibers for biomedical and dental applications. *Materials* **2016**, *9*, 73. [CrossRef] [PubMed]
6. Flemming, R.G.; Murphy, C.J.; Abrams, G.A.; Goodman, S.L.; Nealey, P.F. Effects of synthetic micro- and nano-structured surfaces on cell behavior. *Biomaterials* **1999**, *20*, 573–588. [PubMed]
7. Von Recum, A.F.; Shannon, C.E.; Cannon, C.E.; Long, K.J.; van Kooten, T.G.; Meyle, J. Surface roughness, porosity, and texture as modifiers of cellular adhesion. *Tissue Eng.* **1996**, *2*, 241–253.
8. Green, A.M.; Jansen, J.A.; van der Waerden, J.P.C.M.; Von Recum, A.F. Fibroblast response to microtextured silicone surfaces: Texture orientation into or out of the surface. *J. Biomed. Mater. Res. Part A* **1994**, *28*, 647–653.
9. Mitragotri, S.; Anderson, D.G.; Chen, X.; Chow, E.K.; Ho, D.; Kabanov, A.V.; Karp, J.M.; Kataoka, K.; Mirkin, C.A.; Petrosko, S.H.; et al. Accelerating the translation of nanomaterials in biomedicine. *ACS Nano* **2015**, *9*, 6644–6654.

10. Jiang, L.; Jiang, Y.; Stiadle, J.; Wang, X.; Wang, L.; Li, Q.; Shen, C.; Thibeault, S.L.; Turng, L.-S. Electrospun nanofibrous thermoplastic polyurethane/poly(glycerol sebacate) hybrid scaffolds for vocal fold tissue engineering applications. *Mater. Sci. Eng. C* **2019**, *94*, 740–749. [CrossRef] [PubMed]

11. Campiglio, C.; Marcolin, C.; Draghi, L. Electrospun ECM macromolecules as biomimetic scaffold for regenerative medicine: Challenges for preserving conformation and bioactivity. *AIMS J.* **2017**, *4*, 638–669. [CrossRef]

12. Bölgen, N.; Vargel, I.; Korkusuz, P.; Menceloğlu, Y.Z.; Pişkin, E. In vivo performance of antibiotic embedded electrospun PCL membranes for prevention of abdominal adhesions. *J. Biomed. Mater. Res. Part B Appl. Biomater.* **2010**, *81B*, 530–543.

13. Huang, Z.M.; Yang, C.L.H. Encapsulating drugs in biodegradable ultrafine fibers through co-axial electrospinning. *J. Biomed. Mater. Res. Part A* **2010**, *77A*, 169–179. [CrossRef] [PubMed]

14. Kim, K.; Luu, Y.K.; Chang, C.; Fang, D.; Hsiao, B.S.; Chu, B.; Hadjiargyrou, M. Incorporation and controlled release of a hydrophilic antibiotic using poly(lactide-*co*-glycolide)-based electrospun nanofibrous scaffolds. *J. Control. Release* **2004**, *98*, 47–56. [PubMed]

15. Nie, H.; Wang, C.H. Fabrication and characterization of PLGA/HAp composite scaffolds for delivery of BMP-2 plasmid DNA. *J. Control. Release* **2007**, *120*, 111–121. [CrossRef] [PubMed]

16. Chew, S.Y.; Jie, W.; Yim, E.K.F.; Leong, K.W. Sustained release of proteins from electrospun biodegradable fibers. *Biomacromolecules* **2005**, *6*, 2017–2024. [CrossRef]

17. Sadeghi, A.; Moztarzadeh, F.; Aghazadeh Mohandesi, J. Investigating the effect of chitosan on hydrophilicity and bioactivity of conductive electrospun composite scaffold for neural tissue engineering. *Int. J. Biol. Macromol.* **2019**, *121*, 625–632. [CrossRef]

18. Venugopal, E.; Rajeswaran, N.; Sahanand, K.S.; Bhattacharyya, A.; Rajendran, S. In vitro evaluation of phytochemical loaded electrospun gelatin nanofibers for application in bone and cartilage tissue engineering. *Biomed. Mater.* **2018**, *14*, 015004. [CrossRef]

19. Ding, Y.; Li, W.; Zhang, F.; Liu, Z.; Zanjanizadeh Ezazi, N.; Liu, D.; Santos, H.A. Electrospun fibrous architectures for drug delivery, tissue engineering and cancer therapy. *Adv. Funct. Mater.* **2019**, *29*, 1802852.

20. Sill, T.J.; Von Recum, H.A. Electrospinning: Applications in drug delivery and tissue engineering. *Biomaterials* **2008**, *29*, 1989–2006. [CrossRef]

21. Kenawy, E.R.; Bowlin, G.L.; Mansfield, K.; Layman, J.; Simpson, D.G.; Sanders, E.H.; Wnek, G.E. Release of tetracycline hydrochloride from electrospun poly(ethylene-*co*-vinylacetate), poly(lactic acid), and a blend. *J. Control. Release* **2002**, *81*, 57–64. [CrossRef]

22. Park, K.; Ju, Y.M.; Son, J.S.; Ahn, K.D.; Dong, K.H. Surface modification of biodegradable electrospun nanofiber scaffolds and their interaction with fibroblasts. *J. Biomater. Sci. Polym. Ed.* **2007**, *18*, 369–382. [CrossRef]

23. Ye, K.; Liu, D.; Kuang, H.; Cai, J.; Chen, W.; Sun, B.; Xia, L.; Fang, B.; Morsi, Y.; Mo, X. Three-dimensional electrospun nanofibrous scaffolds displaying bone morphogenetic protein-2-derived peptides for the promotion of osteogenic differentiation of stem cells and bone regeneration. *J. Colloid Interface Sci.* **2019**, *534*, 625–636. [CrossRef]

24. Chen, R.; Wang, J.; Liu, C. Biomaterials act as enhancers of growth factors in bone regeneration. *Adv. Funct. Mater.* **2016**, *26*, 8810–8823. [CrossRef]

25. Zhao, P.; Jiang, H.H.; Zhu, K.; Chen, W. Biodegradable fibrous scaffolds composed of gelatin coated poly(epsilon-caprolactone) prepared by coaxial electrospinning. *J. Biomed. Mater. Res. A* **2010**, *83A*, 372–382. [CrossRef] [PubMed]

26. Zhang, Y.Z.; Wang, X.; Feng, Y.; Li, J.; Lim, C.T.; Ramakrishna, S. Coaxial electrospinning of (fluorescein isothiocyanate-conjugated bovine serum albumin)-encapsulated poly(epsilon-caprolactone) nanofibers for sustained release. *Biomacromolecules* **2006**, *7*, 1049–1057. [CrossRef]

27. Yan, L.I. A facile technique to prepare biodegradable coaxial electrospun nanofibers for controlled release of bioactive agents. *J. Control. Release* **2005**, *108*, 237–243.

28. Su, Y.; Li, X.; Wang, H.; He, C.; Mo, X. Fabrication and characterization of biodegradable nanofibrous mats by mix and coaxial electrospinning. *J. Mater. Sci. Mater. Med.* **2009**, *20*, 2285–2294. [CrossRef]

29. Prado-Prone, G.; Silva-Bermudez, P.; Almaguer-Flores, A.; García-Macedo, J.A.; García, V.I.; Rodil, S.E.; Ibarra, C.; Velasquillo, C. Enhanced antibacterial nanocomposite mats by coaxial electrospinning of polycaprolactone fibers loaded with Zn-based nanoparticles. *Nanomed. Nanotechnol. Biol. Med.* **2018**, *14*, 1695–1706. [CrossRef]

30. He, P.; Zhong, Q.; Ge, Y.; Guo, Z.; Tian, J.; Zhou, Y.; Ding, S.; Li, H.; Zhou, C. Dual drug loaded coaxial electrospun PLGA/PVP fiber for guided tissue regeneration under control of infection. *Mater. Sci. Eng. C* **2018**, *90*, 549–556. [CrossRef]

31. Yan, S.; Li, X.; Liu, S.; Mo, X.; Ramakrishna, S. Controlled release of dual drugs from emulsion electrospun nanofibrous mats. *Colloids Surf. B Biointerfaces* **2009**, *73*, 376–381. [CrossRef] [PubMed]

32. Chen, S.; Li, R.; Li, X.; Xie, J. Electrospinning: An enabling nanotechnology platform for drug delivery and regenerative medicine. *Adv. Drug Deliv. Rev.* **2018**, *132*, 188–213. [CrossRef] [PubMed]

33. Chandra, A.; Suliman, A.; Angle, N. Spontaneous dissection of the carotid and vertebral arteries: The 10-year UCSD experience. *Ann. Vasc. Surg.* **2007**, *21*, 178–185. [CrossRef]

34. Schoder, M.; Cartes-Zumelzu, F.; Grabenwöger, M.; Cejna, M.; Funovics, M.; Krenn, C.G.; Hutschala, D.; Wolf, F.; Thurnher, S.; et al. Elective endovascular stent-graft repair of atherosclerotic thoracic aortic aneurysms: Clinical results and midterm follow-up. *AJR Am. J. Roentgenol.* **2003**, *180*, 709–715. [CrossRef] [PubMed]

35. Grabenwöger, M.; Hutschala, D.; Cartes-Zumelzu, F.; Ehrlich, M.; Grimm, M.; Thurnher, S.; Lammer, J.; Wolner, E.; Havel, M. Behandlung von thorakalen Aortenaneurysmen mit selbstexpandierenden endoluminalen Gefäßprothesen. *Acta Chir. Austriaca* **1999**, *31*, 319–322. [CrossRef]

36. Golshani, K.; Ferrel, A.; Lessne, M.; Shah, P.; Chowdhary, A.; Choulakian, A.; Alexander, M.J.; Smith, T.P.; Enterline, D.S.; Zomorodi, A.R. Stent-assisted coil emboilization of ruptured intracranial aneurysms: A retrospective multicenter review. *Surg. Neurol. Int.* **2012**, *3*, 84.

37. Wu, C.; An, Q.; Li, D.; Jing, W.; He, L.; Chen, H.; Yu, L.; Wei, Z.; Mo, X. A novel heparin loaded poly(L-lactide-*co*-caprolactone) covered stent for aneurysm therapy. *Mater. Lett.* **2014**, *116*, 39–42. [CrossRef]

38. Wang, J.; An, Q.; Li, D.; Wu, T.; Chen, W.; Sun, B.; El-Hamshary, H.; Al-Deyab, S.S.; Zhu, W.; Mo, X. Heparin and vascular endothelial growth factor loaded poly(L-lactide-*co*-caprolactone) nanofiber covered stent-graft for aneurysm treatment. *J. Biomed. Nanotechnol.* **2015**, *11*, 1947–1960. [CrossRef]

39. Feng, W.; Liu, P.; Yin, H.; Gu, Z.; Wu, Y.; Zhu, W.; Liu, Y.; Zheng, H.; Mo, X. Heparin and rosuvastatin calcium loaded ploy(L-lactide-*co*-caprolactone) nanofiber covered stent-graft for aneurysm treatment. *New J. Chem.* **2017**, *41*, 9014–9023. [CrossRef]

40. Raimondo, S.; Fornaro, M.; Tos, P.; Battiston, B.; Giacobini-Robecchi, M.G.; Geuna, S. Perspectives in regeneration and tissue engineering of peripheral nerves. *Ann. Anat.* **2011**, *193*, 334–340.

41. Evans, G.R.D.; Brandt, K.; Widmer, M.S.; Lu, L.; Meszlenyi, R.K.; Gupta, P.K.; Mikos, A.G.; Hodges, J.; Williams, J.; Gürlek, A. In vivo evaluation of poly(L-lactic acid) porous conduits for peripheral nerve regeneration. *Biomaterials* **1999**, *20*, 1109–1115.

42. Hsu, C.-C.; Serio, A.; Amdursky, N.; Besnard, C.; Stevens, M.M. Fabrication of hemin-doped serum albumin-based fibrous scaffolds for neural tissue engineering applications. *ACS Appl. Mater. Interfaces* **2018**, *10*, 5305–5317. [CrossRef] [PubMed]

43. Shao, Z. Application of self-assembling peptide nanofiber scaffold in nerve tissue engineering. *Chin. J. Repar. Reconstr. Surg.* **2009**, *23*, 861–863.

44. Chun-Yang, W.; Jun-Jian, L.; Cun-Yi, F.; Xiu-Mei, M.; Hong-Jiang, R.; Feng-Feng, L. The effect of aligned core-shell nanofibres delivering NGF on the promotion of sciatic nerve regeneration. *J. Biomater. Sci. Polym. Ed.* **2012**, *23*, 167–184.

45. Zhang, K.; Wang, C.; Fan, C.; Mo, X. Aligned SF/P(LLA-CL)-blended nanofibers encapsulating nerve growth factor for peripheral nerve regeneration. *J. Biomed. Mater. Res. Part A* **2014**, *102*, 2680–2691.

46. Su, Y.; Li, X.; Tian, L.; Chen, H.; Xiumei, M. Poly(L-lactide-*co*-ε-caprolactone) electrospun nanofibers for encapsulating and sustained releasing proteins. *Polymer* **2009**, *50*, 4212–4219.

47. Sun, B.; Wu, T.; He, L.; Zhang, J.; Yuan, Y.; Huang, X.; El-Hamshary, H.; Al-Deyab, S.S.; Xu, T.; Mo, X. Development of dual neurotrophins-encapsulated electrosupun nanofibrous scaffolds for peripheral nerve regeneration. *J. Biomed. Nanotechnol.* **2016**, *12*, 1987–2000. [PubMed]

48. Bhutto, M.A.; Wu, T.; Sun, B.; Ei-Hamshary, H.; Al-Deyab, S.S.; Mo, X. Fabrication and characterization of vitamin B5 loaded poly (L-lactide-*co*-caprolactone)/silk fiber aligned electrospun nanofibers for Schwann cell proliferation. *Colloids Surf. B Biointerfaces* **2016**, *144*, 108–117.

49. Tong, W.; Li, D.; Wang, Y.; Sun, B.; Li, D.; Morsi, Y.; Hamshary, H.A.E.; Al-Deyab, S.S.; Mo, X.M. Laminin-coated nerve guidance conduits based on poly(L-lactide-*co*-glycolide) fibers and yarns for promoting Schwann cells proliferation and migration. *J. Mater. Chem. B* **2017**, *5*, 3186–3194.

50. Junka, R.; Valmikinathan, C.M.; Kalyon, D.M.; Yu, X. Laminin functionalized biomimetic nanofibers for nerve tissue engineering. *J. Biomater. Tissue Eng.* **2013**, *3*, 494–502.

51. Liu, C.; Wang, C.; Zhao, Q.; Li, X.; Xu, F.; Yao, X.; Wang, M. Incorporation and release of dual growth factors for nerve tissue engineering using nanofibrous bicomponent scaffolds. *Biomed. Mater.* **2013**, *13*, 044107. [CrossRef] [PubMed]

52. Canver, C.C. Conduit options in coronary artery bypass surgery. *Chest* **1995**, *108*, 1150–1155. [CrossRef] [PubMed]

53. Chlupác, J.; Filová, E.; Bacáková, L. Vascular prostheses: 50 years of advancement from synthetic towards tissue engineering and cell therapy. *Rozhledy* **2010**, *89*, 85–94.

54. Huang, C.; Wang, S.; Qiu, L.; Ke, Q.; Zhai, W.; Mo, X. Heparin loading and pre-endothelialization in enhancing the patency rate of electrospun small-diameter vascular grafts in a canine model. *ACS Appl. Mater. Interfaces* **2013**, *5*, 2220–2226. [CrossRef] [PubMed]

55. Chen, X.; Wang, J.; An, Q.; Li, D.; Liu, P.; Zhu, W.; Mo, X. Electrospun poly(L-lactic acid-*co*-ε-caprolactone) fibers loaded with heparin and vascular endothelial growth factor to improve blood compatibility and endothelial progenitor cell proliferation. *Colloids Surf. B Biointerfaces* **2015**, *128*, 106–114. [CrossRef] [PubMed]

56. Yin, A.; Bowlin, G.L.; Luo, R.; Zhang, X.; Wang, Y.; Mo, X. Electrospun silk fibroin/poly(L-lactide-ε-caplacton) graft with platelet-rich growth factor for inducing smooth muscle cell growth and infiltration. *Regen. Biomater.* **2016**, *3*, 239–245.

57. Kuang, H.; Wang, Y.; Hu, J.; Wang, C.; Lu, S.; Mo, X. A method for preparation of an internal layer of artificial vascular graft co-modified with Salvianolic acid B and heparin. *ACS Appl. Mater. Interfaces* **2018**, *10*, 19365–19372.

58. Guex, A.G.; Hegemann, D.; Giraud, M.N.; Tevaearai, H.T.; Popa, A.M.; Rossi, R.M.; Fortunato, G. Covalent immobilisation of VEGF on plasma-coated electrospun scaffolds for tissue engineering applications. *Colloids Surf. B Biointerfaces* **2014**, *123*, 724–733.

59. Gurtner, G.C.; Sabine, W.; Yann, B.; Longaker, M.T. Wound repair and regeneration. *Nature* **2008**, *453*, 314–321.

60. Zahedi, P.; Rezaeian, I.; Ranaei-Siadat, S.O.; Jafari, S.H.; Supaphol, P. A review on wound dressings with an emphasis on electrospun nanofibrous polymeric bandages. *Polym. Adv. Technol.* **2010**, *21*, 77–95. [CrossRef]

61. Zeng-Xiao, C.; Xiu-Mei, M.; Kui-Hua, Z.; Lin-Peng, F.; An-Lin, Y.; Chuang-Long, H.; Hong-Sheng, W. Fabrication of chitosan/silk fibroin composite nanofibers for wound-dressing applications. *Int. J. Mol. Sci.* **2010**, *11*, 3529–3539.

62. Alhusein, N.; Blagbrough, I.S.; De Bank, P.A. Electrospun matrices for localised controlled drug delivery: Release of tetracycline hydrochloride from layers of polycaprolactone and poly(ethylene-*co*-vinyl acetate). *Drug Deliv. Transl. Res.* **2012**, *2*, 477–488. [CrossRef]

63. Alhusein, N.; Blagbrough, I.S.; Beeton, M.L.; Bolhuis, A.; De Bank, P.A. Electrospun zein/PCL fibrous matrices release tetracycline in a controlled manner, killing *Staphylococcus aureus* both in biofilms and ex vivo on pig skin, and are compatible with human skin cells. *Pharm. Res.* **2016**, *33*, 237–246. [CrossRef] [PubMed]

64. Alhusein, N.; Blagbrough, I.S.; De Bank, P.A. Zein/polycaprolactone electrospun matrices for localised controlled delivery of tetracycline. *Drug Deliv. Transl. Res.* **2013**, *3*, 542–550. [CrossRef] [PubMed]

65. Ghosal, K.; Agatemor, C.; Thomas, S.; Kny, E. Electrospinning tissue engineering and wound dressing scaffolds from polymer–titanium dioxide nanocomposites. *Chem. Eng. J.* **2019**, *358*, 1262–1278. [CrossRef]

66. Li, J.; Zhai, D.; Lv, F.; Yu, Q.; Ma, H.; Yin, J.; Yi, Z.; Liu, M.; Chang, J.; Wu, C. Preparation of copper-containing bioactive glass/eggshell membrane nanocomposites for improving angiogenesis, antibacterial activity and wound healing. *Acta Biomater.* **2016**, *36*, 254–266. [CrossRef] [PubMed]

67. Eming, S.A.; Martin, P.; Tomic-Canic, M. Wound repair and regeneration: Mechanisms, signaling, and translation. *Sci. Transl. Med.* **2014**, *6*, 265sr6. [CrossRef]

68. Gaoxing Luo, M.D.; Jin, T.M.; He, W.; Jun Wu, M.D.; Bing, M.M.; Xihua Wang, M.D.; Chen, X.; Yi, S.; Zhang, X.; Li, X. Antibacterial effect of dressings containing multivalent silver ion carried by zirconium phosphate on experimental rat burn wounds. *Wound Repair Regen.* **2010**, *16*, 800–804.

69. Brett, B.; Sampson, E.M.; Schultz, G.S.; Parnell, L.K.S. Wound dressing components degrade proteins detrimental to wound healing. *Int. Wound J.* **2010**, *5*, 543–551.

70. Ignatova, M.; Manolova, N.; Rashkov, I. Electrospinning of poly(vinyl pyrrolidone)–iodine complex and poly(ethylene oxide)/poly(vinyl pyrrolidone)–iodine complex—A prospective route to antimicrobial wound dressing materials. *Eur. Polym. J.* **2007**, *43*, 1609–1623. [CrossRef]

71. Alhusein, N.; De Bank, P.A.; Blagbrough, I.S.; Bolhuis, A. Killing bacteria within biofilms by sustained release of tetracycline from triple-layered electrospun micro/nanofibre matrices of polycaprolactone and poly(ethylene-co-vinyl acetate). *Drug Deliv. Transl. Res.* **2013**, *3*, 531–541. [CrossRef]

72. Román-Doval, R.; Tellez-Cruz, M.M.; Rojas-Chávez, H.; Cruz-Martínez, H.; Carrasco-Torres, G.; Vásquez-Garzón, V.R. Enhancing electrospun scaffolds of PVP with polypyrrole/iodine for tissue engineering of skin regeneration by coating via a plasma process. *J. Mater. Sci.* **2019**, *54*, 3342–3353. [CrossRef]

73. Sheng, X.; Fan, L.; He, C.; Zhang, K.; Mo, X.; Wang, H. Vitamin E-loaded silk fibroin nanofibrous mats fabricated by green process for skin care application. *Int. J. Biol. Macromol.* **2013**, *56*, 49–56. [CrossRef]

74. El-Aassar, M.R.; El Fawal, G.F.; El-Deeb, N.M.; Hassan, H.S.; Mo, X. Electrospun polyvinyl alcohol/ pluronic F127 blended nanofibers containing titanium dioxide for antibacterial wound dressing. *Appl. Biochem. Biotechnol.* **2015**, *178*, 1–15.

75. Lv, F.; Wang, J.; Xu, P.; Han, Y.; Ma, H.; Xu, H.; Chen, S.; Chang, J.; Ke, Q.; Liu, M. A conducive bioceramic/polymer composite biomaterial for diabetic wound healing. *Acta Biomater.* **2017**, *60*, 128–143. [CrossRef] [PubMed]

76. Bagnaninchi, P.O.; Yang, Y.; El Haj, A.J.; Maffulli, N. Tissue engineering for tendon repair. *Br. J. Sports Med.* **2007**, *41*, e10. [CrossRef]

77. Yang, C.; Deng, G.; Chen, W.; Ye, X.; Mo, X. A novel electrospun-aligned nanoyarn-reinforced nanofibrous scaffold for tendon tissue engineering. *Colloids Surf. B Biointerfaces* **2014**, *122*, 270–276. [CrossRef] [PubMed]

78. Cai, J.; Wang, J.; Ye, K.; Li, D.; Ai, C.; Sheng, D.; Jin, W.; Liu, X.; Zhi, Y.; Jiang, J. Dual-layer aligned-random nanofibrous scaffolds for improving gradient microstructure of tendon-to-bone healing in a rabbit extra-articular model. *Int. J. Nanomed.* **2018**, *13*, 3481–3492. [CrossRef] [PubMed]

79. Xu, Y.; Dong, S.; Zhou, Q.; Mo, X.; Song, L.; Hou, T.; Wu, J.; Li, S.; Li, Y.; Li, P. The effect of mechanical stimulation on the maturation of TDSCs-poly(L-lactide-*co*-ε-caprolactone)/collagen scaffold constructs for tendon tissue engineering. *Biomaterials* **2014**, *35*, 2760–2772. [CrossRef] [PubMed]

80. Sahoo, S.; Ang, L.T.; Goh, J.C.H.; Toh, S.-L. Growth factor delivery through electrospun nanofibers in scaffolds for tissue engineering applications. *J. Biomed. Mater. Res. A* **2010**, *93A*, 1539–1550.

81. Ye, Y.J.; Zhou, Y.Q.; Jing, Z.Y.; Liu, Y.Y.; Yin, D.C. Electrospun heparin-loaded core-shell nanofiber sutures for achilles tendon regeneration in vivo. *Macromol. Biosci.* **2018**, *18*, 1800041. [CrossRef] [PubMed]

82. Xu, Y.; Wu, J.; Wang, H.; Li, H.; Di, N.; Song, L.; Li, S.; Li, D.; Xiang, Y.; Liu, W. Fabrication of electrospun poly(L-lactide-*co*-ε-caprolactone)/collagen nanoyarn network as a novel, three-dimensional, macroporous, aligned scaffold for tendon tissue engineering. *Tissue Eng. Part C Methods* **2013**, *19*, 925–936. [CrossRef] [PubMed]

83. Riggin, C.N.; Qu, F.; Dong, H.K.; Huegel, J.; Steinberg, D.R.; Kuntz, A.F.; Soslowsky, L.J.; Mauck, R.L.; Bernstein, J. Electrospun PLGA nanofiber scaffolds release ibuprofen faster and degrade slower after in vivo implantation. *Ann. Biomed. Eng.* **2017**, *45*, 2348–2359. [CrossRef]

84. Tellado, S.F.; Balmayor, E.R.; Griensven, M.V. Strategies to engineer tendon/ligament-to-bone interface: Biomaterials, cells and growth factors. *Adv. Drug Deliv. Rev.* **2015**, *94*, 126–140. [CrossRef] [PubMed]

85. Sahoo, S.; Toh, S.L.; Goh, J.C.H. A bFGF-releasing silk/PLGA-based biohybrid scaffold for ligament/tendon tissue engineering using mesenchymal progenitor cells. *Biomaterials* **2010**, *31*, 2990–2998. [CrossRef]

86. Manning, C.N.; Schwartz, A.G.; Liu, W.; Xie, J.; Havlioglu, N.; Sakiyamaelbert, S.E.; Silva, M.J.; Xia, Y.; Gelberman, R.H.; Thomopoulos, S. Controlled delivery of mesenchymal stem cells and growth factors using a nanofiber scaffold for tendon repair. *Acta Biomater.* **2013**, *9*, 6905–6914. [CrossRef]

87. Ren, J.; Blackwood, K.; Doustgani, A.; Poh, P.; Steck, R.M.; Stevens, M.; Woodruff, M. Melt-electrospun polycaprolactone strontium-substituted bioactive glass scaffolds for bone regeneration. *J. Biomed. Mater. Res. A* **2014**, *102*, 3140–3153. [CrossRef]

88. Yao, Q.; Cosme, J.G.; Xu, T.; Miszuk, J.M.; Picciani, P.H.; Fong, H.; Sun, H. Three dimensional electrospun PCL/PLA blend nanofibrous scaffolds with significantly improved stem cells osteogenic differentiation and cranial bone formation. *Biomaterials* **2016**, *115*, 115–127. [CrossRef] [PubMed]

89. Poologasundarampillai, G.; Wang, D.; Li, S.; Nakamura, J.; Bradley, R.; Lee, P.D.; Stevens, M.M.; McPhail, D.S.; Kasuga, T.; Jones, J.R. Cotton-wool-like bioactive glasses for bone regeneration. *Acta Biomater.* **2014**, *10*, 3733–3746. [CrossRef]

90. Xu, T.; Miszuk, J.M.; Zhao, Y.; Sun, H.; Fong, H. Electrospun polycaprolactone 3D nanofibrous scaffold with interconnected and hierarchically structured pores for bone tissue engineering. *Adv. Healthc. Mater.* **2015**, *4*, 2238–2246. [CrossRef] [PubMed]

91. Chen, W.; Chen, S.; Morsi, Y.; Elhamshary, H.; El-newehy, M.; Fan, C.; Mo, X. Superabsorbent 3D scaffold based on electrospun nanofibers for cartilage tissue engineering. *ACS Appl. Mater. Interfaces* **2016**, *8*, 24415–24425. [CrossRef]

92. Si, Y.; Yu, J.; Tang, X.; Ge, J.; Ding, B. Ultralight nanofibre-assembled cellular aerogels with superelasticity and multifunctionality. *Nat. Commun.* **2014**, *5*, 5802. [CrossRef]

93. Rose, F.R.; Hou, Q.; Oreffo, R.O. Delivery systems for bone growth factors—The new players in skeletal regeneration. *J. Pharm. Pharmacol.* **2004**, *56*, 415–427. [CrossRef]

94. Lieberman, J.R.; Daluiski, A.; Einhorn, T.A. The role of growth factors in the repair of bone. Biology and clinical applications. *JBJS* **2002**, *84-A*, 1032–1044. [CrossRef]

95. Su, Y.; Su, Q.; Liu, W.; Lim, M.; Venugopal, J.R.; Mo, X.; Ramakrishna, S.; Al-Deyab, S.S.; El-Newehy, M. Controlled release of bone morphogenetic protein 2 and dexamethasone loaded in core–shell PLLACL–collagen fibers for use in bone tissue engineering. *Acta Biomater.* **2012**, *8*, 763–771. [CrossRef]

96. Shimer, A.L.; Öner, F.C.; Vaccaro, A.R. Spinal reconstruction and bone morphogenetic proteins: Open questions. *Injury* **2009**, *40*, S32–S38. [CrossRef]

97. Lin, Z.Y.; Duan, Z.X.; Guo, X.D.; Li, J.F.; Lu, H.W.; Zheng, Q.X.; Quan, D.P.; Yang, S.H. Bone induction by biomimetic PLGA-(PEG-ASP)$_n$ copolymer loaded with a novel synthetic BMP-2-related peptide in vitro and in vivo. *J. Control. Release* **2010**, *144*, 190–195. [CrossRef] [PubMed]

98. Suzuki, Y.; Tanihara, M.; Suzuki, K.; Saitou, A.; Sufan, W.; Nishimura, Y. Alginate hydrogel linked with synthetic oligopeptide derived from BMP-2 allows ectopic osteoinduction in vivo. *J. Biomed. Mater. Res. Part B Appl. Biomater.* **2015**, *50*, 405–409. [CrossRef]

99. Weng, L.; Boda, S.K.; Wang, H.; Teusink, M.J.; Shuler, F.D.; Xie, J. Novel 3D hybrid nanofiber aerogels coupled with BMP-2 peptides for cranial bone regeneration. *Adv. Healthc. Mater.* **2018**, *7*, 1701415. [CrossRef]

100. Zhou, X.; Feng, W.; Qiu, K.; Chen, L.; Wang, W.; Nie, W.; Mo, X.; He, C. BMP-2 derived peptide and dexamethasone incorporated mesoporous silica nanoparticles for enhanced osteogenic differentiation of bone mesenchymal stem cells. *ACS Appl. Mater. Interfaces* **2015**, *7*, 15777–15789. [CrossRef] [PubMed]

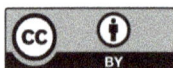

pharmaceutics

MDPI

Article

The Effect of Molecular Properties on Active Ingredient Release from Electrospun Eudragit Fibers

Kieran Burgess, Heyu Li, Yasmin Abo-zeid, Fatimah and Gareth R. Williams *

UCL School of Pharmacy, University College London, 29-39 Brunswick Square, London WC1N 1AX, UK;
kieran.burgess.16@ucl.ac.uk (K.B.); heyu.li@ucl.ac.uk (H.L.); y.abozeid@ucl.ac.uk (Y.A.-z.);
fatimah.14@ucl.ac.uk (F.)
* Correspondence: g.williams@ucl.ac.uk; Tel.: +44-207-753-5868

Received: 16 March 2018; Accepted: 16 May 2018; Published: 24 July 2018

Abstract: The formation of nanoscale fibers from pH-sensitive polymers is a route which has been widely explored for targeted drug delivery. In particular, the Eudragit L100 and S100 families of polymers have received significant attention for this purpose. However, while in some cases it is shown that making drug-loaded Eudragit polymers effectively prevents drug release in low-pH media where the polymer is insoluble, this is not always the case, and other studies have reported significant amounts of drug release at acidic pHs. In this study, we sought to gain insight into the factors influencing the release of active ingredients from Eudragit S100 (ES100) fibers. A family of materials was prepared loaded with the model active ingredients (AIs) benzoic acid, 1-naphthoic acid, 1-naphthylamine, and 9-anthracene carboxylic acid. Analogous systems were prepared with an AI-loaded core and an ES100 sheath. The resultant fibers were smooth and cylindrical in the majority of cases, and X-ray diffraction and differential scanning calorimetry showed them to comprise amorphous solid dispersions. When AI release from the monolithic fibers was probed, it was found that there was significant release at pH 1 in all cases except with 9-anthracene carboxylic acid. Analysis of the results indicated that both the molecular weight of the AI and its acidity/basicity are important in controlling release, with lower molecular weight AIs and basic species released more quickly. The same release trends are seen with the core/shell fibers, but AI release at pH 1 is attenuated. The most significant change between the monolithic and core/shell systems was observed in the case of 1-naphthylamine. Mathematical equations were devised to connect molecular properties and AI release under acidic conditions.

Keywords: electrospinning; Eudragit; nanofibers; drug release

1. Introduction

Electrospinning is a technique which has attracted great attention in the pharmaceutical technology field [1,2]. It most commonly involves the preparation of a polymer solution in a volatile solvent. This is loaded into a syringe and is slowly ejected through a narrow bore needle (the spinneret). A high voltage power supply is used to charge the needle, and the solution expelled towards a grounded collector plate. The application of the electrical energy causes drawing of the polymer solution into a fine jet, and ultimately results in the production of fibers with diameters typically on the nanoscale. The inclusion of a drug molecule in the solution generally yields drug-loaded fibers in the form of amorphous solid dispersions. In the simplest embodiment of the experiment, a single liquid is processed, but more advanced derivatives including coaxial electrospinning (which uses two needles nested concentrically one inside the other to process two liquids) and triaxial spinning (three needles, three solutions) have also been reported. The use of coaxial spinnerets results in core/shell structures, and triaxial spinnerets give three-compartment architectures.

Electrospun nanofibers have been explored for a wide range of drug delivery applications, including preparing fast-dissolving oral drug delivery systems designed for very rapid release in the mouth [3,4], extended release systems allowing the drug cargo to be freed over a number of hours or weeks [5–8], and systems able to respond to external stimuli such as temperature [9–12]. Given that the pH of the human gastrointestinal tract varies from 1–3 in the stomach, 6–8 in the small intestine, and 4–7 in the large intestine, materials able to respond to changes in pH are particularly useful for oral delivery systems. A range of polymers exist which are selectively soluble above or below a particular pH. One clinically used family of such polymers is the Eudragits, methacrylate-based polymers with tunable pH sensitivity. Eudragit L100-55 is soluble above pH 5.5, L100 above pH 6, and S100 above pH 7. This allows different sections of the intestinal tract to be targeted depending on the polymer chosen to fabricate a formulation. A number of authors have explored the electrospinning of Eudragits, as well as other pH-sensitive polymers such as shellac [13,14].

The studies in the literature exploring Eudragit have investigated both monolithic fibers from monoaxial electrospinning and core/shell materials. Shen et al. were the first to electrospin Eudragit, preparing L100-55 fibers loaded with diclofenac sodium [15]. They found that drug release at pH 1.0 was below 3%, confirming that pH-sensitive fibers can be produced. Other studies have built on this and reported similar conclusions, for instance with Eudragit fibers containing mebeverine HCl [16], ketoprofen [17], indomethacin [18] and helicid [19]. However, it is not always the case that simply making a drug-loaded Eudragit fiber formulation prevents drug release in the acidic pHs typical of the stomach. For instance, Karthikeyan et al. reported blend fibers of zein and Eudragit S100 (ES100) loaded with pantoprazole and aceclofenac gave 25% release of the latter after 2 h immersion in 0.1 M HCl [20]. The same has been shown to be true for spironolactone-loaded Eudragit FS fibers (up to 30% release at pH 1.2) [21], and 5-fluorouracil (5-FU)-loaded ES100 fibers, which showed some 80% release at pH 1 [22].

Analogous findings have been found when preparing core/shell systems. Whilst in some instances it is reported that drug release at pH 1–3 can be virtually completely obviated in fibers with a Eudragit shell and drug-loaded core (for instance containing a Gd-based contrast agent or indomethacin [23,24]), similar fibers containing 5-FU in the core release up to 70% of their drug loading under these conditions [22]. The reasons behind the different findings reported in the literature are not completely clear, but it seems that both the molecular weight and acidity or basicity of the drug incorporated are important. Most recently, Jia et al. prepared fibers with an ES100 shell and a poly(ethylene oxide) core containing either mebeverine HCl or indomethacin (model basic and acidic drugs with similar molecular weights (MWs)) [25]. It was observed that release of both the basic mebeverine and acidic indomethacin at pH 1.2 was restrained by the presence of the ES100 shell, but that there was a noticeably greater extent of release in the former case (up to 20%) than the latter (ca. 1%).

In this work, we sought to obtain a fundamental understanding of the factors underlying drug release from Eudragit fibers at acidic pHs. To do this, we assembled a training set of four model active ingredients (AIs; Figure 1). While none has any direct applications in drug delivery, the incremental variation in their structures is ideal for a fundamental study of this type. Benzoic acid (BA), 1-naphthoic acid (NA) and 9-anthracene carboxylic acid (ACA) all contain one carboxylic acid functional group and have similar pK$_a$s (BA: 4.20; NA: 3.67; ACA: 3.68), but the number of aromatic rings in the series increases from one to three. 1-Naphthylamine (NAm) has an identical structure to NA except that the carboxylic acid is replaced by an amine group; the pK$_a$ of NAm conjugate acid is very similar to that of NA at 3.92, and thus the influence of acidity/basicity can be elucidated through this molecule pair.

A series of ES100-based fibers was prepared containing the training set AIs, using both monoaxial electrospinning to generate monolithic composites and also coaxial spinning to produce core/shell systems with the AI confined to the core. The fibers were subject to a detailed examination of their physicochemical properties, and AI release explored at pH 1.0 and 6.8 following pharmacopoeia protocols. Correlations between molecular properties and the release profiles were sought.

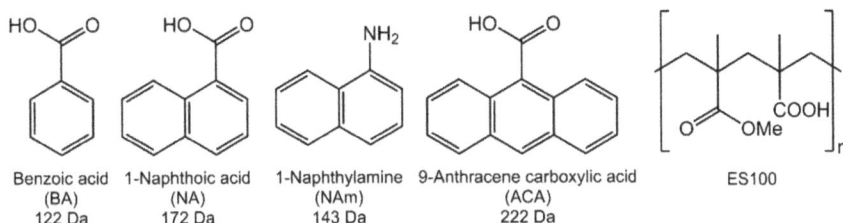

Figure 1. The chemical structures of the active ingredients used in this work and their molecular weights, together with the structure of the polymer ES100. BA: Benzoic acid; NA: 1-naphthoic acid; NAm: 1-Naphthylamine; ACA: 9-anthracene carboxylic acid; ES100: Eudragit S100.

2. Materials and Methods

2.1. Materials

Benzoic acid (BA), 1-naphthoic acid (NA), 1-naphthylamine (NAm), 9-anthracene carboxylic acid (ACA), absolute ethanol and dimethylacetamide (DMAc) were purchased from Sigma-Aldrich (Gillingham, UK). Eudragit S100 (ES100) was a kind gift from Evonik GmbH (Darmstadt, Germany). Analytical grade hydrochloric acid and trisodium phosphate dodecahydrate were obtained from Fisher Scientific (Loughborough, UK). All water was deionised before use.

2.2. Methods

2.2.1. Monoaxial Electrospinning

Following a series of optimisation experiments, a solvent mixture of ethanol/water/DMAc (15/1/4 *v/v/v*) was selected as the most appropriate for electrospinning. A series of solutions was then prepared for monoaxial electrospinning (see Table 1). 1.2 g of ES100 and 0.1 g of the AI of interest were dissolved in 10 mL of the ethanol/water/DMAc solvent system. These were magnetically stirred for a minimum of 24 h to ensure a homogenous solution was formed.

Table 1. Details of the electrospun formulations prepared in this work.

ID	Active Ingredient (AI)	Theoretical Fiber AI Loading (% *w/w*) [a]	Observed Fiber AI Loading (% *w/w*) [b]	Entrapment Efficiency (%) [c]	Fiber Diameter (nm)
Monoaxial electrospinning					
S-BA	Benzoic acid	7.69	9.04 ± 0.13	118 ± 2	483 ± 145
S-NA	1-Naphthoic acid	7.69	7.05 ± 1.02	92 ± 13	129 ± 102
S-NAM	1-Naphthylamine	7.69	6.69 ± 0.27	91 ± 4	214 ± 105
S-ACA	9-Anthracene carboxylic acid	7.69	6.54 ± 0.38	85 + 5	585 ± 158
Coaxial electrospinning					
C-BA	Benzoic acid	2.70	3.42 ± 0.27	127 ± 10	591 ± 189
C-NA	1-Naphthoic acid	2.70	2.38 ± 0.07	88 ± 2	664 ± 171
C-NAM	1-Naphthylamine	2.70	2.20 ± 0.37	81 ± 14	547 ± 124
C-ACA	9-Anthracene carboxylic acid	2.70	2.45 ± 0.16	91 ± 6	621 ± 140

[a] Calculated based on the relative masses of the polymer and drug in the system. [b] Determined experimentally through dissolution of the fibers (mean ± S.D.; $n = 3$). [c] Calculated as the percentage of the theoretical loading observed to be incorporated (mean ± S.D.; $n = 3$).

The solutions were loaded into a 5 mL Terumo syringe, with great care taken to avoid the formation of bubbles. The syringe was then fitted with a blunt-tipped metal needle (internal diameter 0.61 mm; Nordson EFD, Aylesbury, UK), and the positive electrode of a high-voltage power supply (HCP 35–35000, FuG Elektronik, Schechen, Germany) connected to the tip of the needle via a crocodile clip. The grounded collector comprised a flat piece of steel coated with aluminium foil. Liquid was dispensed using a syringe pump (KDS100, Cole Parmer, London, UK). Electrospinning was performed at ambient conditions (25 $\pm$ 3 °C; relative humidity 38 $\pm$ 6%), and processing parameters were as follows: voltage 16 kV; flow rate 0.5 mL h^{-1}; collection distance 18 cm. After fabrication, the fiber products were stored in a desiccator over silica beads.

2.2.2. Coaxial Electrospinning

A 12% *w/v* Eudragit S100 solution in ethanol/water/DMAc (15/1/4 *v/v/v*) was used as the shell liquid for coaxial electrospinning. The core solutions were the same as those used for monoaxial electrospinning (see Table 1). The applied voltage for coaxial spinning was 21 kV, the collection distance 18 cm, and experiments were performed under ambient conditions (25 $\pm$ 3 °C; relative humidity 38 $\pm$ 6%). The core and sheath solutions were independently dispensed through a coaxial spinneret (Linari Engineering, Pisa, Italy) using two separate KDS100 syringe pumps. The spinneret had internal/external diameters for the inner needle of 0.51/0.83 mm and for the outer needle at 1.37/1.83 mm. The core and shell flow rates were 0.4 and 0.8 mL/h respectively. After production, the fiber products were stored in a desiccator over silica beads.

2.3. Characterisation

2.3.1. Electron Microscopy

Small samples (ca. 0.5 $\times$ 0.5 cm) were cut from each fiber mat for scanning electron microscopy (SEM). These were sputter coated with gold and then imaged using a Quanta 200F instrument (FEI, Hillsboro, OR, USA). The fiber diameters were quantified at 100 points for each sample, using the ImageJ software (v1.48; National Institutes of Health, Bethesda, MD, USA). The coaxial materials were also studied with transmission electron microscopy (TEM) on a CM 120 Bio-Twin instrument (Philips, Amsterdam, The Netherlands). For this, fibers were directly spun onto carbon-coated TEM grids (TAAB, Aldermaston, UK).

2.3.2. Physical Form Characterisation

X-ray diffraction (XRD) patterns were collected on a MiniFlex 600 diffractometer (Rigaku, Tokyo, Japan) supplied with Cu Kα radiation. Data were collected over the 2θ range 3 to 35° at a rate of 5° min^{-1}. Differential scanning calorimetry (DSC) was performed on a Q2000 instrument (TA Instruments, New Castle, DE, USA). Samples weighing between 4–7 mg were placed into T-zero aluminium pans, sealed, and pinholed. Samples were equilibrated at 0 °C, heated to 100 °C at 10 °C min^{-1}, and then cooled to 0 °C again. A second heating run (to 200 °C in most cases) was finally performed at 10 °C min^{-1}. All DSC experiments were undertaken under a nitrogen purge of 50 mL min^{-1}. IR spectra were obtained with a Spectrum 100 spectrometer (Perkin Elmer, Waltham, MA, USA) over the wavenumber range 650–4000 cm^{-1} and with resolution of 1 cm^{-1}.

2.3.3. Active Ingredient Loading

After the fibers had been left to dry to remove any residual solvent, samples (ca. 10 mg) were cut from each sample and dissolved in a mixture of ethanol/water/DMAc (15/1/4 *v/v/v*). Calibration curves for each active ingredient (AI) were prepared using a 7315 spectrophotometer (Jenway, Stone, UK), and the AI loading determined (*n* = 3).

2.4. Dissolution Studies

Calibration curves were constructed for each AI at pH 1.0 (0.1 M HCl) and 6.8 (phosphate buffered saline; PBS) with the aid of a 7315 spectrophotometer (Jenway, Stone, UK). Dissolution studies were then undertaken following the USPII method on an automated instrument (Caleva, Dorchester, UK). The dissolution vessels were initially charged with 750 mL of 0.1 M HCl and equilibrated at 37 $\pm$ 0.5 °C under stirring at 50 rpm. Lids on each vessel prevented evaporation. Capsule sinkers were manually filled with ca. 60 mg of a fiber mat and placed into the vessel. Aliquots (5 mL) were periodically withdrawn from the vessels, and replaced with 5 mL of preheated 0.1 M HCl to maintain a constant volume. After 2 h of operation, 250 mL of preheated 0.2 M trisodium phosphate dodecahydrate was added to each vessel, yielding 1 L of a buffer at pH 6.8. Again, 5 mL aliquots were withdrawn at specific time points, and replenished with 5 mL of preheated PBS at pH 6.8. The AI concentrations in each aliquot were quantified with a 7315 spectrophotometer (Jenway, Stone, UK), and cumulative release percentages calculated from these.

3. Results

3.1. Monolithic Fibers

Scanning electron microscopy (SEM) images of the monolithic fibers are presented in Figure 2. In all cases, cylindrical fibers have clearly been formed. In the cases of S-BA and S-ACA, the fibers are homogenous and well formed, with diameters around 500–600 nm (see Table 1). In contrast, the S-NA and S-NAM materials clearly contain two populations of fibers, with a number of very small branched fibers visible, likely due to there being some jet instability during spinning. As a result, the average diameter is rather smaller for these fibers, at 129 ± 102 nm for S-NA and 214 ± 105 nm for S-NAM, and there is a proportionally greater deviation in the diameters.

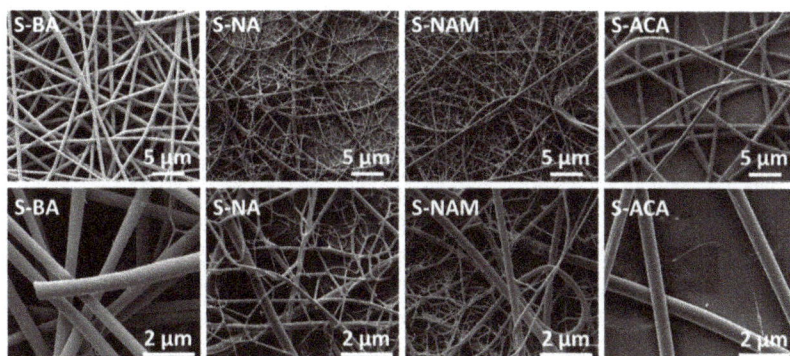

Figure 2. SEM images of the monolithic fibers (top: 10,000× magnification; bottom 40,000× magnification).

The physical form of the AI in the fibers was explored using XRD and DSC (Figure 3). The XRD data in Figure 3a demonstrate that the AIs are crystalline materials, with numerous Bragg reflections visible in their patterns. ES100 is amorphous, and only a broad halo is present in its pattern. No Bragg reflections can be observed for the fibers, showing them to be amorphous solid dispersions. The DSC data (Figure 3b,c) concur with these findings. While the AIs exhibit sharp melting endotherms in their thermograms, these are lacking for ES100 and all the fiber formulations. It should be noted that the DSC experiments were stopped at 200 °C with the fibers, since in preliminary experiments degradation was observed to start just above this temperature (data not shown). Thus, the melting of ACA would not be seen in the data even if crystalline material were present. However, T_g events are present between 100 and 125 °C for all the fibers, confirming their amorphous nature.

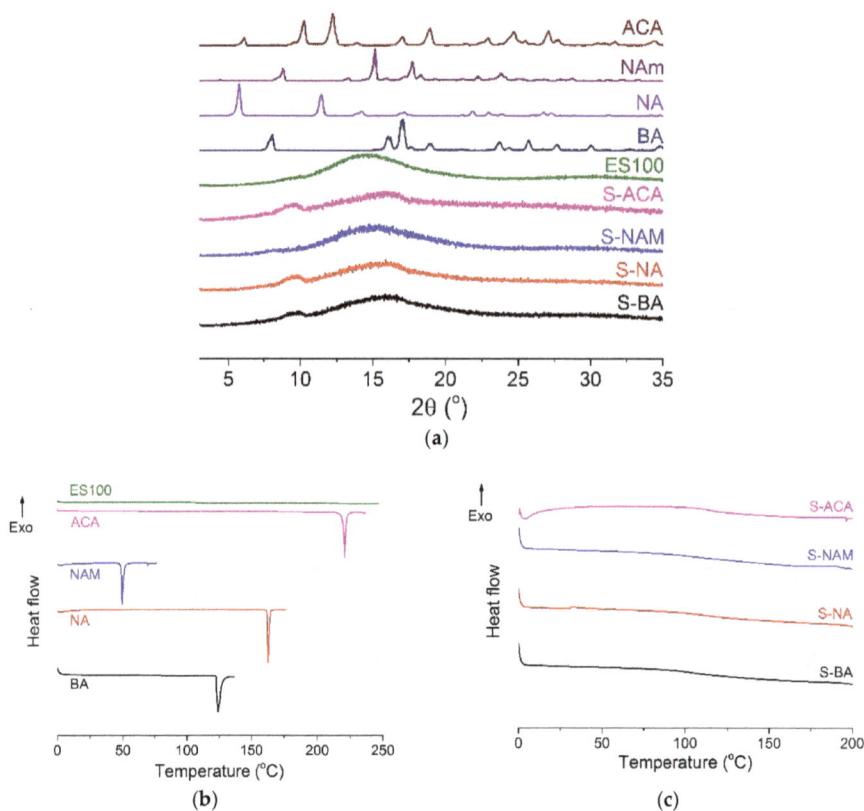

Figure 3. (a) XRD data and DSC data on (b) the raw materials and (c) formulations from monoaxial electrospinning. The data in (a) are normalized for ease of comparison.

IR spectra are given in Figure 4. ES100 has characteristic peaks at 2950–3000 cm^{-1} (CH$_2$ stretching), 1727 cm^{-1} (C=O stretching), and 1150–1275 cm^{-1} (C–O–C stretching). The spectra of the AI-loaded fibers are very similar to that of ES100, as expected given that the AI loading is relatively low (theoretical loading: 7.69%). However, some subtle changes can be observed. The C=O stretch of pure BA is found at 1678 cm^{-1}, and merges with the ES100 C=O stretch in the S-BA fibers to form a single peak at 1725 cm^{-1}. This shift might be attributed to the formation of intermolecular bonding interactions (e.g., H-bonding) between BA and ES100. Similarly, NA and ACA display a C=O stretch at 1667 and 1674 cm^{-1} while the S-NA and S-ACA fibers display single C=O bands at 1727 and 1726 cm^{-1} respectively. No shoulders are visible on these peaks, suggesting again that intermolecular interactions cause the bands to merge. In the case of S-NAM, the N–H stretching vibrations of NAm (at 3411 and 3341 cm^{-1}) are not visible in the fibers, which might be indicative of intermolecular bonding or simply the low AI loading in the formulations.

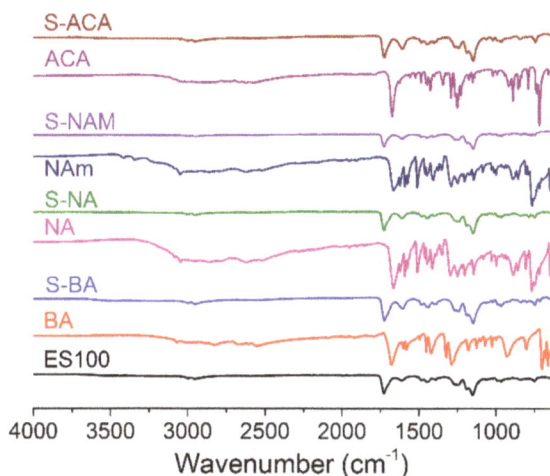

Figure 4. IR spectra of the monolithic fibers.

The AI loading (Table 1) is close to 100% of the theoretical content (>85% in all cases). The differences observed can be attributed to losses of AI during electrospinning (e.g., through small amounts of precipitation or adherence to the syringe walls), the presence of some residual solvent in the fibers, or small inaccuracies in the quantification method.

3.2. Core/Shell Fibers

Core/shell fibers were prepared with an ES100 shell and a core comprising ES100 and the AI. SEM images of these are given in Figure 5. The fibers are, in general, smooth and homogeneous, with average diameters of around 550–700 nm as detailed in Table 1. For C-BA and C-ACA there are a few very fine fibers present as well as the bulk at ca. 600 nm. For C-NA, what appear to be particles can be seen on the fiber surfaces, suggesting some phase separation may have occurred.

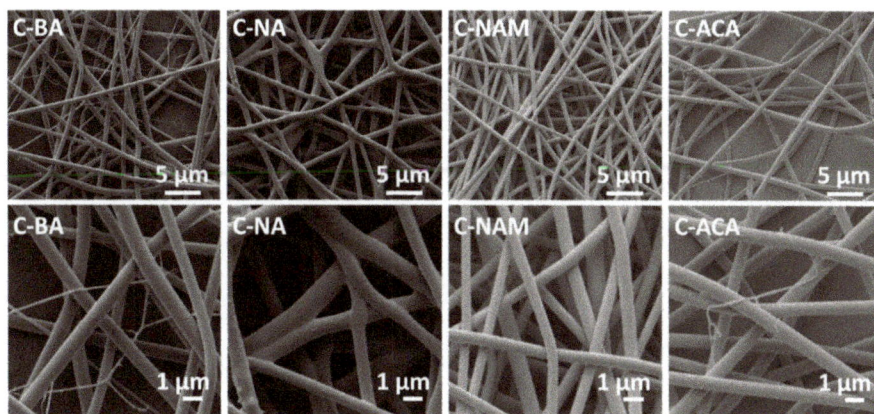

Figure 5. SEM images of the coaxial fibers.

TEM images of the fibers from coaxial electrospinning are depicted in Figure 6. The two solutions used for the core and shell are very similar in their composition, and hence the contrast between the core and shell is not particularly distinct. However, on close inspection it is clear that the fibers have separate core and shell compartments.

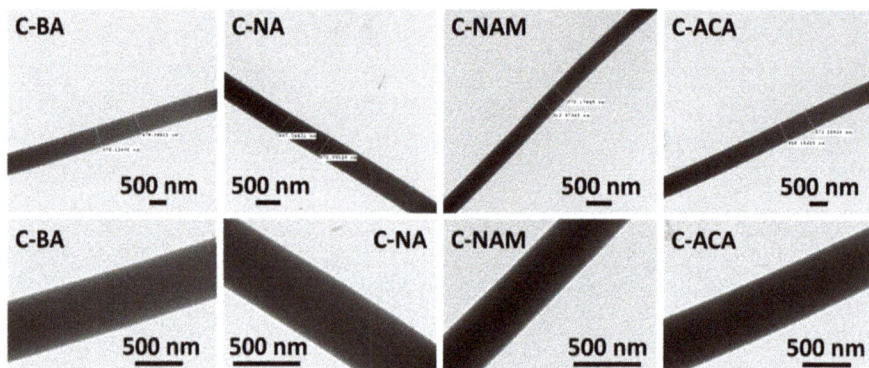

Figure 6. TEM images of the coaxial fibers.

The physical form of the AI in the fibers was probed using XRD and DSC (Figure 7). Similarly to the monolithic fibers, there is no evidence for any crystalline material being present in the products of coaxial electrospinning: the sharp Bragg reflections of the pure AIs are replaced by broad haloes in the XRD patterns of the fibers, consistent with amorphous AI-in-polymer dispersions. The DSC data are also typical of amorphous systems, with no melting endotherms visible but instead clear baseline changes corresponding to T_gs.

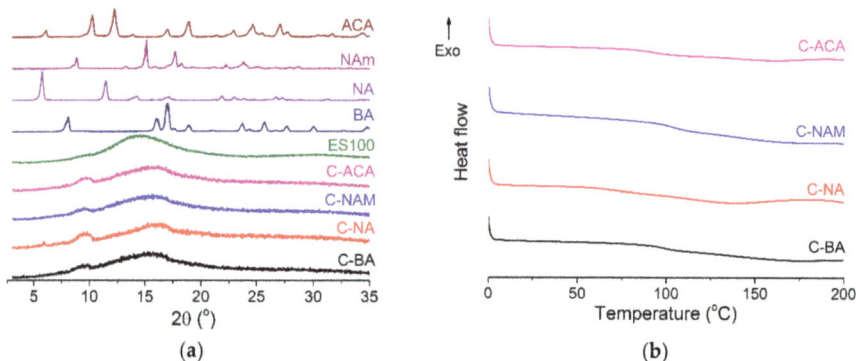

Figure 7. (a) XRD and (b) DSC data for the coaxial fibers. The data in (a) are normalized for ease of comparison.

IR spectra of the core/shell fibers (Figure 8) again are very similar to that of pure ES100, except with some small shifts in peak position (for instance, the C=O peak shifts from 1727 cm^{-1} in ES100 to 1725 cm^{-1} in C-BA and C-NA). Given the low AI loadings of these fibers (theoretical loading: 2.70%) it is not possible to draw any firm conclusions relating to physical form from the IR spectra alone, but it appears that intermolecular bonding may be operational here too.

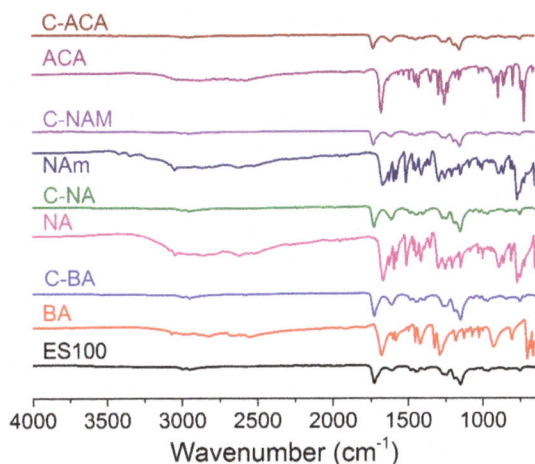

Figure 8. IR spectra of the coaxial fibers.

The AI loadings observed (see Table 1) are again close to 100% of the theoretical content (>80%), with the values close to those found in the monoaxial fibers.

3.3. AI Release

The AI release profiles for the monolithic fibers are shown in Figure 9a. It is clear that the simple fact of making fibers from ES100 does not prevent AI release at pH 1. This is because the AI is able to diffuse through the polymer matrix to reach solution. The extent to which this occurs depends on the nature of the molecule used as the AI: the amount of release in acidic pH decreases in the order S-BA ($86.6 \pm 1.9\%$) > S-NAM ($59.4 \pm 5.7\%$) > S-NA ($25.5 \pm 2.8\%$) > S-ACA ($7.1 \pm 4.5\%$). Both molecular weight (MW) and the acidity/basicity of the AIs are thus important: the lower MW BA (122 Da) releases more quickly and to a greater extent than the intermediate NAm (143 Da) and NA (172 Da) and higher MW ACA (222 Da). S-NAM releases markedly more than S-NA, presumably due to the basic nature of NAm favoring dissolution in the low pH environment in the former case.

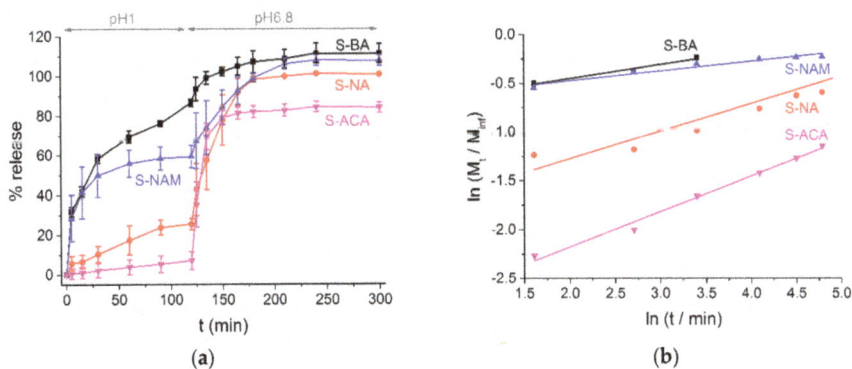

Figure 9. (a) AI release from the monolithic formulations, with data given as mean ± S.D. from three independent experiments; (b) fitting the Korsmeyer-Peppas model to the experimental data obtained at pH 1. Percentages are given relative to the theoretical AI loading in the fibers.

This hypothesis is supported by a Korsmeyer-Peppas analysis of the release data at pH 1 (Figure 9b and Table 2). This model takes the form $M_t/M_{inf} = kt^n$, where M_t is the amount of AI released at time t, M_{inf} is the theoretical AI loading of the fibers, k is a rate constant, and n is an exponent providing information on the reaction mechanism. For all the monolithic fibers, n is <0.45, indicating that Fickian diffusion is the predominant reaction mechanism. The calculated k values fall in the same order as the extent of release data, as would be expected.

Considering the release observed at pH 6.8, all the formulations rapidly release the majority of their remaining AI content after the pH is elevated, with maximum release attained after ca. 60 min immersion in PBS. S-BA, S-NA and S-NAM all reach approximately 100% release, while for S-ACA the plot levels off at around 84%. This can be attributed to the larger MW and lower solubility of ACA compared to the other AIs, as well as the reduced entrapment efficiency noted for S-ACA (calculated to be 85% of the theoretical loading). There are insufficient datapoints for a Peppas analysis of the release data at pH 6.8 but the slopes of plots of ln (M_t/M_{inf}) vs. ln t are much steeper than at acidic pH, indicating that polymer swelling and dissolution are the dominant release mechanisms in neutral conditions.

Table 2. Values extracted from Kormeyer-Peppas analysis of the AI release data at pH 1.

Formulation	n	k (min^{-1})
S-BA	0.14	0.48
S-NA	0.28	0.16
S-NAM	0.10	0.51
S-ACA	0.36	0.055
C-BA	0.11	0.47
C-NA	0.25	0.18
C-NAM	0.22	0.27
C-ACA	NC	NC

NC = not calculated. The release percentages obtained for C-ACA at pH 1 were all very close to zero, and hence mathematical analysis could not be undertaken.

AI release from the coaxial fibers shows similar trends to the monoaxial analogues (Figure 10a). The presence of a blank ES100 shell clearly reduces the amount of AI release seen at pH 1, with C-BA releasing only 57.4 ± 1.7% of its AI loading, cf. 86.6 ± 1.9% in the case of the monolithic systems. Similar results are seen for C-NAM vs. S-NAM (50.9 ± 2.8% and 59.4 ± 5.7% release, respectively) and the ACA-loaded formulations (C-ACA 1.5 ± 0.8%; S-ACA 7.1 ± 4.5%). C-NA and S-NA behave very similarly (C-NA 26.6 ± 1.5%; S-NA 25.5 ± 2.8%). It is evident in all cases bar ACA that a significant proportion of the AI is freed into acidic solution, even though the ES100 sheath is insoluble.

Korsmeyer-Peppas analysis of the pH 1 release data (Figure 10b and Table 2) indicates that, as for the monolithic materials, AI release is diffusion controlled, with n < 0.45. Looking at the rate constants (k), only for C-NAM is there any noticeable change from the monolithic fibers. This is potentially attributable to the basic nature of NAm: NAm has a pKa of 3.92, and so will be fully ionized at pH 1. This will cause it to be highly soluble, providing a thermodynamic driver for the molecules to diffuse out of the polymer matrix and into solution. The other three AIs are acidic, and will be 100% unionized at pH 1. It should be noted that the Korsmeyer-Peppas equation is really only suitable for release from monolithic systems however, and thus some caution must be exercised in considering the results.

When the pH is raised to 6.8, as for the monolithic materials the rate of AI release accelerates noticeably. Both C-NAM and C-NA release 100% of their AI cargo, while C-ACA releases around 81% of the theoretical loading (again consistent with the lower entrapment efficiency of this formulation (91%)). Interesting, C-BA behaves more similarly to the C-ACA material than the naphthalene analogues. It is not obvious why this should be, but it may be that BA forms strong H-bonds with the ES100 carrier as it dissolves, resulting in the formation of AI-polymer aggregates which are removed by filtration before the release percentage is quantified. The maximum extent of release in all cases is reached more slowly than for the monolithic systems, at around 2 h after the elevation of pH.

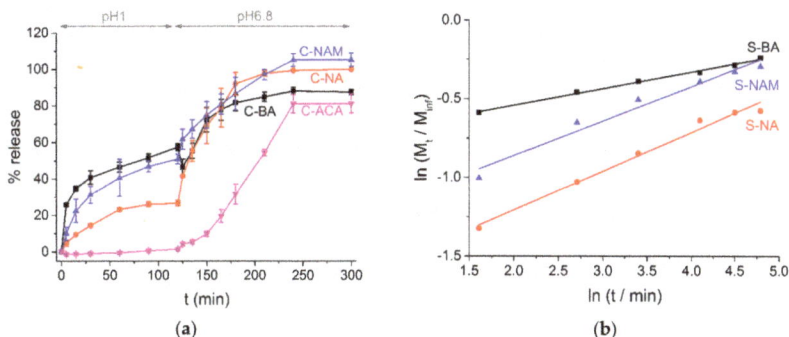

Figure 10. (**a**) AI release from the core/shell formulations, with data given as mean ± S.D. from three independent experiments; (**b**) fitting the Korsmeyer-Peppas model to the experimental data obtained at pH 1. Percentages are given relative to the theoretical AI loading in the fibers.

It proved possible to develop relationships between the molecular weight and the percentage release attained at pH 1 (Figure 11a). It should be noted that some caution is necessary in extracting these, since they are based on data from only a small number of formulations, but nevertheless some trends are clear. We attempted to fit both simple linear and exponential relationships to the percentage release data. For the monolithic fibers, the best fit to the data is obtained with an exponential relationship taking the form % release = $-6.07 + 92.7e^{-(MW-122)/51.3}$, whereas for the coaxial fibers a more simple linear equation gives the best fit: % release = $126 - 0.561MW$. The influence of MW on the release percentage after 2 h at pH 1 is thus dulled by the addition of the blank polymer shell. Considering the Korsmeyer-Peppas rate constants (Figure 11b), an exponential equation of the form $k = 0.146 + 0.324e^{-(MW-122)/22.3}$ gives the best fit to the experimental data for the coaxial systems. In contrast, with the monolithic systems such a relationship can only be constructed for the three carboxylic acids, for which we find $k = 0.00372 + 0.476e^{-(MW-122)/44.9}$. The S-NAM datapoint clearly does not fit on this trendline, indicating that the basicity of the AI has a major influence on the rate constant in the case of the monolithic formulations.

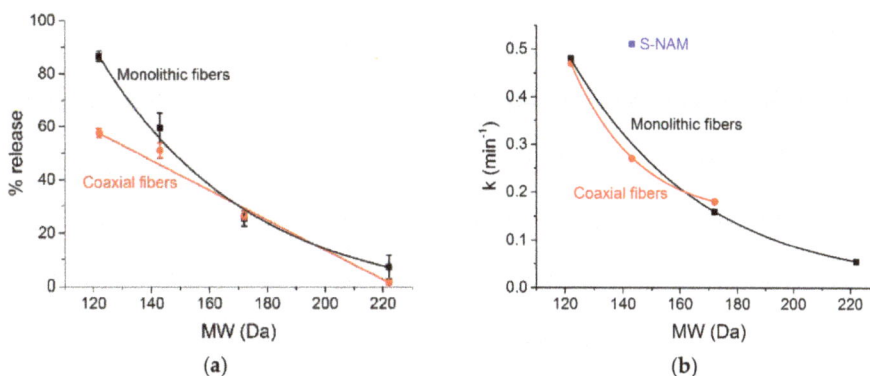

Figure 11. The relationships between AI MW and (**a**) percentage release after 2 h immersion in a pH 1 solution; and (**b**) the Korsmeyer-Peppas rate constant.

4. Discussion

We show in this work that both the molecular weight and the acidity/basicity of an AI are crucial in determining the extent to which release occurs from Eudragit S100 fibers in acidic media. The nanoscale nature of the fiber diameters means that they have very large surface area-to-volume ratios, and thus simply making a fiber from an insoluble polymer does not preclude AI release in conditions where the polymer is insoluble [22,26]. Rather, it is necessary to consider also the ability of the AI to diffuse through the matrix, and the thermodynamic solubility driver for this to happen. It has previously been speculated that lower molecular weight species and those which are more basic will release to a greater extent at acidic pHs [22,25], and in this work we confirm this to be the case.

For coaxial fibers with AI located in the core only, it is demonstrated that the molecular weight of the AI is a good predictor for the percentage and rate of release seen at pH 1, and mathematical relationships can be constructed linking these. For the monolithic fibers, the situation is more complex and although it is possible to elucidate a mathematical relationship between percentage release and AI MW, this does not hold true for the rate of release. For the latter, there is a clear linkage with the MW for the acidic carboxylate AIs considered, but this breaks down for the basic species included in the study. It thus appears that for the coaxial systems, the rate of diffusion through the polymer shell, which will be directly correlated with the MW of the AI, is the dominant factor governing release. For the monolithic analogues, while it is clear that diffusion through the polymer matrix is important, the solubility of the AI in the release milieu is also vital to consider.

5. Conclusions

We report new insights into the factors governing the release of active ingredients (AIs) from electrospun Eudragit S100 (ES100) fibers. Monolithic fibers loaded with benzoic acid, 1-naphthoic acid, 1-naphthylamine, and 9-anthracene carboxylic acid were generated, along with analogous systems with an AI-loaded core and an ES100 shell. The fibers were smooth and cylindrical in the main, and comprised amorphous solid dispersions. There was significant release at pH 1 with all of the monolithic fibers except for those containing 9-anthracene carboxylic acid. Both the molecular weight of the AI and its acidity/basicity are important in controlling release from such materials, with lower molecular weight AIs and basic species freed from the fibers more quickly. With the coaxial fibers, since the AI is present only in the core the acidity/basicity appears to be a less important factor, and the molecular weight, and thus the rate of diffusion through the polymer matrix, is found to be the rate limiting step in release. Mathematical equations could be constructed to predict the release obtained in acidic conditions with AIs of differing molecular properties.

Author Contributions: K.B., H.L, F. and G.R.W. conceived and designed the experiments; K.B. and Y.A.-z. performed the experiments; K.B., H.L., Y.A.-z., F. and G.R.W. analyzed the data; K.B. and G.R.W. wrote the manuscript.

Acknowledgments: We thank the China Scholarship Council for funding H.L.'s work in UCL, the British Council and Egyptian Sciences and Technology Development Fund for awarding a Newton-Mosharafa Researcher Links Travel Grant to Y.A.-z., and the Indonesia Endowment Fund for Education for the award of a PhD studentship to Fatimah.

Conflicts of Interest: The authors declare no conflict of interest.

References

1. Sebe, I.; Szabo, P.; Kallai-Szabo, B.; Zelko, R. Incorporating small molecules or biologics into nanofibers for optimized drug release: A review. *Int. J. Pharm.* **2015**, *494*, 516–530. [CrossRef] [PubMed]
2. Xie, J.; Jiang, J.; Davoodi, P.; Srinivasan, M.P.; Wang, C.H. Electrohydrodynamic atomization: A two-decade effort to produce and process micro-/nanoparticulate materials. *Chem. Eng. Sci.* **2015**, *125*, 32–57. [CrossRef] [PubMed]

3. Yu, D.G.; Shen, X.X.; Branford-White, C.; White, K.; Zhu, L.M.; Bligh, S.W. Oral fast-dissolving drug delivery membranes prepared from electrospun polyvinylpyrrolidone ultrafine fibers. *Nanotechnology* **2009**, *20*, 055104. [CrossRef] [PubMed]

4. Illangakoon, U.E.; Gill, H.; Shearman, G.C.; Parhizkar, M.; Mahalingam, S.; Chatterton, N.P.; Williams, G.R. Fast dissolving paracetamol/caffeine nanofibers prepared by electrospinning. *Int. J. Pharm.* **2014**, *477*, 369–379. [CrossRef] [PubMed]

5. Lu, H.; Wang, Q.; Li, G.; Qiu, Y.; Wei, Q. Electrospun water-stable zein/ethyl cellulose composite nanofiber and its drug release properties. *Mater. Sci. Eng. C* **2017**, *74*, 86–93. [CrossRef] [PubMed]

6. Meng, Z.X.; Zheng, W.; Li, L.; Zheng, Y.F. Fabrication, characterization and in vitro drug release behavior of electrospun PLGA/chitosan nanofibrous scaffold. *Mater. Chem. Phys.* **2011**, *125*, 606–611. [CrossRef]

7. Jia, X.; Zhao, C.; Li, P.; Zhang, H.; Huang, Y.; Li, H.; Fan, J.; Feng, W.; Yuan, X.; Fan, Y. Sustained release of VEGF by coaxial electrospun dextran/PLGA fibrous membranes in vascular tissue engineering. *J. Biomater. Sci. Polym. Ed.* **2011**, *22*, 1811–1827. [CrossRef] [PubMed]

8. Xie, J.; Wang, C.H. Electrospun micro- and nanofibers for sustained delivery of paclitaxel to treat C6 glioma in vitro. *Pharm. Res.* **2006**, *23*, 1817–1826. [CrossRef] [PubMed]

9. Li, H.; Williams, G.R.; Wu, J.; Lv, Y.; Sun, X.; Wu, H.; Zhu, L.M. Thermosensitive nanofibers loaded with ciprofloxacin as antibacterial wound dressing materials. *Int. J. Pharm.* **2017**, *517*, 135–147. [CrossRef] [PubMed]

10. Li, H.; Williams, G.R.; Wu, J.; Wang, H.; Sun, X.; Zhu, L.M. Poly(*N*-isopropylacrylamide)/poly(L-lactic acid-*co*-caprolactone) fibers loaded with ciprofloxacin as wound dressing materials. *Mater. Sci. Eng. C* **2017**, *79*, 245–254. [CrossRef] [PubMed]

11. Hu, J.; Li, H.-Y.; Williams, G.R.; Yang, H.-H.; Tao, L.; Zhu, L.-M. Electrospun poly(*N*-isopropylacrylamide)/ethyl cellulose nanofibers as thermoresponsive drug delivery systems. *J. Pharm. Sci.* **2016**, *105*. [CrossRef]

12. Lin, X.; Tang, D.; Cui, W.; Cheng, Y. Controllable drug release of electrospun thermoresponsive poly(*N*-isopropylacrylamide)/poly(2-acrylamido-2-methylpropanesulfonic acid) nanofibers. *J. Biomed. Mater. Res. A* **2012**, *100*, 1839–1845. [CrossRef] [PubMed]

13. Wang, X.; Yu, D.G.; Li, X.Y.; Bligh, S.W.; Williams, G.R. Electrospun medicated shellac nanofibers for colon-targeted drug delivery. *Int. J. Pharm.* **2015**, *490*, 384–390. [CrossRef] [PubMed]

14. Salehi, R.; Irani, M.; Eskandani, M.; Nowruzi, K.; Davaran, S.; Haririan, I. Interaction, controlled release, and antitumor activity of doxorubicin hydrochloride from pH-sensitive p(NIPAAm-MAA-VP) nanofibrous scaffolds prepared by green electrospinning. *Int. J. Polym. Mater.* **2014**, *63*, 609–619. [CrossRef]

15. Shen, X.; Yu, D.; Zhu, L.; Branford-White, C.; White, K.; Chatterton, N.P. Electrospun diclofenac sodium loaded Eudragit(R) L 100-55 nanofibers for colon-targeted drug delivery. *Int. J. Pharm.* **2011**, *408*, 200–207. [CrossRef] [PubMed]

16. Illangakoon, U.E.; Nazir, T.; Williams, G.R.; Chatterton, N.P. Mebeverine-loaded electrospun nanofibers: Physicochemical characterization and dissolution studies. *J. Pharm. Sci.* **2014**, *103*, 283–292. [CrossRef] [PubMed]

17. Yu, D.-G.; Williams, G.R.; Wang, X.; Liu, X.-K.; Li, H.-L.; Bligh, S.W.A. Dual drug release nanocomposites prepared using a combination of electrospraying and electrospinning. *RSC Adv.* **2013**, *3*, 4652. [CrossRef]

18. Akhgari, A.; Heshmati, Z.; Afrasiabi Garekani, H.; Sadeghi, F.; Sabbagh, A.; Sharif Makhmalzadeh, B.; Nokhodchi, A. Indomethacin electrospun nanofibers for colonic drug delivery: In vitro dissolution studies. *Colloids Surf. B* **2017**, *152*, 29–35. [CrossRef] [PubMed]

19. Yu, D.-G.; Liu, F.; Cui, L.; Liu, Z.-P.; Wang, X.; Bligh, S.W.A. Coaxial electrospinning using a concentric Teflon spinneret to prepare biphasic-release nanofibers of helicid. *RSC Adv.* **2013**, *3*, 17775–17783. [CrossRef]

20. Karthikeyan, K.; Guhathakarta, S.; Rajaram, R.; Korrapati, P.S. Electrospun zein/eudragit nanofibers based dual drug delivery system for the simultaneous delivery of aceclofenac and pantoprazole. *Int. J. Pharm.* **2012**, *438*, 117–122. [CrossRef] [PubMed]

21. Balogh, A.; Farkas, B.; Domokos, A.; Farkas, A.; Démuth, B.; Borbás, E.; Nagy, B.; Marosi, G.; Nagy, Z.K. Controlled-release solid dispersions of Eudragit®FS 100 and poorly soluble spironolactone prepared by electrospinning and melt extrusion. *Eur. Polym. J.* **2017**, *95*, 406–417. [CrossRef]

22. Illangakoon, U.E.; Yu, D.G.; Ahmad, B.S.; Chatterton, N.P.; Williams, G.R. 5-Fluorouracil loaded Eudragit fibers prepared by electrospinning. *Int. J. Pharm.* **2015**, *495*, 895–902. [CrossRef] [PubMed]

23. Jin, M.; Yu, D.G.; Wang, X.; Geraldes, C.F.; Williams, G.R.; Bligh, S.W. Electrospun contrast-agent-loaded fibers for colon-targeted MRI. *Adv. Healthcare Mater.* **2016**, *5*, 977–985. [CrossRef] [PubMed]
24. Jin, M.; Yu, D.G.; Geraldes, C.F.; Williams, G.R.; Bligh, S.W. Theranostic fibers for simultaneous imaging and drug delivery. *Mol. Pharm.* **2016**, *13*, 2457–2465. [CrossRef] [PubMed]
25. Jia, D.; Gao, Y.; Williams, G.R. Core/shell poly(ethylene oxide)/Eudragit fibers for site-specific release. *Int. J. Pharm.* **2017**, *523*, 376–385. [CrossRef] [PubMed]
26. Yu, D.G.; Li, X.Y.; Wang, X.; Yang, J.H.; Bligh, S.W.; Williams, G.R. Nanofibers fabricated using triaxial electrospinning as zero order drug delivery systems. *ACS Appl. Mater. Interfaces* **2015**, *7*, 18891–18897. [CrossRef] [PubMed]

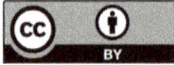

pharmaceutics

MDPI

Article

Fast Dissolving of Ferulic Acid via Electrospun Ternary Amorphous Composites Produced by a Coaxial Process

Weidong Huang [1,2], Yaoyao Yang [3], Biwei Zhao [3], Gangqiang Liang [3], Shiwei Liu [3], Xian-Li Liu [2,*] and Deng-Guang Yu [3,*]

[1] School of Chemistry and Chemical Engineering, Hubei Polytechnic University, Huangshi 435003, China; neweydong@hbpu.edu.cn
[2] Hubei Key Laboratory of Mine Environmental Pollution Control and Remediation, Hubei Polytechnic University, Huangshi 435003, China
[3] School of Materials Science and Engineering, University of Shanghai for Science and Technology, Shanghai 200093, China; yyyang@usst.edu.cn (Y.Y.); 1526410303@st.usst.edu.cn (B.Z.); 1526410214@st.usst.edu.cn (G.L.); 1526410109@st.usst.edu.cn (S.L.)
* Correspondence: liuxianli@hbpu.edu.cn (X.-L.L.); ydg017@usst.edu.cn (D.-G.Y.); Tel.: +86-714-6368937 (X.-L.L.); +86-21-5527-0632 (D.-G.Y.)

Received: 30 May 2018; Accepted: 24 July 2018; Published: 2 August 2018

Abstract: Enhancing the dissolution of insoluble active ingredients comprises one of the most important issues in the pharmaceutical and biomaterial fields. Here, a third generation solid dispersion (3rd SD) of ferulic acid was designed and fabricated by a modified coaxial electrospinning process. A traditional second generation SD (2nd SD) was also prepared by common one-fluid blending electrospinning and was used as a control. With poly(vinyl alcohol) as the fiber matrix and polyvinylpyrrolidone K10 as an additive in the 3rd SDs, the two electrospinning processes were investigated. The prepared 2nd and 3rd SDs were subjected to a series of characterizations, including X-ray diffraction (XRD), scanning electron microscope (SEM), hydrophilicity and in vitro drug dissolving experiments. The results demonstrate that both SDs were monolithic nanocomposites and that the drugs were amorphously distributed within the matrix. However, the 3rd SDs had better morphology with smaller size, narrower size distribution, and smaller water contact angles than the 2nd SDs. Dissolution tests verified that the 3rd SDs could release their loaded cargoes within 60 s, which was over three times faster than the 2nd SDs. Therefore, a combined strategy based on the modified coaxial electrospinning and the logical selections of drug carriers is demonstrated for creating advanced biomaterials.

Keywords: amorphous composite; coaxial electrospinning; fast dissolution; insoluble drug; solid dispersion

1. Introduction

Many drugs are insoluble or poorly water soluble, and improving their dissolution is one of the central challenges in pharmaceutics [1–4]. Among the different kinds of strategies that have been broadly investigated to resolve this problem, drug solid dispersions (SDs) are some of the most promising ways with many commercial products [5–9]. New methods for creating new kinds of high-performance SDs are always desired and are thus becoming a rapidly developing branch of pharmaceutical technologies [10–15].

Over the past half century, first generation SDs (1st SDs) have progressed to second (2nd SDs) and third generation SDs (3rd SDs) [16,17]. Figure 1 is a schematic of the differences in their characteristics. Often, 1st and 2nd SDs are binary systems with the drug distributed in carriers.

In 1st SDs, carriers are mainly crystalline pharmaceutical excipients; in 2nd SDs, amorphous polymers are frequently used as host polymers. The concept of 3rd SDs has gained the interest of researchers in related fields [18]. This new type of SD is typically a ternary or quaternary system with one or two additives (such as surfactants and other polymeric excipients) that, together with the drug and host polymer, are combined to exert a synergistic effect on drug-dissolution improvement [17,18]. The polymer-based SDs are amorphous composites. When an amorphous polymer is exploited not only for drug dissolution but also for controlling drug release, the SD is often termed a 4th generation SD [19,20].

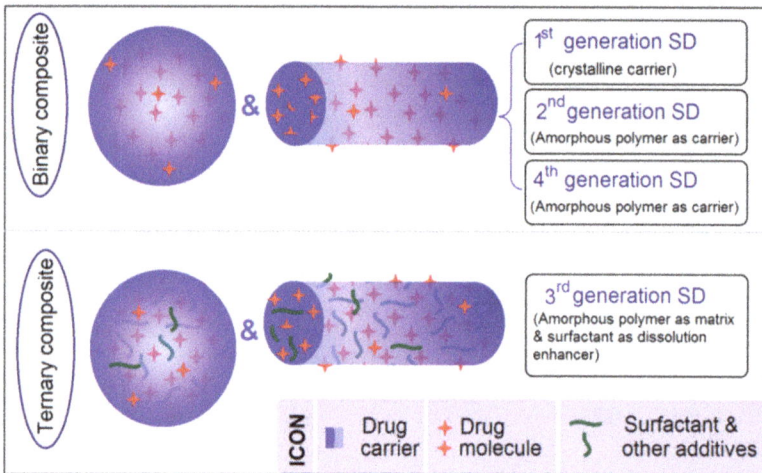

Figure 1. A diagram showing the development of solid dispersions (SDs) from the initial first generation to the third and fourth generations.

Considering the present nano-era, SDs are inevitably advancing to nanoproduction because a fine size always means large surface area for functional performance. Among different pharmaceutical nanotechnologies, electrospinning is distinct from others because of its high effectiveness, easy implementation, and low cost for creating polymer nanofibers [21–28]. Electrospinning and also electrospraying are simple, one-step, "top-down" electrohydrodynamic atomization (EHDA) processes that have quickly developed from the traditional one-fluid blending process to two-fluid (side-by-side and coaxial) processes, and also to tri-axial processes [29–33]. Some studies have demonstrated that single-fluid EHDA and traditional coaxial EHDA are powerful tools for creating SDs [34,35].

For SDs produced from a co-dissolving solution using the one-fluid blending process, several amorphous water-soluble polymers have been investigated. These polymers include poly(ethylene oxide), polyvinylpyrrolidone (PVP), poly(vinyl alcohol) (PVA), gelatin, and some other natural products, e.g., water-soluble polysaccharides [36,37]. Among them, PVA has wide-ranging applications in the pharmaceutical, cosmetic, food, medical and packaging industries. In the field of biomaterials, PVA gels are exploited as drug carriers directly or in the form of particles added to other carriers for tablet formulation. However, these studies have focused only on drug-sustained release; cross-linking is often carried out for creating insoluble nonwoven mats [36]. For SDs, the role of the carrier in forming SDs is very important [38,39]. PVA, as a highly water soluble, highly biocompatible and nontoxic polymer, is a good candidate carrier for promoting drug dissolution [36,37].

Ferulic acid (FA), an abundant polyphenol in maize bran and vegetables, was utilized as a model of a poorly water-soluble drug. It has been explored for a wide variety of potential applications such as age-related diseases, cancer, cardiovascular diseases and diabetes [40]. However, its poor solubility has greatly limited its oral bioavailability [41]. Thus, based on our previous work on the fabrication of SD using traditional coaxial electrospinning [42], here, the usage of advanced modified coaxial electrospinning to prepare 3rd SDs was investigated for the first time.

2. Materials and Methods

2.1. Materials

PVA (M_w = 170,000 g/mol; 88% hydrolyzed) was bought from Shanghai Meimengjia Chemical Co., Ltd. (Shanghai, China). FA (purity > 99%) was purchased from Shanghai Rong-Chuang Biotechnology Co., Ltd. (Shanghai, China). PVP K10 with a molecular weight of 10,000 g/mol was obtained from Sigma-Aldrich Co., Ltd. (Shanghai, China). Anhydrous ethanol and methylene blue were bought from Shanghai Chemical Reagents Co., Ltd. (Shanghai, China).

2.2. Electrospinning

The electrospinning system had the following four parts: a power supply (ZGF60kV-2mA, Wuhan Hua-Tian Corp., Wuhan, China), two fluid drivers (KDS100 and KDS200, Cole-Parmer, Vernon Hills, IL, USA), a collector and a homemade concentric spinneret. After some optimization experiments, the preparation conditions were determined as follows: an applied voltage of 14 kV, a spinneret-collector distance of 15 cm, and a fixed core fluid flow rate of 1.0 mL/h. The environmental temperature and humidity were 21 ± 4 °C and 51 ± 5%, respectively. The properties of the working fluids, including conductivity, surface tension and viscosity were measured using a conductivity meter (DDS-11, Shanghai Rex Co-perfect Instrument Co., Ltd., Shanghai, China), a surface tension tensiometer (BZY-1, Shanghai Hengping Instrument & Meter Factory, Shanghai, China), and a rotary viscometer (NDJ 279, Machinery & Electronic Factory of Tongji University, Shanghai, China), respectively. All the experiments were repeated three times.

2.3. Morphology

The nanofibers' morphologies were studied with the aid of a Quanta FEG450 scanning electron microscope (FE-SEM; FEI Corporation, Hillsboro, OR, USA). Samples were platinum sputter-coated under a nitrogen atmosphere for 100 s prior to visualization. Fiber diameters were calculated using the ImageJ software (National Institutes of Health, Bethesda, MD, USA) to measure the fibers at 100 different points.

2.4. Physical Form and Compatibility

X-ray diffraction (XRD) patterns were collected on a D/Max-BR diffractometer (Rigaku, Tokyo, Japan) over the 2θ range 5 to 60°. The instrument was supplied with Cu Kα radiation at 40 mV and 30 mA. Differential scanning calorimetry (DSC) was carried out using an MDSC 2910 differential scanning calorimeter (TA Instruments Co., New Castle, DE, USA). Sealed samples were heated at 10 °C·min^{-1} from 21 to 250 °C. The nitrogen gas flow rate was kept at 40 mL·min^{-1}. Fourier transform infrared (FTIR) spectroscopy was carried out on a Nicolet-Nexus 670 FTIR spectrometer (Nicolet Instrument Corporation, Madison, WI, USA) at a range of 500 to 4000 cm^{-1} and a resolution of 2 cm^{-1}.

2.5. Property and Functional Performances

A DSA100 drop analysis instrument (Krüss GmbH, Hamburg, Germany) was exploited to measure the surface contact angle (WCA) of nanofiber mats. Distilled water droplets (3 µL) were placed onto the sample's surface. Six different regions of each surface were measured, and the obtained data were averaged.

FA has a maximum UV absorbance at λ_{max} = 321 nm and a shoulder at 278 nm. A calibration curve was thus constructed at 321 nm with the aid of a Lambda 750S spectrophotometer (Perkin Elmer,

Waltham, MA, USA). This took the form $C = 17.74A + 0.14$ ($R^2 = 0.9996$), where C is the concentration of FA ($\mu g/mL$) and A is the absorbance (linear range: 1–20 $\mu g/mL$).

Drug release was quantified following the Chinese Pharmacopoeia Method II (a paddle method) on RCZ-8A dissolution apparatus (Tianjin University Radio Factory, Tianjin, China) at 50 rpm and 37 °C. Then, 30 mg of each sample was placed into 600 mL of phosphate buffered saline (PBS, pH = 7.0, 0.1 M). At predetermined time points, 5 mL aliquots were withdrawn, and 5 mL of fresh preheated PBS was added to maintain a constant volume. The absorbance of the aliquots at $\lambda_{max} = 321$ nm was used to determine the amount of FA released at each time point (with suitable dilution performed where required, to ensure the absorbance lay within the calibration range). Dissolution tests for each sample were performed six times.

2.6. Statistical Method

All experiments for statistical analysis were repeated with a minimum of $n = 6$. Statistical analysis was performed using two-way analysis of variance (ANOVA). Statistically significant values were defined at $\alpha = 0.05$.

3. Results and Discussion

3.1. One System but Two Different Electrospinning Processes

Figure 2 is a schematic of the homemade electrospinning system that can be used to implement both one-fluid blending electrospinning and two-fluid coaxial processes. When the sheath fluid flow rate (Fs) was turned off, i.e., $Fs = 0$ mL/h, it was a typical one-fluid blending spinning process; when $Fs > 0$ mL/h, it became a two-fluid coaxial spinning process. In the literature, almost all single-fluid electrospinning processes are carried out using a metal capillary as a spinneret, and all double coaxial processes are carried out using a concentric spinneret [17,32]. In the present study, one system with a key component (concentric spinneret) was used for both processes. An image of the working system is shown in Figure 3a. The system consisted of two syringe pumps, a collector, a concentric spinneret (inset of Figure 3a), and a power supply. The power supply was connected with the spinneret through an crocodile clip (Figure 3b).

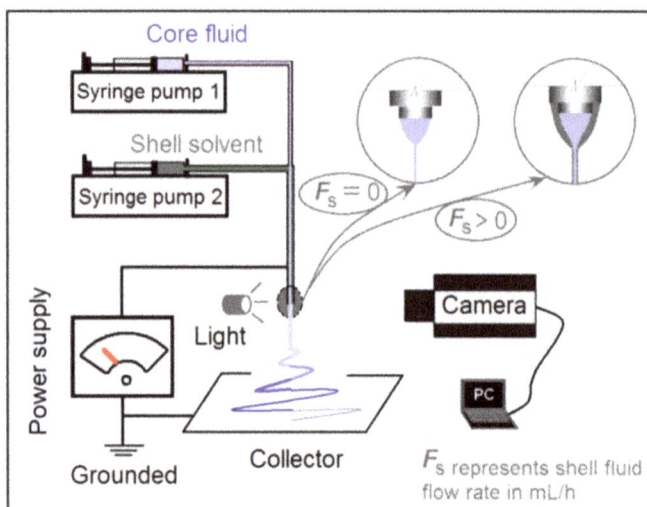

Figure 2. Schematic of the electrospinning system.

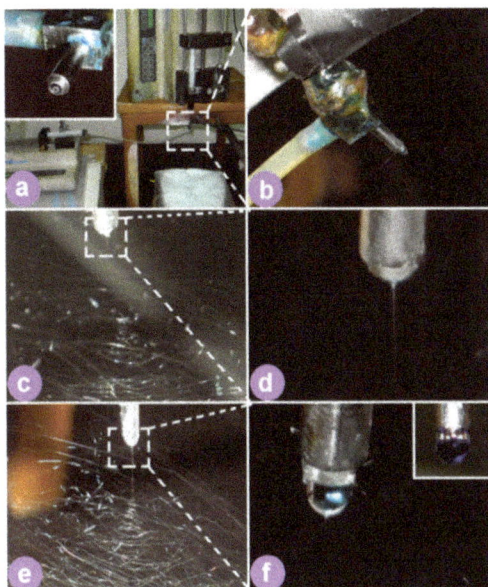

Figure 3. Two electrospinning processes. (**a**) An image of the working system; the inset is the concentric spinneret. (**b**) The connection between the spinneret and the power supply. (**c**) An image of the one-fluid electrospinning process. (**d**) An enlarged image of the Taylor cone in a single-fluid process. (**e**) An image of the coaxial process. (**f**) An enlarged image of the Taylor cone in a two-fluid coaxial process.

In the preparation of 2nd SDs, a blending solution composed of 13% (w/v) PVA and 2.0% (w/v) FA in 50% (v/v) aqueous ethanol was used as the working fluid for the one-fluid blending electrospinning. In the preparation of 3rd SDs using the modified coaxial process, 50% (v/v) aqueous ethanol was used as the sheath fluid. A co-dissolving solution composed of 13% (w/v) PVA, 2% (w/v) PVP K10, and 2% (w/v) FA in 50% (v/v) aqueous ethanol was exploited as the core working liquid. For observing the experimental processes, methylene blue (5 ng/mL in 50% (v/v) aqueous ethanol) was mixed into the core solutions. Details for the preparation are included in Table 1.

Table 1. Parameters for solid dispersion (SD) preparations.

No.	Electrospinning	Sheath Fluid	Core Fluid	Flow Rate (mL/h)	
				Sheath	Core
2nd	Blending	–	13% (w/v) PVA and 2% (w/v) FA in 50% (v/v) aqueous ethanol	–	1.0
3rd	Modified coaxial process	50% (v/v) aqueous ethanol	13% (w/v) PVA, 2% (w/v) PVP K10 and 2% (w/v) FA in 50% (v/v) aqueous ethanol	0.2	1.0

Abbreviation: PVP = polyvinylpyrrolidone, PVA = poly(vinyl alcohol), and FA = Ferulic acid.

Figure 3c shows a single-fluid electrospinning process, where a Taylor cone (Figure 3d) was adjacent to a straight fluid jet and to bending and whipping loops for drawing the fluid jets. Similarly, when coaxial electrospinning was carried out (Figure 3e), a straight fluid jet was ejected out from a compound Taylor cone (Figure 3f), which was followed by a series of enlarged loops. The inset of Figure 3f shows an initial droplet before applying a high voltage, suggesting an easy diffusion of the methylene blue dye from the core solution to the sheath solvent in the static state.

As shown in Table 2, the addition of PVP K10 into the PVA and FA co-dissolving solutions increased their viscosity and slightly elevated their surface tension and conductivity. These changes had little influence on their filament-forming property. However, when the sheath solvent mixture was exploited to surround the core spinnable fluid, it generated a significant influence on the working processes. The coaxial working process was initiated more easily, the Taylor cone was rounder, and the straight fluid jet was shorter than the cases in the single-fluid process, which is obvious from a comparison of Figure 3c,d with Figure 3e,f. In the electrical field, the electronic energy always gathered on the surface of fluid jets. The small viscosity and surface tension of the sheath solvent mixture (Table 2) played their positive roles for a stable and continuous electrospinning process, offsetting the negative influences of a small conductivity.

Table 2. The properties of the three working fluids during the electrospinning processes ($n = 6$).

Electrospinning Working Fluid	Viscosity	Surface Tension	Conductivity
	(cp)	($N \cdot m^{-1} \times 10^{-3}$)	($\mu S \cdot cm^{-1}$)
Fluid for the blending process	212.4 ± 4.5	87.6 ± 1.2	57.4 ± 0.5
Core fluid of the coaxial process	343.7 ± 6.8	93.3 ± 0.7	57.8 ± 0.5
Sheath fluid of the coaxial process	2.87 ± 0.04	27.5 ± 0.4	0.87 ± 0.02

3.2. Morphology

One-fluid and modified coaxial processes were both able to create composite nanofibers that were assessed by SEM. All of them had a linear morphology without any discernible bead or spindle. However, the differences in the two types of nanofibers were significant. As shown in Figure 4a,b, the 2nd SDs had an average diameter of 560 ± 140 nm (Figure 4c). The 3rd SDs from the modified coaxial process (Figure 4d,e) had an average diameter of 220 ± 40 nm (Figure 4f), meaning a higher quality than the 2nd SDs in terms of a smaller diameter and more concentrated size distribution. The sheath solvents in the modified coaxial process retained a stable and robust spinning process and enabled a longer time drawing on the fluid jets to further downsize the nanofibers.

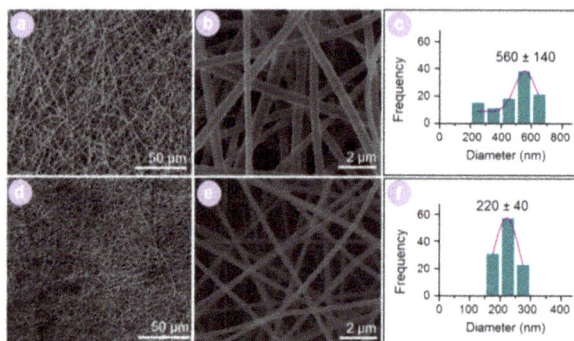

Figure 4. Scanning electron microscope (SEM) images of electrospun nanofibers and their size distributions. (**a,b**) Morphology of 2nd SDs with different magnifications. (**c**) Diameter distribution of 2nd SDs. (**d,e**) Morphology of 3rd SDs with different magnifications. (**f**) Diameter distribution of 3rd SDs.

3.3. Physical Forms

The X-ray powder diffraction (XRD) patterns of the crude materials (FA, PVA, and PVP K10), 2nd SDs, and 3rd SDs are shown in Figure 5a. The numerous sharp peaks in the patterns of FA suggest that the raw FA particles were crystalline. In sharp contrast, the two halos in the patterns of PVP

K10 suggest that the raw PVP particles were an amorphous polymer matrix. The semi-crystalline, hydrophilic nature of PVA was demonstrated by the single blunt peak. However, both binary and ternary SDs had no sharp peak of the drug and had only one clear hump. These results suggest that both of them were monolithic and amorphous regardless of the two or three components present within the nanofibers. DSC thermograms of the crude powders (FA, PVA, and PVP K10), 2nd SDs, and 3rd SDs are shown in Figure 5b. These data concur with the XRD results. FA and PVA each had a single melting point at 174 and 231 °C, respectively. PVP had a blunt dehydrated endothermic peak before 100 °C, followed by a small conversion slope from the glass state to a rubber state around 170 °C (the inset of Figure 5b). However, in the curves of 2nd SDs and 3rd SDs, no peaks of FA could be detected along with the peaks from PVP and PVA, suggesting that FA was completely converted into an amorphous state. Meanwhile, the drug FA generated some plasticization effects on PVA, moving the melting points from 231 °C to 228 °C and 227 °C for 2nd SDs and 3rd SDs, respectively.

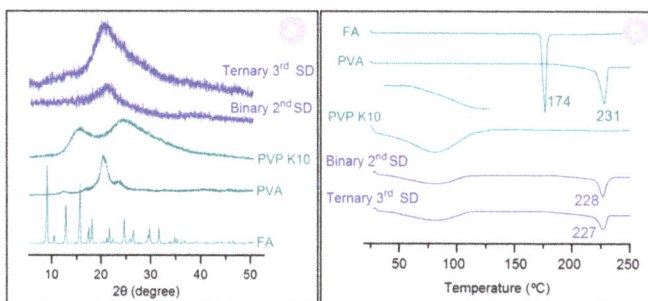

Figure 5. (a) XRD patterns; (b) DSC thermograms.

Shown in Figure 6a are the FTIR spectra of the crude powders (FA, PVA, and PVP K10) and their binary 2nd SDs and ternary 3rd SDs. Their molecular formulae are shown in Figure 6b. The FTIR spectra of FA powders have a series of sharp peaks, such as 1689 and 1663 cm^{-1} (Figure 6a). These peaks should result from the stretching vibration of C=O groups, giving a hint that they were in a different crystal lattice (Figure 6b). FA molecules have both OH and C=O groups, PVA molecules have numerous OH groups and PVP molecules have numerous C=O groups. When electrospun into binary 2nd SDs or ternary 3rd SDs, they were compatible because of the favorable secondary interactions between the drug and the polymers.

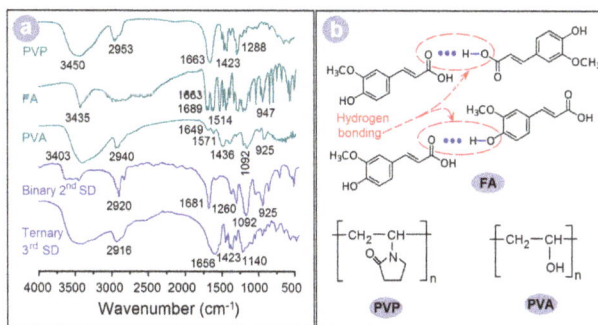

Figure 6. (a) FTIR spectra; (b) The molecular formula of the raw materials, ferulic acid (FA), polyvinylpyrrolidone (PVP), and poly(vinyl alcohol) (PVA).

In the spectra of binary 2nd SDs, there is, only one, sharp peak at 1681 cm^{-1} due to the stretching vibration of C=O groups, suggesting that FA lost its original crystal state in the binary nanocomposites with PVA. In the spectra of binary 3rd SDs, the large peak at 1656 cm^{-1} was a combined result from the stretching vibration of C=O groups both in the FA and also PVP molecules, similarly suggesting that FA was amorphous in the ternary nanocomposites. Meanwhile, the intensities of several sharp peaks in the fingerprint region of FA spectra were greatly decreased or had totally disappeared, giving hints about the formation of amorphous composites between FA and PVA in the binary 2nd SDs and between PVA and PVP in the ternary 3rd SDs.

3.4. Property and Functional Performance

PVA is a highly water-soluble polymer. Both types of electrospun nanofibers were highly hydrophilic. The water droplets rapidly receded after they were placed on the fibers' surfaces. Thus, to differentiate the hydrophilicity of SDs, WCA was recorded after a water droplet was placed on their surface for 2 s. Average Water Contact Angle (WCA) values ($n = 6$) and typical images are shown in Figure 7a. The 3rd SDs had an average value of 31.7° ± 5.2°, smaller than that of 2nd SDs, which had an average value of 53.3° ± 7.8°. This difference suggests that the 3rd SDs had better hydrophilicity than their counterpart due to the third additive PVP K10 and also their smaller diameter.

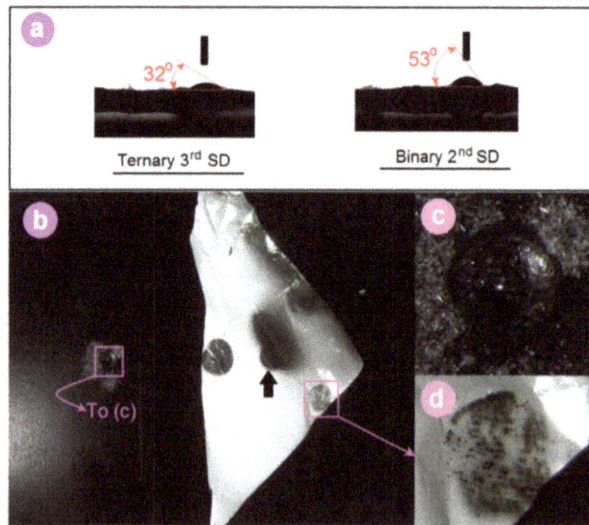

Figure 7. (a) Water contact angles (WCA). (b) Digital images when water droplet was dripped on the FA powders and the electrospun ternary SDs; (c) An enlarged image of the drop of water on the powder; (d) A fingermark on the electrospun nanofibers due to moisture.

Figure 7b shows an intuitive impression on the hydrophilic properties of the raw FA powders and the FA-loaded ternary nanofiber film. FA is a poorly water-soluble drug. Thus, the droplet of water stood on the powders without any discernible dissolution (Figure 7c). In sharp contrast, the FA-loaded film was dissolved at once, as indicated by the arrow in Figure 7b. When a finger was pressed on the fiber film, a clear fingermark appeared because of the moisture (Figure 7d). These phenomena demonstrate that the electrospun nanofibers had fine hydrophilicity, and the ternary SDs were better than the binary SDs.

Figure 8 shows the in vitro drug release profiles of raw FA powders and the 2nd and 3rd SDs. After 5 min, only 5.7 ± 2.4% of the raw FA powders were freed into the dissolution media. The 2nd

SDs released all their cargoes after 220 s, whereas the 3rd SDs needed only 60 s. Although both of them were amorphous and monolithic electrospun nanofibers, their functional applications in enhancing drug dissolution significantly differed. This could be attributed to the fact that the 3rd SDs had better hydrophilicity than their counterparts and they also had a smaller diameter.

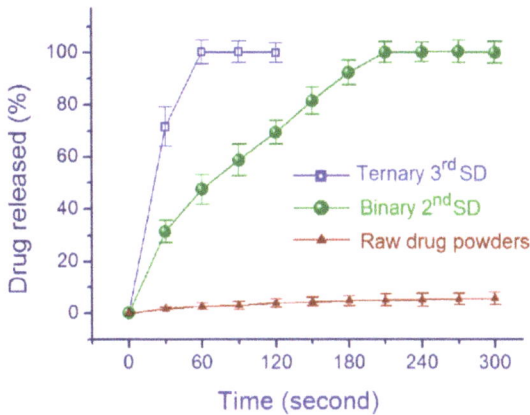

Figure 8. Drug-release profiles of the raw FA powders, the 2nd SDs and 3rd SDs.

Figure 9 is a schematic of the nanostructures of the two SDs and their dissolution processes. The 2nd and 3rd SDs had average diameters of 560 and 220 nm, respectively. For the nanofibers with a cylindrical shape, their volume (V) can be achieved according to the equation of $V = r^2 \pi L$, where L and r are the length of fiber and the radius of its cross-section. The nanofiber's surface area (S) can be obtained by the equation $S = 2\pi r L$. Based on the same volume of nanofibers of 2nd SDs ($V_1 = r_1^2 \pi L_1$) and 3rd SDs ($V_4 = r_4^2 \pi L_4$), the following relationship can be deduced: $r_2^2 \pi L_2 = r_3^2 \pi L_3$, i.e., $L_3/L_2 = r_2^2/r_3^2$. Thus, the surface area ratio of 3rd SDs to 2nd SDs can be calculated as follows:

$$S_3/S_2 = (2\pi r_3 L_3)/(2\pi r_2 L_2)$$

$$= r_3/r_2 \cdot L_3/L_2$$

$$= r_3/r_2 \cdot r_2^2/r_3^2 = r_2/r_3$$

$$= 560/220 = 2.5$$

This is to say that the reduction in nanofiber diameter from 560 nm for 2nd SDs to 220 nm for 3rd SDs resulted in a significant increase in the fiber's total surface area by 2.5-fold. The smaller diameter meant double nano effects for drug dissolution, one was a larger surface area and the other was a shorter distance for the water/drug molecules to diffuse in/out of the bulk dissolution media.

However, the most important reason should be the presence of PVP in the PVA matrix, which effectively promoted the disintegration of PVA gels owing to PVP's relatively small molecular weight, high solubility in water, and high permeation ability. The dissolution of a polymer always experiences water absorbance, swelling, and disentanglement of the polymer chains before the polymeric molecules enter the dissolution media. Shown in Figure 9, the PVP K10 molecules completely revised the dissolution processes of PVA molecules. It made the 3rd SDs nanofibers swell more quickly than the 2nd SDs nanofibers. Meanwhile, it promoted the 3rd SDs to dissolve in a disintegration manner, getting rid of the traditional layer-by-layer dissolution model that happens in the 2nd SDs. Certainly, during these processes, the water and also the drug molecules were able to diffuse more easily into and out of the gel regions formed by the PVA matrix within the 3rd SDs than the 2nd SDs.

The generation of electrospun nanofibers on a large scale is drawing increasing attention in both the scientific research and industrial fields [43]. The ternary amorphous nanocomposites hold great promises for further developing fast dissolution drug delivery systems, which is popular for the administration of many active ingredients [44]. In future, these medicated nanofibers can be converted into different kinds of dosage forms, such as tablets, membranes, and also capsules [45].

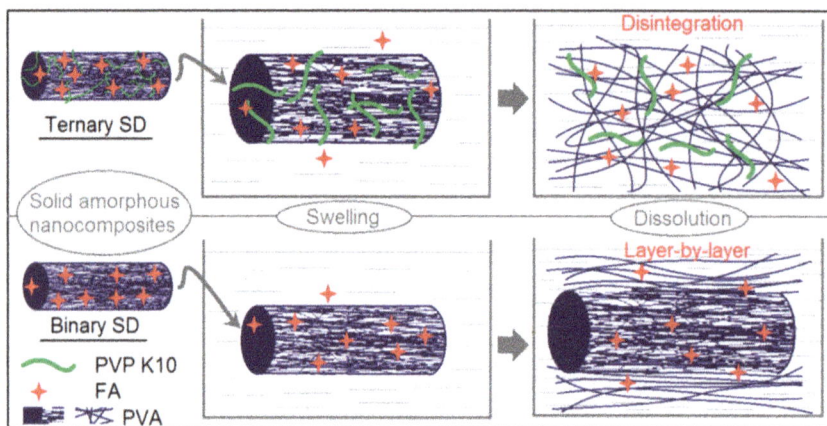

Figure 9. A diagram comparing the dissolution process of the 2nd SDs and 3rd SDs.

4. Conclusions

We successfully prepared 2nd and 3rd SDs by a one-fluid blending electrospinning process and a two-fluid coaxial process, respectively. Both processes were conducted smoothly and continuously, and the resulting nanofibers had fine linear morphology without any discernible bead or spindle. Although XRD patterns demonstrated that both SD types were monolithic and amorphous nanoproducts, 3rd SDs showed over three times faster drug-release rate than 2nd SDs. The added third component PVP, the smaller diameter and corresponding larger surface, the shorter water/drug molecule diffusion distance, and the improved hydrophilicity exerted a combined effect to result in the better performance of 3rd SDs. This study has provided a new protocol for designing and developing new kinds of functional biomaterials as an alternative solution to the problem of insoluble drugs.

Author Contributions: X.-L.L. and D.-G.Y. conceived and designed the experiments; W.H., Y.Y., B.Z., G.L. and S.L. performed the experiments and analyzed the data; W.H. and D.-G.Y. wrote the paper.

Funding: This research was funded by the Hubei Provincial Department of Education (Nos.B2013060 and 2012107) and the USST College Student Innovation Project (Nos. XJ10252324-330 and SH10252194).

Conflicts of Interest: The authors declare no conflict of interest.

References

1. Singh, A.; Van den Mooter, G. Spray drying formulation of amorphous solid dispersions. *Adv. Drug Deliv. Rev.* **2016**, *100*, 27–50. [CrossRef] [PubMed]
2. Lauer, M.E.; Maurer, R.; Paepe, A.T.; Stillhart, C.; Jacob, L.; James, R.; Kojima, Y.; Rietmann, R.; Kissling, T.; van den Ende, J.A.; et al. A miniaturized extruder to prototype amorphous solid dispersions: Selection of plasticizers for hot melt extrusion. *Pharmaceutics* **2018**, *10*, 58. [CrossRef] [PubMed]

3.   Feng, D.; Peng, T.; Huang, Z.; Singh, V.; Shi, Y.; Wen, T.; Lu, M.; Quan, G.; Pan, X.; Wu, C. Polymer-surfactant system based amorphous solid dispersion: Precipitation inhibition and bioavailability enhancement of itraconazole. *Pharmaceutics* **2018**, *10*, 53. [CrossRef] [PubMed]

4.   Chen, L.; Okuda, T.; Lu, X.Y.; Chan, H.K. Amorphous powders for inhalation drug delivery. *Adv. Drug Deliv. Rev.* **2016**, *100*, 102–115. [CrossRef] [PubMed]

5.   Ponnammal, P.; Kanaujia, P.; Yani, Y.; Ng, W.K.; Tan, R.B.H. Orally disintegrating tablets containing melt extruded amorphous solid dispersion of tacrolimus for dissolution enhancement. *Pharmaceutics* **2018**, *10*, 35. [CrossRef] [PubMed]

6.   Ousset, A.; Chavez, P.F.; Meeus, J.; Robin, F.; Schubert, M.A.; Somville, P.; Dodou, K. Prediction of phase behavior of spray-dried amorphous solid dispersions: Assessment of thermodynamic models, standard screening methods and a novel atomization screening device with regard to prediction accuracy. *Pharmaceutics* **2018**, *10*, 29. [CrossRef] [PubMed]

7.   Huang, S.; Mao, C.; Williams, R.O.; Yang, C.Y. Solubility advantage (and disadvantage) of pharmaceutical amorphous solid dispersions. *J. Pharm. Sci.* **2016**, *105*, 3549–3561. [CrossRef] [PubMed]

8.   Li, J.; Patel, D.; Wang, G. Use of spray-dried dispersions in early pharmaceutical development: Theoretical and practical challenges. *AAPS J.* **2016**, *2016*, 1–13. [CrossRef] [PubMed]

9.   Chiou, W.L.; Riegelman, S. Pharmaceutical applications for solid dispersion systems. *J. Pharm. Sci.* **1971**, *60*, 1281–1302. [CrossRef] [PubMed]

10.   Mishra, J.; Rades, T.; Löbmann, K.; Grohganz, H. Influence of solvent composition on the performance of spray-dried co-amorphous formulations. *Pharmaceutics* **2018**, *10*, 47. [CrossRef] [PubMed]

11.   Saleh, A.; McGarry, K.; Chaw, C.S.; Elkordy, A.A. Feasibility of using gluconolactone, trehalose and hydroxy-propyl gamma cyclodextrin to enhance bendroflumethiazide dissolution using lyophilisation and physical mixing techniques. *Pharmaceutics* **2018**, *10*, 22. [CrossRef] [PubMed]

12.   Balogh, A.; Farkas, B.; Pálvölgyi, Á.; Domokos, A.; Démuth, B.; Marosi, G.; Nagy, Z.K. Novel alternating current electrospinning of hydroxypropylmethylcellulose acetate succinate (HPMCAS) nanofibers for dissolution enhancement: The importance of solution conductivity. *J. Pharm. Sci.* **2017**, *106*, 1634–1643. [CrossRef] [PubMed]

13.   Balogh, A.; Farkas, B.; Domokos, A.; Farkas, A.; Démuth, B.; Borbás, E.; Nagy, B.; Marosi, G.; Nagy, Z.K. Controlled-release solid dispersions of Eudragit® FS 100 and poorly soluble spironolactone prepared by electrospinning and melt extrusion. *Eur. Polym. J.* **2017**, *95*, 406–417. [CrossRef]

14.   Borbás, E.; Nagy, Z.K.; Nagy, B.; Balogh, A.; Farkas, B.; Tsinman, O.; Tsinman, K.; Sinkó, B. The effect of formulation additives on in vitro dissolution-absorption profile and in vivo bioavailability of telmisartan from brand and generic formulations. *Eur. J. Pharm. Sci.* **2018**, *114*, 310–317. [CrossRef] [PubMed]

15.   Van Duong, T.; Van den Mooter, G. The role of the carrier in the formulation of pharmaceutical solid dispersions. Part II: Amorphous carriers. *Expert Opin. Drug Deliv.* **2016**, *13*, 1681–1694. [CrossRef] [PubMed]

16.   Vasconcelos, T.; Sarmento, B.; Costa, P. Solid dispersions as strategy to improve oral bioavailability of poor water soluble drugs. *Drug Discov. Today* **2007**, *12*, 1068–1075. [CrossRef] [PubMed]

17.   Kenawy, E.R.; Abdel-Hay, F.I.; El-Newehy, M.H.; Wnek, G.E. Controlled release of ketoprofen from electrospun poly (vinyl alcohol) nanofibers. *Mater. Sci. Eng. A* **2007**, *459*, 390–396. [CrossRef]

18.   Le-Ngoc Vo, C.; Park, C.; Lee, B.J. Current trends and future perspectives of solid dispersions containing poorly water-soluble drugs. *Eur. J. Pharm. Biopharm.* **2013**, *85*, 799–813.

19.   Zhang, Z.; Li, W.; Wang, G.; Qu, Y.; Yu, D.G. Electrospun 4th generation solid dispersions of poorly water-soluble drug utilizing two different processes. *J. Nanomater.* **2018**, *2018*, 2012140. [CrossRef]

20.   Hallouard, F.; Mehenni, L.; Lahiani-Skiba, M.; Anouar, Y.; Skiba, M. Solid dispersions for oral administration: An overview of the methods for their preparation. *Curr. Pharm. Des.* **2016**, *22*, 4942–4958. [CrossRef] [PubMed]

21.   Wang, K.; Wen, H.F.; Yu, D.G.; Yang, Y.; Zhang, D.F. Electrosprayed hydrophilic nanocomposites coated with shellac for colon-specific delayed drug delivery. *Mater. Des.* **2018**, *143*, 248–255. [CrossRef]

22.   Yang, Y.; Zhang, M.; Wang, K.; Yu, D.G. pH-sensitive polymer nanocoating on hydrophilic composites fabricated using modified coaxial electrospraying. *Mater. Lett.* **2018**, *227*, 93–96. [CrossRef]

23. Liu, Z.P.; Zhang, L.L.; Yang, Y.Y.; Wu, D.; Jiang, G.; Yu, D.G. Preparing composite nanoparticles for immediate drug release by modifying electrohydrodynamic interfaces during electrospraying. *Powder Technol.* **2018**, *327*, 179–187. [CrossRef]

24. Yang, Y.Y.; Zhang, M.; Liu, Z.P.; Wang, K.; Yu, D.G. Meletin sustained-release gliadin nanoparticles prepared via solvent surface modification on blending electrospray. *Appl. Surf. Sci.* **2018**, *434*, 1040–1047. [CrossRef]

25. Liu, X.K.; Shao, W.Y.; Luo, M.Y.; Bian, J.Y.; Yu, D.G. Electrospun blank nanocoating for improved sustained release profiles from medicated gliadin nanofibers. *Nanomaterials* **2018**, *8*, 184.

26. Xu, Y.; Li, J.J.; Yu, D.G.; Williams, G.R.; Yang, J.H.; Wang, X. Influence of the drug distribution in electrospun gliadin fibers on drug-release behavior. *Eur. J. Pharm. Sci.* **2017**, *106*, 422–430. [CrossRef] [PubMed]

27. Li, X.Y.; Zheng, Z.B.; Yu, D.G.; Liu, X.K.; Qu, Y.L.; Li, H.L. Electrosprayed sperical ethylcellulose nanoparticles for an improved sustained-release profile of anticancer drug. *Cellulose* **2017**, *24*, 5551–5564. [CrossRef]

28. Liu, Z.P.; Zhang, Y.Y.; Yu, D.G.; Wu, D.; Li, H.L. Fabrication of sustained-release zein nanoparticles via modified coaxial electrospraying. *Chem. Eng. J.* **2018**, *334*, 807–816. [CrossRef]

29. Yu, D.G.; Li, X.Y.; Wang, X.; Yang, J.H.; Annie Bligh, S.W.; Williams, G.R. Nanofibers fabricated using triaxial electrospinning as zero order drug delivery systems. *ACS Appl. Mater. Interfaces* **2015**, *7*, 18891–18897. [CrossRef] [PubMed]

30. Yu, D.G.; Li, J.J.; Zhang, M.; Williams, G.R. High-quality janus nanofibers prepared using three-fluid electrospinning. *Chem. Commun.* **2017**, *53*, 4542–4545. [CrossRef] [PubMed]

31. Wang, Q.; Yu, D.G.; Zhang, L.L.; Liu, X.K.; Deng, Y.C.; Zhao, M. Electrospun hypromellose-based hydrophilic composites for rapid dissolution of poorly water-soluble drug. *Carbohydr. Polym.* **2017**, *174*, 617–625. [CrossRef] [PubMed]

32. Yang, Y.Y.; Liu, Z.P.; Yu, D.G.; Wang, K.; Liu, P.; Chen, X.H. Colon-specific pulsatile drug release provided by electrospun shellac nanocoating on hydrophilic amorphous composites. *Int. J. Nanomed.* **2018**, *13*, 2395–2404. [CrossRef] [PubMed]

33. Wang, K.; Liu, X.K.; Chen, X.H.; Yu, D.G.; Yang, Y.Y.; Liu, P. Electrospun hydrophilic janus nanocomposites for the rapid onset of therapeutic action of helicid. *ACS Appl. Mater. Interfaces* **2018**, *10*, 2859–2867. [CrossRef] [PubMed]

34. Agarwal, S.; Greiner, A.; Wendorff, J.H. Functional materials by electrospinning of polymers. *Prog. Polym. Sci.* **2013**, *38*, 963–991. [CrossRef]

35. Wang, Q.; Yu, D.G.; Zhou, S.Y.; Li, C.; Zhao, M. Fabrication of amorphous electrospun medicated-nanocomposites using a Teflon-based concentric spinneret. *e-Polymer* **2018**, *18*, 3–11. [CrossRef]

36. Tang, C.; Saquing, C.D.; Harding, J.R.; Khan, S.A. In situ cross-linking of electrospun poly (vinyl alcohol) nanofibers. *Macromolecules* **2009**, *43*, 630–637. [CrossRef]

37. Li, X.; Kanjwal, M.A.; Lin, L.; Chronakis, I.S. Electrospun polyvinyl-alcohol nanofibers as oral fast-dissolving delivery system of caffeine and riboflavin. *Colloid Surf. B* **2013**, *103*, 182–188. [CrossRef] [PubMed]

38. Démuth, B.; Galata, D.L.; Szabó, E.; Nagy, B.; Farkas, A.; Balogh, A.; Hirsch, E.; Pataki, H.; Rapi, Z.; Bezúr, L.; et al. Investigation of deteriorated dissolution of amorphous itraconazole: Description of incompatibility with magnesium stearate and possible solutions. *Mol. Pharm.* **2017**, *14*, 3927–3934. [CrossRef] [PubMed]

39. Gately, N.M.; Kennedy, J.E. The development of a melt-extruded shellac carrier for the targeted delivery of probiotics to the colon. *Pharmaceutics* **2017**, *9*, 38. [CrossRef] [PubMed]

40. Barone, E.; Calabrese, V.; Mancuso, C. Ferulic acid and its therapeutic potential as a hormetin for age-related diseases. *Biogerontology* **2009**, *10*, 97–108. [CrossRef] [PubMed]

41. Yu, D.G.; Yang, J.M.; Branford-White, C.; Lu, P.; Zhang, L.; Zhu, L.M. Third generation solid dispersions of ferulic acid in electrospun composite nanofibers. *Int. J. Pharm.* **2010**, *400*, 158–164. [CrossRef] [PubMed]

42. Yu, D.G.; Zhu, L.M.; Branford-White, C.; Yang, J.H.; Wang, X.; Li, Y.; Qian, W. Solid dispersions in the form of electrospun core-sheath nanofibers. *Int. J. Nanomed.* **2011**, *6*, 3271–3280. [CrossRef] [PubMed]

43. Szabó, E.; Démuth, B.; Nagy, B.; Molnár, K.; Farkas, A.; Szabó, B.; Balogh, A.; Hirsch, E.; Marosi, G.; Nagy, Z.K. Scaled-up preparation of drug-loaded electrospun polymer fibres and investigation of their continuous processing to tablet form. *Express Polym. Lett.* **2018**, *12*, 436–451. [CrossRef]

44. Ono, A.; Ito, S.; Sakagami, S.; Asada, H.; Saito, M.; Quan, Y.S.; Kamiyama, F.; Hirobe, S.; Okada, N. Development of novel faster-dissolving microneedle patches for transcutaneous vaccine delivery. *Pharmaceutics* **2017**, *9*, 59. [CrossRef] [PubMed]
45. Démuth, B.; Nagy, Z.K.; Balogh, A.; Vigh, T.; Marosi, G.; Verreck, G.; Van Assche, I.; Brewster, M.E. Downstream processing of polymer-based amorphous solid dispersions to generate tablet formulations. *Int. J. Pharm.* **2015**, *486*, 268–286. [CrossRef] [PubMed]

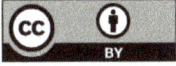

pharmaceutics

MDPI

Article

Development of A New Delivery System Based on Drug-Loadable Electrospun Nanofibers for Psoriasis Treatment

Leticia Martínez-Ortega [†], **Amalia Mira, Asia Fernandez-Carvajal, C. Reyes Mateo, Ricardo Mallavia** * **and Alberto Falco** *,[†]

Institute of Research, Development and Innovation in Biotechnology of Elche (IDiBE) and Molecular and Cellular Biology Institute (IBMC), Miguel Hernández University (UMH), 03202 Elche, Spain; leticia.martinez@goumh.umh.es (L.M.-O.); a.mira@umh.es (A.M.); asia.fernandez@umh.es (A.F.-C.); rmateo@umh.es (C.R.M.)
* Correspondence: r.mallavia@umh.es (R.M.); alber.falco@umh.es (A.F.)
† These authors contributed equally to this work.

Received: 12 November 2018; Accepted: 23 December 2018; Published: 4 January 2019

Abstract: Psoriasis is a chronic autoimmune systemic disease with an approximate incidence of 2% worldwide; it is commonly characterized by squamous lesions on the skin that present the typical pain, stinging, and bleeding associated with an inflammatory response. In this work, poly(methyl vinyl ether-*alt*-maleic ethyl monoester) (PMVEMA-ES) nanofibers have been designed as a delivery vehicle for three therapeutic agents with palliative properties for the symptoms of this disease (salicylic acid, methyl salicylate, and capsaicin). For such a task, the production of these nanofibers by means of the electrospinning technique has been optimized. Their morphology and size have been characterized by optical microscopy and scanning electron microscopy (SEM). By selecting the optimal conditions to achieve the smallest and most uniform nanofibers, approximate diameters of up to 800–900 nm were obtained. It was also determined that the therapeutic agents that were used were encapsulated with high efficiency. The analysis of their stability over time by GC-MS showed no significant losses of the encapsulated compounds 15 days after their preparation, except in the case of methyl salicylate. Likewise, it was demonstrated that the therapeutic compounds that were encapsulated conserved, and even improved, their capacity to activate the transient receptor potential cation channel 1 (TRPV1) channel, which has been associated with the formation of psoriatic lesions.

Keywords: PMVE/MA; electrospinning; nanofibers; capsaicin; psoriasis; TRPV1

1. Introduction

Psoriasis is a chronic immune-mediated disease that affects 2% of the population, comprising different clinical manifestations, which are mainly characterized by skin disorders such as erythematous papules or scaly teardrop-like lesions associated with the characteristic pain, stinging, and even bleeding of an inflammatory process. The most affected areas are usually the elbows, knees, scalp, and lower back [1,2].

The immune system plays a crucial role in the pathogenesis of the disease, and particularly, the deregulation of the crosstalk between the innate and adaptive immune system within the interleukin-23 (IL23)/T helper cell 17 (Th17) axis [1,3,4]. Thus, the therapeutic treatments focus on targeting the Th17 response, either as local or systemic non-specific immunosuppressors (conventional therapies) such as dermocorticoids and methotrexate. The side effects produced by these treatments have boosted the use of antibody-based systemic treatments that recognize, bind, and block the activity of those cytokines involved in the Th17 response (biological therapies), such as IL17A (Ixekizumab,

Taltz™; Secukinumab, Cosentyx™), IL23 (Guselkumab, Tremfya™), IL23 and IL12 (Ustekinumab, Stelara™), and TNF-α (Adalimumab, Humira™; Etanercept, Enbrel™; Infliximab, Remicade™) [1,5,6]. However, despite the promising results offered by this type of treatment, they also have limitations such as their high cost, some adverse effects, a loss of efficacy due to the development of anti-drug antibodies, and the inability to avoid occasional symptomatic outbreaks or to act on some poorly accessible locations [1,7–9]. Therefore, there is still a need to use therapeutic agents to alleviate the discomfort derived from the symptoms caused by the psoriatic lesions [1,6,10].

The main palliative agents for the dermal symptomatology of the disease are keratolytics, to reduce the generation of scales, and analgesics, to relieve the painful and itching sensation. Among the keratolytics, salicylic acid stands out, which acts by lowering the pH of the stratum corneum and thus preventing the adhesion of keratinocytes [11]. In turn, it also improves the absorption of other topical treatments by reducing the stiffness of the stratum, and also reduces the pruritus [12].

In terms of analgesic therapy, one of the most common targets in topical applications is the transient receptor potential cation channel 1 (TRPV1), commonly called the capsaicin receptor. This receptor is mainly found in the nociceptive neurons of the peripheral nervous system, although they have also been described in other non-neuronal tissues, including skin cells. TRPV1 is a non-selective tetrameric cation channel with high permeability to calcium (Ca^{2+}) that has been involved in the transmission and modulation of pain when triggered by different physical and chemical stimuli such as temperatures above 43 °C, acidic pH, capsaicin, and some endogenous mediators of inflammation [13–15]. Capsaicin, an alkaloid present in several species in the genus *Capsicum*, and some of its derivatives act as analgesic agents by producing TRPV1 desensitization [13,16]. Additionally, this family of compounds hold other biological properties such as cardiovascular stimulator, antioxidant, and anticancer, as well as anti-inflammatory, by for instance suppressing the inducement of TNF-α, which is also a psoriasis mediator [17–20]. Methyl salicylate, which is derived from salicylic acid, is another analgesic agent. This compound belongs to the family of non-steroidal anti-inflammatory drugs (NSAIDs), and has also been reported to activate TRPV1 [21,22]. In addition, it is easily absorbed through the skin, and is already used for the treatment of inflammation and pain [22].

However, for the maximization of the expected benefits of their combined delivery, it would be necessary to have a suitable system for their topical application, and desirably, an encapsulation procedure that allows combining all three compounds together without losing their activity, in addition to being simple and scalable to industrial production. In this sense, recent advances in nanotechnology applied to the field of medicine offer an alternative that meets all these requirements, i.e., polymer nanofibers produced by the electrospinning technique [23–25]. In addition, the correct choice of the integrating materials would allow the development of nanostructures with appropriate release properties according the particular dosage needs of their load, which in the specific case of capsaicin should be sustained in order to keep TRPV1 desensitized for a prolonged period.

In this work, based on the progress made in our previous study [26], the production process of electrospun nanofibers loaded with all three compounds described above is optimized using poly(methyl vinyl ether-*alt*-maleic ethyl monoester) (PMVEMA-ES) as the polymeric material. Such a biodegradable, biocompatible, bioadhesive, and low-toxic polymer is already commercialized, and used in other biomedical applications, and has already shown its suitability for the creation of these nanostructured systems with the appropriate release characteristics [26–30]. Additionally, this polymer not only allows the possibility of being used as the main building polymer for the creation of nanofibers, but also allows combining with other materials, such as fluorene-based copolymers [31,32], in order to combine functional properties within the same nanostructure [26,33,34]. The morphological characterization of these nanofibers, together with their encapsulation capacity, stability over time, and activity of the encapsulated compounds are also analyzed in this study.

2. Materials and Methods

2.1. Polymers, Solvents, Drugs, and Common Materials

The copolymer of poly(methyl vinyl ether-*alt*-maleic acid) monoethyl ester (PMVEMA-ES) (M_w: ~130 kg/mol) was supplied in a 50% w/w solution in ethanol (Sigma-Aldrich, Saint Louis, MO, USA).

The solvents used were dichloromethane, acetone, ethanol (Merck KGaA, Darmstadt, Germany), methanol (VWR International, Radnor, PA, USA), sulfuric acid, and anhydrous dimethyl sulfoxide (DMSO) (Sigma-Aldrich).

The reagents used were salicylic acid, capsaicin, ruthenium red (RR) (Sigma-Aldrich), magnesium sulfate anhydrous (Honeywell Fluka, Morris Plains, NJ, USA), sodium hydroxide (Panreac AppliChem—ITW Reagents, Cinisello Balsamo, Milan, Italy), and ferric chloride (Sigma-Aldrich). Although it is considered in the text as a unique therapeutic agent, according to the supplier's analysis certificate, the purity of the commercial capsaicin used in this work was 61.1%, and it contained 31.2% of dihydrocapsaicin, which is a derivative with very similar chemical and biological properties to capsaicin.

Methyl salicylate was synthesized from the esterification of salicylic acid in a solution of methanol and sulfuric acid by following the method proposed by Carrillo-Arcos *et al.* (2016) [35]. Briefly, the 2-hydroxybenzoic acid (28.96 mmol) was dissolved in 60 mL of methanol, and then sulfuric acid (98%, 2 mL) was added dropwise to the solution, and the mixture was stirred at reflux for 18 h. Next, the solvent of the reaction was removed by vacuum rotary-evaporation, and the crude product was neutralized to pH 5–6 with a solution of NaOH (1 M, 50 mL), which was extracted three times with dichloromethane (3 × 50 mL). The combined organic phases were dried (magnesium sulfate) and concentrated (rotavap). The crude oil was distilled in a Kugelrohr B-585 glass furnace (Büchi, Flawil, Switzerland) to finally obtain a colorless oil (yield of 75%).

2.2. Electrospinning

The preparation of nanofibers was performed by means of the methodology described before by Mira *et al.* (2017) [26]. After optimization, an electrospinnable solution containing 25% w/w of PMVE/MA-ES in ethanol was selected. As for the active agents, a combination of 1.5% salicylic acid, 1% capsaicin (2:1 together with dihydrocapsaicin), and 1% methyl salicylate, all w/w with respect to the polymer weight, was used.

The electrospinning process was performed on a device that included a two-mL Discardit II syringe (Becton Dickinson, Franklin Lakes, NJ, USA) through which the polymer solution was introduced, and from which it was pumped through a blunt-end stainless steel hypodermic needle 316 of 20 Gauge (101.6 mm in length, external diameter 0.902 mm, and internal diameter 0.584 mm) (Sigma-Aldrich) at a sustained flow controlled by a KDS 100 infusion pump (KD Scientific, Holliston, MA, USA). The needle and the aluminum foil collector, faced vertically, are connected to a Series FC high voltage source (Glassman High Voltage Inc., Whitehouse Station, NJ, USA), which provides the voltage responsible for the generation of the jet to be deposited on the collector located at a settled distance. Any material that is intended to be covered with a mat of electrospun nanofibers, as for example in this work, the adhesive dressings, would be placed on the aluminum collector. After the optimization of the operational parameters (see corresponding section for further details), values were selected for the elaboration of the batches of nanofibers for the following experiments.

2.3. Microscopy

For the observation in optical microscopy, the nanofibers were electropun on a microscope slide (Deltalab, Barcelona, Spain) arranged on top of the aluminum collector. The inverted fluorescence optical microscope that was used was a Microsystems DMI3000B (Leica, Bensheim, Germany) equipped with a Leica EL6000 compact light source and a Leica DFC 3000G digital camera. The images were taken with a 63× objective in phase contrast, and the image processing was done manually using the program Leica Application Suite AF 6000 Module Systems. By this methodology, an initial screening, and then a more exhaustive screening, were carried out.

After the optimization of the electrospinning parameters, selected nanofiber samples were also analyzed by scanning electron microscopy (SEM), without metal coating, in a JSM-6360 LV device (Jeol, Tokyo, Japan). In both cases, from the images obtained for each sample, a total of 100 measurements of nanofiber diameters were taken and analyzed by using the Image J software (National Institutes of Health, NIH, Bethesda, MD, USA).

2.4. Gas Chromatography and Mass Spectrometry (GC-MS)

The amount of the therapeutic agents contained in the nanofibers, which are necessary for analyzing the encapsulation efficiency and the stability of the encapsulation over time, was determined by means of a gas chromatograph coupled to a mass spectrometer, in particular, a GCMS-QP2010 SE equipment with quadrupole detector supplemented with a thermal TD-20 adsorption attachment and an AOC-20i/s automatic sample injector (Shimadzu, Kyoto, Japan). The employed GC column was an Agilent J&W capillary HP-5MS UI (5% diphenyl–95% dimethylpolysiloxane, 30 m × 0.25 mm id, film thickness 0.25 μm) (Agilent Technologies Inc., Santa Clara, CA, USA).

The procedure of this analytical methodology is based on a previous study [36]. Briefly, the temperatures of the injector and detector were 250 °C and 210 °C, respectively. Helium was used as a carrier gas at a flow rate of 1.5 mL/min. The chosen program was 40 °C for two minutes; then, the temperature was raised at a speed of 10 °C/min to 240 °C and, thereafter, at a rate of 5 °C/min up to 270 °C, which was finally maintained for five minutes.

In each experiment, a calibration curve was created for each of the analyzed compounds whose concentration ranges were between 0.018–1.420 mg/mL for capsaicin, 0.009–0.720 mg/mL for dihydrocapsaicin, 0.04–3.22 mg/mL for methyl salicylate, and 0.161–3.22 mg/mL for salicylic acid. All of the values that were provided for each curve corresponded to the area under the curve that was obtained for each concentration of the corresponding compound. In this way, the curves were preferably adjusted to a quadratic equation correlating area with concentration R^2 coefficients greater than 0.99 in all of the cases (see Figure S1 in supplementary information).

The analyzed samples corresponded to two independent productions of nanofibers loaded with the three therapeutic agents as described above. Each sample of nanofibers was analyzed when just prepared and at 5 and 15 days post-production. These samples were stored in a drawer, uncovered, protected from light, and at room temperature. Immediately prior to their analysis, the samples were dissolved in dichloromethane, filtered with 0.2-μm nylon membranes (Millipore, Bedford, OH, USA) and injected at a concentration of 10 mg/mL *w/v*. As controls, nanofibers without encapsulated compounds and fresh polymer solutions (made just prior to the electrospinning process) were used.

2.5. Cell Culture

For *in vitro* cell assays, human embryonic kidney cells stably expressing TRPV1 (HEK293-VR1) were used. The cells were maintained in Dulbecco's modified Eagle's medium (DMEM) supplemented with 10% *v/v* fetal bovine serum (FBS) (Sigma-Aldrich) and 50 μg/mL gentamicin (Thermo Fisher Scientific, Waltham, MA, USA). Cells were cultured in 25-cm^2 flasks at 37 °C in a humidified atmosphere with 5% CO_2, and for their harvest they were detached with 0.25% trypsin-EDTA solution. For the assays, cells were seeded in opaque 96-well plates with transparent bottoms (Corning Incorporated, Corning, NY, USA) at a cell density of 40,000 cells three days before treatment.

2.6. TRPV1 Channel Activity Assays

Since the TRPV1 channel allows the non-selective passage of cations such as Ca^{2+} when activated, a Ca^{2+} fluorescence probe has been used to indirectly quantify such activation, which might be induced by the experimental treatments. Thus, Ca^{2+} fluorography assays were performed by using the probe Fluo-4 NW (Molecular Probes-Thermo Fisher Scientific, Waltham, MA, USA) supplemented with

2.5 mM of probenecid, which improves the permeation of the probe in the cells and inhibits losses of fluorescence by avoiding its exit to the cellular exterior, as was recently reported by Serafini *et al.* (2018) [37].

Briefly, in cell plates prepared as described in the previous section, the culture medium was removed, and 100 µL/well of probe solution was added and incubated for 30 min at 37 °C followed by 30 min at 30 °C, always in the dark. Then, the fluorescence measurements were taken (excitation at 485 nm and emission at 535 nm) with a POLARstar Omega plate reader (BMG LABTECH GmbH, Offenburg, Germany) for 20 cycles (each one corresponding to a period of 156 s) and at a constant internal temperature of 30 °C. After the third cycle, one µL/well of each formulation that had been previously dissolved in DMSO at the corresponding concentration was added manually in order to reach the expected treatment doses in the well. In this sense, nanofibers were dissolved at 50 mg/mL in order to treat cells with 54 µM, 33 µM, and 10 µM of salicylic acid, methyl salicylate, and capsaicin, respectively. A solvent control (DMSO), capsaicin as agonist compound at 10 µM [38], and RR as a non-competitive inhibitor [39] at 10 µM were also included. Then, the measurements continued until cycle 20. After cycle 10, one µL of 10 µM capsaicin in DMSO was added to some wells that had been previously treated with RR in order to check the stability and selectivity of the system. Calibration curves for capsaicin and methyl salicylate were also included (range 0.1–30 µM and 15–120 µM, respectively). Each sample was analyzed in triplicate in each assay.

2.7. Preliminary In Vivo Test of Topical Application

An initial *in vivo* study was carried out with three healthy human volunteers to evaluate, when administered topically, the stability time of the experimental nanofibers, as well as to determine the functionality of the encapsulated TRPV1 agonists by analyzing the responsiveness to them. Each volunteer was given an adhesive dressing with electrospun nanofibers on each arm on the skin surface of the deltoid. This test was blind, since for each volunteer, one of the dressings contained empty nanofibers, and the other contained drug-loaded ones, but they were assigned randomly to each of their arms. Each dressing contained approximately 25 mg of nanofibers distributed over a surface area of 20 cm^2. The duration of the treatment was eight hours. The surface of the dressing was kept protected from light throughout the full period. Every two hours, photographs were taken of each dressing to determine the state of the nanofibers and treated skin. At the end of the trial, each volunteer was asked which dressing they thought contained the TRPV1 agonists. This study was approved by the Project Evaluation Board of Miguel Hernández University (approval no. 2018.12.05.FPRL).

2.8. Data Analysis and Graphics

Data were analyzed by either GraphPad Prism v6 and Microsoft Excel software. Both of them were used for creating the graphs. Statistical analysis was performed with GraphPad Prism v6 specifically. Applied statistical methods are stated together with the analyzed data in the Results section.

3. Results and Discussion

3.1. Optimization of PMVE/MA-ES Nanofibers Encapsulating Three Therapeutic Agents

Initially, we proceeded to the optimization of the morphology and size of the nanofibers without the encapsulated agent. For this, the operational values of the electrospinning procedure were modulated within a range that had been estimated from our previous study [26]. They included a concentration of PMVEMA-ES (20–28% w/w), pumping flow (0.25–1.35 mL/h), voltage (6–17.5 kV), and distance between the needle and collector (8–30 cm).

The concentration of polymer was shown to be determinant for the morphology and size of the final nanofibers. Independently of the other parameters, the values of greater uniformity and smaller fiber diameter were obtained with a concentration of 25% w/w of PMVE/MA-ES (as in our previous study [26]). Therefore, the concentration of polymer was fixed at this value for the analysis of the rest of the operational parameters, which were shown to be inversely proportional to the size of the nanofibers until reaching a critical value at which abrupt increases in size or the appearance of morphological aberrations could be observed. In short, the combination of values with which the smallest uniform fibers (810 ± 141 nm) were obtained were 15.5 kV, 12 cm, and 0.25 mL/h (Figure 1). However, when adding the therapeutic agents, nanofibers were significantly larger (about 200 nm more) by using these same parameters; the reason we proceeded to refine them again under these new circumstances was in order to reduce the size of the nanofibers below the micron. Thus, the optimal values to obtain uniform nanofibers of 878 ± 209 nm were 17 kV voltage, an eight cm needle–collector distance, and a flow of 0.25 mL/h (Figure 1).

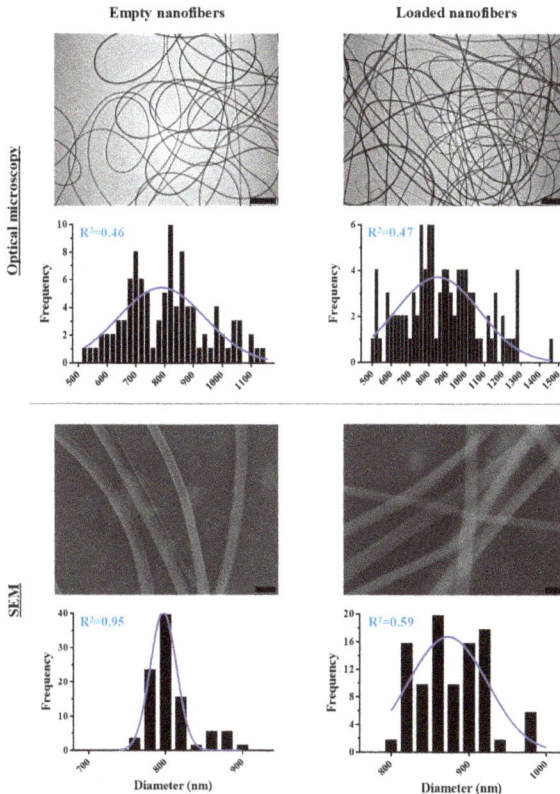

Figure 1. Optical microscopy and SEM analysis of optimized nanofibers. Representative optical microscopy and SEM images that include either empty or loaded nanofibers obtained by using optimized electrospinning parameters are shown (scale bars: 25 μm for optical microscopy, and 1 μm for SEM images). Corresponding frequency histograms of their diameters are also included. Each histogram was performed from the data obtained from several images until reaching 100 measurements. Best-fit adjustments (and their R^2) to a Gaussian distribution are indicated in blue.

So far, the analysis of the nanofibers had been done by optical microscopy; however, to analyze the morphology in more detail and with greater precision, the size of the optimized nanofibers was observed by SEM. The measurements obtained by electron microscopy are equivalent to those obtained by optical microscopy: 808 ± 31 nm for empty nanofibers, and 875 ± 49 nm for those with encapsulated therapeutic content (Figure 1).

The low amount of encapsulated drug that was used in this work (3.5% all together) does not explain the increase in size that was observed in the loaded nanofibers, even more considering that loading percentages are usually much higher for molecules that have a similar complexity, which even reduces nanofiber diameters [40,41]. Neither did an incompatibility in solubility, since all three compounds are soluble in the polymer-solvent system that was used. In fact, this aspect has been reported as critical, as well as the adequate selection of the solvent [42,43], for the morphology of fibers [44]. In this sense, from a broad perspective, the factors influencing fiber morphology are classified into two main groups: the processing and solution ones (briefly reviewed in [45]). Thus, while the processing factors are associated with the electrospinning mechanical set-up and environmental conditions, such as relative humidity, the solution factors refer to the physicochemical characteristics of the electrospinning solution, and, among them, some of the relevant ones are the conductivity and viscosity, according to several authors [41,45,46]. Therefore, if the addition of a compound, or a combination of them, is significantly affecting the final morphology of fibers, it might be as a consequence of modifying such solution parameters. Given that, as reported in studies, within moderate drug-loading ranges, fiber diameters generally increase with decreasing conductivity or increasing viscosity values [40,41,45,47,48], the combination of compounds that was used in the present work may be affecting the electrospinning solution either way, but most probably by increasing the viscosity of the solution, since none of the molecules employed was either a salt or a polyelectrolyte [40,41].

3.2. Determination of the Encapsulated Content and Its Stability over Time

To quantify the amount of encapsulated therapeutic agent, they were separated by gas chromatography, and then identified with mass spectrometry. In the calibration process, the elution times were precisely determined for the four compounds: methyl salicylate, 12.5 min; salicylic acid, 14.0 min; capsaicin, 29.0 min; and dihydrocapsaicin, 29.3 min (for further details in this regard, see Figure S1 in the supplementary information).

By following this procedure, the encapsulation efficiency was calculated for each therapeutic agent, which was found to be approximately 100% (in comparison to theoretical full encapsulation) in all cases when measuring right after the production of nanofibers ($t = 0$, data not shown). Such value was used as a reference for calculating the encapsulated content over time (Figure 2). Regarding the permanence of the encapsulated content, the obtained results indicate that methyl salicylate is lost over time; specifically, after 15 days, just $60.2 \pm 7.8\%$ of methyl salicylate remained in fibers. Regarding the other agents, there seemed to be a tendency to decrease the quantity of encapsulated compound, but these changes were not significant in the period of time that was analyzed (0–15 days).

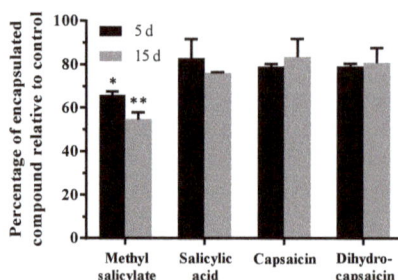

Figure 2. Stability of the loaded compounds over time. The graph indicates the percentage of compound that remained encapsulated in the nanofibers 5 and 15 days (d) after they were produced. Compound content was determined by GC-MS. Values are relative to the content measured right after the production of the nanofibers. Statistical analysis comprised multiple *t* test corrected for multiple comparisons by using the Holm–Sidak method. Significant changes in the content of each compound over time with respect to the corresponding initial values are indicated as: *, $p < 0.05$ and **, $p < 0.01$.

Thus, by adjusting the operational parameters, it is possible to load the nanofibers described here with approximately 100% efficiency by using a concentration of 3.5% w/w of the three compounds, all together. In addition, the absence of significant changes in size and shape suggests that their encapsulation capacity might be higher. In this sense, by using the same nanostructured system, they were loaded with up to 16.6% w/w of 5-aminolevulinic acid in PMVE/MA-ES and Ac nanofibers [26]. Other evidence of electrospun nanofibers made of a blend of other polymers and PMVE/MA were shown to be able to be loaded with even zinc oxide-containing nanoparticles [33] and silver nanoparticles [34]. Indeed, the electrospinning technique allows loadability concentrations of up to 60% w/w in some cases [49] and encapsulation yields close to full efficiency levels [26,50].

Regarding the concentration of each therapeutic agent proposed, salicylic acid is usually used at concentrations of 0.5–60% w/w for the treatment of psoriasis [51]. The concentration that was chosen in this work was 1.5% w/w, which is similar to the concentrations used in acne creams [52]. The use of methyl salicylate in nanostructures has not been described yet, but it is in other topical applications to treat pain in general, especially musculoskeletal pain [21]. The concentrations of this compound used in creams are usually 10–30% w/w (*Bengay* and *Icy Hot* creams) and even 45% in the case of the *Reflex* gel. In the case of capsaicin, it has been used at 1% w/w, as in the present study, with respect to the base polymer in nanofibers and nanoparticles for topical use in psoriasis [53,54]. In addition, there is a commercial patch of 8% capsaicin, *Qutenza Astellas*, which is used to treat neuropathic pain.

One of the most surprising results was the loss of product observed for methyl salicylate, which seems to be due to the increase in surface area with respect to the volume that occurs in one-dimensional materials when they are nanostructured, which increases the evaporation of the encapsulated substances [55]. This effect would also be increased in those more volatile molecules, such as in the case of methyl salicylate, which is liquid at room temperature (melting point (mp): −9 °C), while capsaicin and salicylic acid are solid (mp: 62 and 159 °C, respectively). In any case, this loss of compound could be avoided or delayed by packaging the nanofiber mats tightly and hermetically, as is done for other similar products with volatile compounds. On the contrary, this might be an advantage for topical applications because of the possibility of gradually alternating the release of different compounds. From the *in vitro* skin permeability studies performed in our previous work to evaluate the potential of this polymeric family for topical applications [26], it was concluded that nanofibers made with this same material can achieve both fast and high rates of transdermal release of a non-volatile compound (90% of 5-ALA release in two hours by following a Higuchi kinetic model). However, under these conditions that mimic those existing in the human dermal surface (high humidity and 32.5 °C), the diffusion of a more volatile compound, such as methyl salicylate, should be faster, anticipating its treatment with respect to the less volatile ones.

3.3. Assessment of the Activation Capacity of TRPV1 by the Encapsulated Agents

The activity of the TRPV1 agonist compounds encapsulated in the experimental nanofibers (only methyl salicylate and capsaicin, not salicylic acid), alone or in combination with the other two agents (i.e., all three compounds), was assessed by treating HEK293-VR1 cells. These results were represented in percentages relative to the highest value obtained for the activation induced by capsaicin at 10 μM and using the lowest one after inoculating RR as the baseline.

Firstly, in Figure 3A, records of values induced by control samples to check the validity of the system are shown. As can be observed, both methyl salicylate and capsaicin are able to activate TRPV1 by inducing an increase of fluorescence because of the internal increase of Ca^{2+} after being inoculated in cycle three. The graph also shows that TRPV1 is highly activated right after the inoculation of each agent and remains at high levels, which even increase in the case of capsaicin. The specificity of the system is checked by the blocking of the channel with RR, which is even able to desensitize it to a subsequent stimulation with capsaicin (cycle 10). Figure 3 also shows that the activation of TRPV1 is concentration-dependent for both compounds (Figure 3B and 3C for methyl salicylate and capsaicin, respectively), considering the highest value from each time-course analysis for the calculations. In the specific case of methyl salicylate, this curve seems to plateau within the range of concentrations used, from 60 µM in particular.

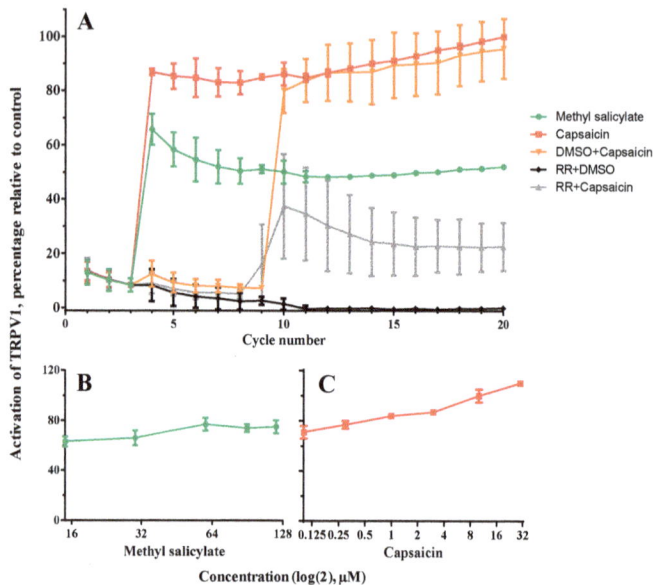

Figure 3. Functional analysis of transient receptor potential cation channel 1 (TRPV1) *in vitro* and calibration of its agonists. (**A**) TRPV1 activation dynamics were determined by performing fluorescence time-course assays in cells stably expressing TRPV1 after treatment with agonists (30 µM of methyl salicylate and 10 µM of capsaicin) and antagonist (ruthenium red, RR). TRPV1 activation was observed once agonists were added, while the inoculation of the antagonist attenuated this response. (**B,C**) Additionally, concentrations of agonists lower and higher than those to be tested from produced nanofibers under these experimental conditions were assayed in order to better assess the functionality of the compounds when they were encapsulated. For all analysis, the level of activation is calculated as the percentage relative to the highest value from the time-course in cells treated with 10 µM of capsaicin, and relative to the lowest value from RR treatment as the baseline.

For the comparison of the activity of the agonist compounds on TRPV1 when they are encapsulated in nanofibers, alone or together with the other therapeutic agents, the same above-described procedure was followed, but including experimental nanofibers that were previously dissolved in DMSO. In these *in vitro* cell assays (Figure 4), although the obtained values were moderately higher when the agent was encapsulated, no significant changes were found between the encapsulated and non-encapsulated compounds, and only significant variations were found, as expected, when comparing each compound among them (two-way ANOVA corrected with Tukey's test for multiple comparisons; $F(3, 8) = 15.59$; $p = 0.0011$), meaning that the encapsulation process did not affect the chemical properties of the encapsulated agents. Some activation of TRPV1 was also observed when treating with empty nanofibers.

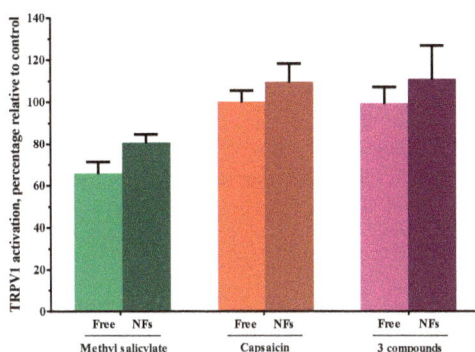

Figure 4. Effect of the encapsulation on the ability of the experimental compounds to activate TRPV1. Fluorescence time-course assays were performed on cells stably expressing TRPV1 and treated with the agonist compounds employed either alone or in combination, and also including salicylic acid (three compounds). These samples included compound-containing nanofibers (NFs) and non-encapsulated compounds (Free). The level of activation is calculated as the percentage relative to the highest value from the time-course in cells treated with 10 µM of capsaicin and the lowest value from RR treatment. Statistical analysis comprised two-way ANOVA corrected with Tukey's test for multiple comparisons (Free vs. NFs) and no significant differences were found between the experimental and control samples.

The combination of different compounds within the same formulation generally pursues a synergistic effect that could allow the reduction of the concentration of each one, and thus their potential adverse effects; however, other benefits from such an approach might be the combination of other functional properties such as, in this case, the ones introduced previously, which are also related to treating psoriasis and other factors such as their antimicrobial activities [56,57].

Finally, but also related to the assessment of the ability of the developed nanofibers to activate TRPV1, it has been possible to successfully electrospin the experimental nanofibers on adhesive dressings for topical application and preliminarily check their gradual degradation by visual observation, as well as their content release by assessing the typical reddening reaction of the capsaicin in the skin (Figure 5). Both effects were evident eight hours after the application of the patch covered with loaded nanofibers on the skin from volunteers' arms. In this sense, no effects were either observed or detected on skin when treating with control patches based on empty nanofibers. Future studies will be aimed at describing the release and dermal absorption of this system, as well as at revealing the possible effect of the polymers on TRPV1.

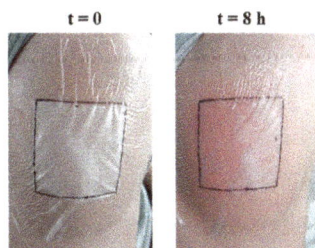

Figure 5. Preliminary assessment of the feasibility of transdermal patches based on experimental nanofibers. Dressings for topical applications produced by electrospinning experimental nanofibers onto adhesive patches were developed and tested for up to eight hours on volunteers' arms. Representative pictures of their application are shown at both the beginning and the end of the test. After eight hours of treatment, the degradation of the nanofibers and the typical reddening of the skin as a consequence of the action of capsaicin on the surface of the skin were observed.

4. Conclusions

In this work, it has been possible to optimize the electrospinning parameters to create PMVE/MA-ES nanofibers loaded with a combination of three compounds with therapeutic activity to alleviate the dermal symptoms of psoriasis (salicylic acid, methyl salicylate, and capsaicin at a concentration of 3.5% w/w all together with respect to the amount of polymer), with an encapsulation efficiency of approximately 100%. The stability studies of the content encapsulated over time (up to 15 days after its production) showed significant losses especially of methyl salicylate, which were probably due to its higher volatility. *In vitro* studies revealed that the TRPV1 agonist compounds maintained their channel-activating capacity at the expected levels after being encapsulated. Finally, it was found that the proposed nanofibers are suitable for the creation of skin adhesive dressings and allow the release of the encapsulated compounds by the disintegration of the nanostructure. In this study, the effect of those compounds with the capacity to activate TRPV1 was checked *in vivo*.

Supplementary Materials: The following are available online at http://www.mdpi.com/1999-4923/11/1/14/s1, Figure S1: GC-MS chromatograms and calibration curves.

Author Contributions: Conceptualization, R.M. and A.F.; methodology, L.M.-O., A.M., A.F.-C and A.F.; software, L.M.-O. and A.F.; validation, A.F.-C.; formal analysis, R.M. and A.F.; investigation, L.M.-O., A.M. and A.F.; resources, C.R.M. and R.M.; data curation, A.F.; writing—original draft preparation, A.F.; writing—review and editing, A.F.-C., C.R.M., R.M. and A.F.; visualization, A.F.; supervision, R.M. and A.F.; project administration, C.R.M. and R.M.; funding acquisition, C.R.M. and R.M.

Funding: This research was funded by the Spanish Ministerio de Economía y Competitividad grant numbers MAT-2017-86805-R and MAT-2014-53282-R.

Acknowledgments: We thank Elisa Pérez and Irene Mudarra-Fraguas for technical assistance. It is also appreciated the collaboration of the volunteers in the preliminary topical test.

Conflicts of Interest: The authors declare no conflict of interest.

References

1. Boehncke, W.H.; Schon, M.P. Psoriasis. *Lancet* **2015**, *386*, 983–994. [CrossRef]
2. Christophers, E. Psoriasis—Epidemiology and clinical spectrum. *Clin. Exp. Dermatol.* **2001**, *26*, 314–320. [CrossRef] [PubMed]
3. Nickoloff, B.J.; Qin, J.Z.; Nestle, F.O. Immunopathogenesis of psoriasis. *Clin. Rev. Allergy Immunol.* **2007**, *33*, 45–56. [CrossRef] [PubMed]
4. Nickoloff, B.J. Cracking the cytokine code in psoriasis. *Nat. Med.* **2007**, *13*, 242–244. [CrossRef] [PubMed]
5. Di Cesare, A.; Di Meglio, P.; Nestle, F.O. The IL-23/Th17 axis in the immunopathogenesis of psoriasis. *J. Investig. Dermatol.* **2009**, *129*, 1339–1350. [CrossRef] [PubMed]
6. MacDonald, A.; Burden, A.D. Psoriasis: Advances in pathophysiology and management. *Postgrad. Med. J.* **2007**, *83*, 690–697. [CrossRef]
7. Wozel, G. Psoriasis treatment in difficult locations: Scalp, nails, and intertriginous areas. *Clin. Dermatol.* **2008**, *26*, 448–459. [CrossRef]
8. Raut, A.S.; Prabhu, R.H.; Patravale, V.B. Psoriasis clinical implications and treatment: A review. *Crit. Rev. Ther. Drug Carrier Syst.* **2013**, *30*, 183–216. [CrossRef]
9. Hsu, L.; Snodgrass, B.T.; Armstrong, A.W. Antidrug antibodies in psoriasis: A systematic review. *Br. J. Dermatol.* **2014**, *170*, 261–273. [CrossRef]
10. Ryan, C.; Korman, N.J.; Gelfand, J.M.; Lim, H.W.; Elmets, C.A.; Feldman, S.R.; Gottlieb, A.B.; Koo, J.Y.; Lebwohl, M.; Leonardi, C.L.; et al. Research gaps in psoriasis: Opportunities for future studies. *J. Am. Acad. Dermatol.* **2014**, *70*, 146–167. [CrossRef]
11. Fluhr, J.W.; Cavallotti, C.; Berardesca, E. Emollients, moisturizers, and keratolytic agents in psoriasis. *Clin. Dermatol.* **2008**, *26*, 380–386. [CrossRef]
12. Dawn, A.; Yosipovitch, G. Treating itch in psoriasis. *Dermatol. Nurs.* **2006**, *18*, 227.
13. Caterina, M.J.; Schumacher, M.A.; Tominaga, M.; Rosen, T.A.; Levine, J.D.; Julius, D. The capsaicin receptor: A heat-activated ion channel in the pain pathway. *Nature* **1997**, *389*, 816–824. [PubMed]

14. Ferrer-Montiel, A.; García-Martínez, C.; Morenilla-Palao, C.; García-Sanz, N.; Fernández-Carvajal, A.; Fernández-Ballester, G.; Planells-Cases, R. Molecular architecture of the vanilloid receptor. *FEBS J.* **2004**, *271*, 1820–1826.

15. Baumann, T.K.; Martenson, M.E. Extracellular protons both increase the activity and reduce the conductance of capsaicin-gated channels. *J. Neurosci.* **2000**, *20*, RC80. [CrossRef] [PubMed]

16. Anand, P.; Bley, K. Topical capsaicin for pain management: Therapeutic potential and mechanisms of action of the new high-concentration capsaicin 8% patch. *Br. J. Anaesth.* **2011**, *107*, 490–502. [CrossRef] [PubMed]

17. Zhao, J.J.; Hu, Y.W.; Huang, C.; Ma, X.; Kang, C.M.; Zhang, Y.; Guo, F.X.; Lu, J.B.; Xiu, J.C.; Qiu, Y.R.; et al. Dihydrocapsaicin suppresses proinflammatory cytokines expression by enhancing nuclear factor ia in a nf-kappab-dependent manner. *Arch. Biochem. Biophys.* **2016**, *604*, 27–35. [CrossRef]

18. Tang, J.; Luo, K.; Li, Y.; Chen, Q.; Tang, D.; Wang, D.; Xiao, J. Capsaicin attenuates LPS-induced inflammatory cytokine production by upregulation of LXR alpha. *Int. Immunopharmacol.* **2015**, *28*, 264–269. [CrossRef]

19. Reyes-Escogido, M.d.L.; Gonzalez-Mondragon, E.G.; Vazquez-Tzompantzi, E. Chemical and pharmacological aspects of capsaicin. *Molecules* **2011**, *16*, 1253–1270. [CrossRef]

20. Bode, A.M.; Dong, Z. The two faces of capsaicin. *Cancer Res.* **2011**, *71*, 2809–2814. [CrossRef]

21. Ohta, T.; Imagawa, T.; Ito, S. Involvement of transient receptor potential vanilloid subtype 1 in analgesic action of methylsalicylate. *Mol. Pharmacol.* **2009**, *75*, 307–317. [CrossRef] [PubMed]

22. Wu, K.K.-Y. Biochemical pharmacology of nonsteroidal anti-inflammatory drugs. *Biochem. Pharmacol.* **1998**, *55*, 543–547. [PubMed]

23. Xie, J.; Li, X.; Xia, Y. Putting electrospun nanofibers to work for biomedical research. *Macromol. Rapid Commun.* **2008**, *29*, 1775–1792. [CrossRef] [PubMed]

24. Ji, W.; Sun, Y.; Yang, F.; van den Beucken, J.J.; Fan, M.; Chen, Z.; Jansen, J.A. Bioactive electrospun scaffolds delivering growth factors and genes for tissue engineering applications. *Pharm. Res.* **2011**, *28*, 1259–1272. [CrossRef] [PubMed]

25. Bhardwaj, N.; Kundu, S.C. Electrospinning: A fascinating fiber fabrication technique. *Biotechnol. Adv.* **2010**, *28*, 325–347. [CrossRef] [PubMed]

26. Mira, A.; Mateo, C.R.; Mallavia, R.; Falco, A. Poly (methyl vinyl ether-alt-maleic acid) and ethyl monoester as building polymers for drug-loadable electrospun nanofibers. *Sci. Rep.* **2017**, *7*, 17205. [CrossRef] [PubMed]

27. Iglesias, T.; de Cerain, A.L.; Irache, J.; Martín-Arbella, N.; Wilcox, M.; Pearson, J.; Azqueta, A. Evaluation of the cytotoxicity, genotoxicity and mucus permeation capacity of several surface modified poly (anhydride) nanoparticles designed for oral drug delivery. *Int. J. Pharm.* **2017**, *517*, 67–79. [CrossRef]

28. Iglesias, T.; Dusinska, M.; El Yamani, N.; Irache, J.M.; Azqueta, A.; Lopez de Cerain, A. In vitro evaluation of the genotoxicity of poly(anhydride) nanoparticles designed for oral drug delivery. *Int. J. Pharm.* **2017**, *523*, 418–426. [CrossRef]

29. Prieto, E.; Puente, B.; Uixera, A.; Garcia de Jalon, J.A.; Perez, S.; Pablo, L.; Irache, J.M.; Garcia, M.A.; Bregante, M.A. Gantrez an nanoparticles for ocular delivery of memantine: In vitro release evaluation in albino rabbits. *Ophthalmic Res.* **2012**, *48*, 109–117. [CrossRef]

30. Gardner, C.M.; Burke, N.A.; Chu, T.; Shen, F.; Potter, M.A.; Stover, H.D. Poly(methyl vinyl ether-alt-maleic acid) polymers for cell encapsulation. *J. Biomater. Sci. Polym. Ed.* **2011**, *22*, 2127–2145. [CrossRef]

31. Kahveci, Z.; Vazquez-Guillo, R.; Mira, A.; Martinez, L.; Falco, A.; Mallavia, R.; Mateo, C.R. Selective recognition and imaging of bacterial model membranes over mammalian ones by using cationic conjugated polyelectrolytes. *Analyst* **2016**, *141*, 6287–6296. [CrossRef] [PubMed]

32. Vázquez-Guilló, R.; Falco, A.; Martínez-Tomé, M.J.; Mateo, C.R.; Herrero, M.A.; Vázquez, E.; Mallavia, R. Advantageous microwave-assisted suzuki polycondensation for the synthesis of aniline-fluorene alternate copolymers as molecular model with solvent sensing properties. *Polymers* **2018**, *10*, 215. [CrossRef]

33. Chhabra, H.; Deshpande, R.; Kanitkar, M.; Jaiswal, A.; Kale, V.P.; Bellare, J.R. A nano zinc oxide doped electrospun scaffold improves wound healing in a rodent model. *RSC Adv.* **2016**, *6*, 1428–1439. [CrossRef]

34. Xavier, P.; Jain, S.; Chatterjee, K.; Bose, S. Designer porous antibacterial membranes derived from thermally induced phase separation of PS/PVME blends decorated with an electrospun nanofiber scaffold. *RSC Adv.* **2016**, *6*, 10865–10872. [CrossRef]

35. Carrillo-Arcos, U.A.; Rojas-Ocampo, J.; Porcel, S. Oxidative cyclization of alkenoic acids promoted by agoac. *Dalton Trans.* **2016**, *45*, 479–483. [CrossRef] [PubMed]

36. Gonzalez-Penas, E.; Lopez-Alvarez, M.; de Narvajas, F.M.; Ursua, A. Simultaneous gc determination of turpentine, camphor, menthol and methyl salicylate in a topical analgesic formulation (dologex®). *Chromatographia* **2000**, *52*, 245–248. [CrossRef]

37. Serafini, M.; Griglio, A.; Aprile, S.; Seiti, F.; Travelli, C.; Pattarino, F.; Grosa, G.; Sorba, G.; Genazzani, A.A.; Gonzalez-Rodriguez, S.; et al. Targeting transient receptor potential vanilloid 1 (TRPV1) channel softly: The discovery of passerini adducts as a topical treatment for inflammatory skin disorders. *J. Med. Chem.* **2018**, *61*, 4436–4455. [CrossRef]

38. Kim, S.; Kang, C.; Shin, C.Y.; Hwang, S.W.; Yang, Y.D.; Shim, W.S.; Park, M.-Y.; Kim, E.; Kim, M.; Kim, B.-M. TRPV1 recapitulates native capsaicin receptor in sensory neurons in association with Fas-associated factor 1. *J. Neurosci.* **2006**, *26*, 2403–2412. [CrossRef]

39. Dray, A.; Forbes, C.; Burgess, G. Ruthenium red blocks the capsaicin-induced increase in intracellular calcium and activation of membrane currents in sensory neurones as well as the activation of peripheral nociceptors in vitro. *Neurosci. Lett.* **1990**, *110*, 52–59. [CrossRef]

40. Shen, X.; Yu, D.; Zhu, L.; Branford-White, C.; White, K.; Chatterton, N.P. Electrospun diclofenac sodium loaded Eudragit® L 100-55 nanofibers for colon-targeted drug delivery. *Int. J. Pharm.* **2011**, *408*, 200–207. [CrossRef]

41. Samprasit, W.; Akkaramongkolporn, P.; Ngawhirunpat, T.; Rojanarata, T.; Kaomongkolgit, R.; Opanasopit, P. Fast releasing oral electrospun PVP/CD nanofiber mats of taste-masked meloxicam. *Int. J. Pharm.* **2015**, *487*, 213–222. [CrossRef] [PubMed]

42. Moghe, A.; Gupta, B. Co-axial electrospinning for nanofiber structures: Preparation and applications. *Polym. Rev.* **2008**, *48*, 353–377. [CrossRef]

43. Liu, Y.; Ma, G.; Fang, D.; Xu, J.; Zhang, H.; Nie, J. Effects of solution properties and electric field on the electrospinning of hyaluronic acid. *Carbohydr. Polym.* **2011**, *83*, 1011–1015. [CrossRef]

44. Zeng, J.; Xu, X.; Chen, X.; Liang, Q.; Bian, X.; Yang, L.; Jing, X. Biodegradable electrospun fibers for drug delivery. *J. Control. Release* **2003**, *92*, 227–231. [CrossRef]

45. Nezarati, R.M.; Eifert, M.B.; Cosgriff-Hernandez, E. Effects of humidity and solution viscosity on electrospun fiber morphology. *Tissue Eng. Part C Methods* **2013**, *19*, 810–819. [CrossRef] [PubMed]

46. Fong, H.; Chun, I.; Reneker, D. Beaded nanofibers formed during electrospinning. *Polymer* **1999**, *40*, 4585–4592. [CrossRef]

47. Reda, R.I.; Wen, M.M.; El-Kamel, A.H. Ketoprofen-loaded eudragit electrospun nanofibers for the treatment of oral mucositis. *Int. J. Nanomed.* **2017**, *12*, 2335–2351. [CrossRef] [PubMed]

48. Canbolat, M.F.; Celebioglu, A.; Uyar, T. Drug delivery system based on cyclodextrin-naproxen inclusion complex incorporated in electrospun polycaprolactone nanofibers. *Colloids Surf. B* **2014**, *115*, 15–21. [CrossRef]

49. Krogstad, E.A.; Woodrow, K.A. Manufacturing scale-up of electrospun poly (vinyl alcohol) fibers containing tenofovir for vaginal drug delivery. *Int. J. Pharm.* **2014**, *475*, 282–291. [CrossRef]

50. Ball, C.; Woodrow, K.A. Electrospun solid dispersions of maraviroc for rapid intravaginal preexposure prophylaxis of hiv. *Antimicrob. Agents Chemother.* **2014**, *58*, 4855–4865. [CrossRef]

51. Lebwohl, M. The role of salicylic acid in the treatment of psoriasis. *Int. J. Dermatol.* **1999**, *38*, 16–24. [CrossRef] [PubMed]

52. Zheng, Y.; Wan, M.; Chen, H.; Ye, C.; Zhao, Y.; Yi, J.; Xia, Y.; Lai, W. Clinical evidence on the efficacy and safety of an antioxidant optimized 1.5% salicylic acid (SA) cream in the treatment of facial acne: An open, baseline-controlled clinical study. *Skin Res. Technol.* **2013**, *19*, 125–130. [CrossRef] [PubMed]

53. Opanasopit, P.; Sila-on, W.; Rojanarata, T.; Ngawhirunpat, T. Fabrication and properties of capsicum extract-loaded PVA and CA nanofiber patches. *Pharm. Dev. Technol.* **2013**, *18*, 1140–1147. [CrossRef] [PubMed]

54. Gupta, R.; Gupta, M.; Mangal, S.; Agrawal, U.; Vyas, S.P. Capsaicin-loaded vesicular systems designed for enhancing localized delivery for psoriasis therapy. *Artif. Cells Nanomed. Biotechnol.* **2016**, *44*, 825–834. [CrossRef]

55. Sánchez, L.M.D.; Rodríguez, L.; López, M. Electrospinning: La era de las nanofibras. *Rev. Iberoam. Polím.* **2013**, *14*, 10–27.

56. Özçelik, B.; Kartal, M.; Orhan, I. Cytotoxicity, antiviral and antimicrobial activities of alkaloids, flavonoids, and phenolic acids. *Pharm. Biol.* **2011**, *49*, 396–402. [CrossRef]
57. Kantouch, A.; El-Sayed, A.A.; Salama, M.; El-Kheir, A.A.; Mowafi, S. Salicylic acid and some of its derivatives as antibacterial agents for viscose fabric. *Int. J. Biol. Macromol.* **2013**, *62*, 603–607. [CrossRef]

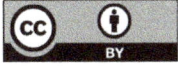

pharmaceutics

MDPI

Article

Homogenization of Amorphous Solid Dispersions Prepared by Electrospinning in Low-Dose Tablet Formulation

Gergő Fülöp [1,2], Attila Balogh [2], Balazs Farkas [2], Attila Farkas [2], Bence Szabó [2], Balázs Démuth [2], Enikő Borbás [2], Zsombor Kristóf Nagy [2,*] and György Marosi [2]

[1]   Gedeon Richter Plc., Formulation R&D, Gyömrői Street 19-21, H-1103 Budapest, Hungary;
       fulop.gergo89@gmail.com
[2]   Department of Organic Chemistry and Technology, Budapest University of Technology and Economics,
       Budafoki út 8. 3, H-1103 Budapest, Hungary; baloghattila5@gmail.com (A.B.);
       farkasbalazs09@gmail.com (B.F.); farkas.attila88@gmail.com (A.F.); szabob@oct.bme.hu (B.S.);
       demuth@oct.bme.hu (B.D.); eniko.borbas@gmail.com (E.B.); gmarosi@mail.bme.hu (G.M.)
*   Correspondence: zsknagy@oct.bme.hu; Tel.: +36-1-463-1424

Received: 15 June 2018; Accepted: 23 July 2018; Published: 2 August 2018

Abstract: Low-dose tablet formulations were produced with excellent homogeneity based on drug-loaded electrospun fibers prepared by single-needle as well as scaled-up electrospinning (SNES and HSES). Carvedilol (CAR), a BCS II class compound, served as the model drug while poly (vinylpyrrolidone-*co*-vinyl acetate) (PVPVA64) was adopted as the fiber-forming polymer. Scanning electron microscopy (SEM) imaging was used to study the morphology of HSES and SNES samples. Different homogenization techniques were compared to maximize homogeneity: mixing in plastic bags and in a high-shear granulator resulting in low-shear mixing (LSM) and high-shear mixing (HSM). Drug content and homogeneity of the tablets were measured by UV-Vis spectrometry, the results revealed acceptably low-dose fluctuations especially with formulations homogenized with HSM. Sieve analysis was used on the final LSM and HSM powder mixtures in order to elucidate the observed differences between tablet homogeneity. Tablets containing drug-loaded electrospun fibers were also studied by Raman mapping demonstrating evenly distributed CAR within the corpus.

Keywords: carvedilol; poly (vinylpyrrolidone-*co*-vinyl acetate); high-speed electrospinning; high-shear mixing; homogenization; Raman mapping; sieve analysis

---

1. Introduction

Tablets are generally regarded as the most popular and accepted dosage forms in pharmaceutical technology. Their ease of manufacturing and high patient compliance make them an ideal choice for both the industry and therapeutics [1]. Tablets are available with doses ranging from very low (micrograms) to very high (1–2 g). In such extreme cases, manufacturing becomes more challenging which is especially true for microgram dosed formulations. Handling low quantities of active pharmaceutical ingredients (APIs) can often lead to decreased drug content and high relative standard deviation (RSD) values in the final batches [2]. Proper content uniformity (CU) among others is one of the basic requirements of tablets by Pharmacopeias across the world [3] ensuring high quality and patient safety.

In terms of formulation development, amorphous solid dispersions (ASD) are getting more recognition since enhanced dissolution and bioavailability can be achieved this way [4]. Techniques capable of manufacturing ASDs on the industrial scale, such as spray drying (SD) [5] and hot-melt extrusion (HME) [6] have already produced FDA approved formulations such as Raplixa [7] and NuvaRing [8]. However, SD generally requires high capital investment for the equipment and its maintenance, while it has a low thermal efficiency due to the large volume of hot air circulating in the drying chamber [9]. HME usually operates at even higher temperatures that should be avoided in case of thermosensitive components and it is not applicable for ASD formation in case of APIs of very high melting points [10].

On the other hand, both SD and HME are continuous technologies, which are heavily encouraged by the leading regulatory agencies [11]. Continuous manufacturing has multiple advantages over traditional batch methods, such as huge improvement in productivity, time-efficiency, less energy requirement and a reduced amount of actual waste [12]. As of today, three products have been produced and approved this way in the following chronological order: Orkambi (lumacaftor/ivacaftor) manufactured by Vertex [13], Prezista (darunavir) produced by Janssen [14] and Symdeko (tezacaftor/ivacaftor and ivacaftor) also developed by Vertex [15].

Electrospinning (ES) is a unique method enabling the production of ASDs from a polymer solution or melt [16,17]. Applying ES polymer fibers are formed in the micro and nanometer scale by the creation and elongation of an electrified fluid jet [18]. In comparison with the aforementioned ASD producing technologies, ES operates at ambient conditions resulting in a gentle drying process at minimal costs [19]. The electrospun fibers have an enormous surface area where the API is often molecularly dispersed in a polymer matrix, producing a nano-amorphous solid dispersion (NASD) [20–23]. ES is also being investigated for various biomedical purposes for its advantages in controlled delivery [24–27], tissue engineering [28,29], wound dressing, enzyme immobilization and biodrug delivery [30].

Regarding scaled-up nanofiber production, the high-speed electrospinning (HSES) technology has the capability to produce approximately half kg of product per hour [31] in accordance with industrial guidelines, while the traditional single-needle electrospinning (SNES) technique can only produce a few grams per hour at best [32,33]. HSES achieves this increased output by combining electrostatic and high-speed rotational jet generation [34,35]. There are also other alternate methods such as pressurized gyration [36], infusion gyration [37] and pressure-coupled infusion gyration [38], that have shown the capability of increased nanofiber output. The latest results and their possible future implications are assembled in a most recent review article [39].

The tableting of electrospun nanofibrous materials is a rather new concept so only a few studies have been reported that tackle this field [40–42]. However, there is no publication dealing with the homogeneity challenges in tablet formulation. Based on our previous experiences, this can be mainly attributed to the flowability concerns during downstream processing of the ES material. Moreover, ensuring homogeneity, and thus, appropriate CU can be a tall order when very low doses are needed especially in the case of tablets based on electrospun fibers [43].

To produce ES-based tablets on the industrial scale at any dose, the homogenization characteristics need to be better comprehended and implemented. This work aimed at developing a suitable technology to provide low-dose tablets with proper homogeneity containing electrospun substance prepared by an industrial HSES process. For this purpose, a direct compression (DC) technology was intended to be applied along with industrial tableting by a tablet rotary press. A model system was selected containing carvedilol (CAR, Figure 1), an antihypertensive drug, and PVPVA64, a copolymer as the matrix forming agent (the model drug was selected for analytical reasons, not for any biological relevance at such a low concentration).

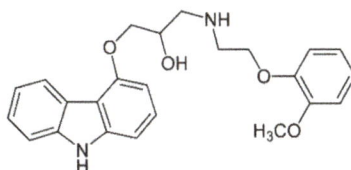

Figure 1. Carvedilol.

2. Materials and Methods

2.1. Materials

Carvedilol (CAR) was provided by Sigma-Aldrich (Budapest, Hungary) with purity ≥ 98% and a melting point of 117 °C. Kollidon VA 64 (Copovidone, PVPVA64) was supplied by BASF (Ludwigshafen, Germany), is a vinylpyrrolidone/vinylacetate amorphous copolymer (6:4) with a molecular weight in the range of 45–70 kDa. Lactose monohydrate (Flowlac 100 mesh) was provided by Meggle Pharma (Wasserburg, Germany), while microcrystalline cellulose (Vivapur 112), Croscarmellose sodium (Vivasol) and sodium stearyl fumarate (Pruv) were supplied by JRS Pharma (Rosenberg, Germany).

2.2. Single-Needle Electrospinning (SNES)

The single-needle electrospinning experiments were carried out using a spinneret equipped with an NT-35 high voltage DC supply (Unitronik Ltd., Nagykanizsa, Hungary). An electric potential of 25 kV was applied to the spinneret electrode. Sample collection was obtained using a grounded aluminum plate completely covered by aluminum foil. The distance of the spinneret from the collector was set at 15 cm, and the experiments were executed at ambient temperature (25 °C). The electrospinnable solution (Table 1) was dosed utilizing a SEP-10S Plus type syringe pump (Aitecs, Vilnius, Lithuania). The feed rate was 6 mL/h.

Table 1. Tablet composition.

Applied Tableting Ingredients	Amount (mg)/Tablet	Amount (%)/Tablet	Total Amount of Materials (Batch Size 5000 Tablets)
Electrospun/Crys. Carvedilol	0.05	0.05	0.25 g
poly (vinylpyrrolidone-*co*-vinyl acetate) (PVPVA64)	4.95	4.95	24.75 g
Flowlac 100 mesh (amorphous lactose)	65.00	65.00	325 g
Microcrystalline cellulose (MCC) 112	25.50	25.50	127.5 g
Croscarmellose sodium (CCS)	3.00	3.00	15.0 g
Sodium stearyl fumarate (Pruv)	1.5	1.50	7.5 g
Σ	100.0	100.0	500.00 g

2.3. High-Speed Electrospinning (HSES)

The scaled-up electrospinning productions were achieved by adopting a high-speed electrostatic spinning setup made up of a stainless steel spinneret with sharp edges and spherical cap geometry controlled by a high-speed motor. The electrospinnable solution was dosed by means of a SEP-10S Plus syringe pump. The flow rate was set at 750 mL/h. A rotational speed of 35,000 rpm was applied to the spinneret, while the voltage was 35 kV through the experiments (NT-65 high voltage DC supply Unitronik Ltd., Nagykanizsa, Hungary). The grounded collector completely covered by aluminum foil was positioned 35 cm from the spinneret in each case. The manufacture of fibers was carried out at ambient temperature (25 °C). More details about HSES can be found in the literature [44].

2.4. Low-Shear and High-Shear Homogenization

Homogenizations were carried out in plastic bags (low-shear mixing, LSM) or in a Diosna P-06 high-shear mixer (HSM). The tablet composition is detailed in Table 1.

A 100-mesh amorphous lactose called Flowlac was used as the filler, microcrystalline cellulose type 112 was applied as the binder, croscarmellose sodium (CCS) was adopted as the superdisintegrant and sodium stearyl fumarate (SSF) was implemented as the lubricant.

In the HSM setup, the chopper blades are set horizontally, which is standard for Diosna high-shear mixers.

In practice, all ingredients except the API and SSF were placed into plastic bags (LSM) or into the HSM, where they were pre-homogenized in 2 min (200 rpm impeller, 600 rpm chopper for HSM). Then the electrospun product or the crystalline CAR was added to the mixture, where it was homogenized in 7 min (200 rpm impeller, 850 rpm chopper for HSM). Upon completion, the mixtures were sieved applying a 500 μm sieve. Finally, SSF was added and blended with the other components in 30 s (200 rpm impeller, 0 rpm chopper for HSM).

2.5. Tableting and in Process Control (IPC) Tests

The average tablet weight was set to 100 mg, with the dose of CAR at 50 μg. Tableting was performed on a Riva Piccola tablet rotary press machine using 8 tablet dies with 6 mm diameter and no markings. Table speed was 40 rpm, Fill-O-Matic was 7 rpm and compression force was between 1–1.5 kN. A reference batch was also produced containing crystalline carvedilol as the API. Each batch consisted of 5000 tablets.

The compressed tablets were evaluated by IPC tests, such as tablet weight, thickness, hardness, friability measurement and time of disintegration. The first 3 were determined by an Erweka MultiCheck apparatus, while friability tests were conducted in a Pharmatest PTFR-A analyzer and disintegration time was measured in a Pharmatest PTZ-Auto disintegration tester. All in all 10 tablets were examined by the MultiCheck, 6 tablets were studied by the PTZ-Auto and tablets with the sum weight of 6.5 g were evaluated by the PTFR-A. Friability tests were made according to the Pharmacopeias with 100 turns in 4 min [45].

2.6. Scanning Electron Microscopy (SEM) and Fiber Diameter Analysis

Sample morphology was studied by applying a JEOL 6380LVa (JEOL, Tokyo, Japan) type scanning electron microscope. Initially, the samples were secured by virtue of a conductive double-sided carbon adhesive tape, then were coated with an alloy consisting of gold-palladium prior to investigation. The applied accelerating voltage was between 15 and 25 kV, while the working distance was in the range of 12–16 mm. A randomized fiber diameter determination method developed in-house was implemented as described in our previous work [46], $n = 100$ measurements were made on each sample.

2.7. Differential Scanning Calorimetry (DSC)

The differential scanning calorimetry (DSC) experiments were made with a DSC 92 Setaram device (Caluire, France). The average sample weight of ~10–15 mg was placed in a closed aluminum pan. A nitrogen purge gas flow of 50 mL/min was used in all experiments. The temperature program started with a preliminary isothermal period that lasted for 1 min at 25 °C. Upon completion, a subsequent linear heating phase ensued from 25 °C to 200 °C at a rate of 10 °C/min. Purified indium standard was applied for calibration.

2.8. Raman Mapping

Raman mapping was performed using Horiba Jobin-Yvon LabRAM-type microspectrometer with external 785 nm diode laser source and Olympus BX-40 optical microscope. The laser beam was focused by an objective of 20 × (NA = 0.4) to the tablet surface. The confocal hole of 1000 μm was used in the confocal system. 950 groove/mm grating monochromator dispersed the backscattered light. The spectral range of 460–1680 cm^{-1} was detected as the relevant range with 5 cm^{-1} resolution. Spectral data were collected from 41 × 41 points with 25 μm step size. The acquisition time was 40 s and two spectra were averaged per point. The classical least squares (CLS) method was applied to calculate the concentration of the different materials. All reference spectra (excipients and ES samples) were recorded and the combination of these was used to approximate the spectra of the maps. The so-obtained coefficients were depicted in the maps.

2.9. Content Uniformity Analysis

Content uniformity (CU) was measured by UV-Vis spectrometry. Ten random tablets were individually put into 10 mL volumetric flasks where they were disintegrated in an acidic buffer (pH 1) within an ultrasonic bath in 15 min. Upon completion they were filtered by a 0.45 μm polytetrafluoroethylene (PTFE) syringe filter and the concentration of CAR in the acidic buffer (pH 1) was determined by a Hewlett-Packard HP 8453G UV-Vis spectrophotometer (Palo Alto, CA, USA) at a wavelength of 241 nm based on a former calibration.

2.10. Sieve Analysis

Sieve analyses were made on the pure ES material and the final powder mixtures by a Fritsch Analysette 3 Pro Vibratory Sieve Shaker (Idar-Oberstein, Germany). A total weight of 25 g was investigated in each case. The pure ES material and the final powder mixtures were sieved for 10 min with the amplitude set at 0.5. Upon completion, the sieved fractions were weighed and evaluated.

3. Results and Discussion

As briefly mentioned at the beginning of this paper, the goal was to achieve highly homogenous NASD containing tablets with low doses of API. By doing so, we could develop a standard method for producing high-quality electrospun products, which meet the requirements of the Pharmacopeias. Fiber morphology of the HSES fibers was studied and compared with SNES samples by SEM. CU was evaluated by UV-Vis spectrometry, while API distribution in the tablets was also studied with Raman mapping and final powder mixture homogeneity was evaluated by sieve analysis.

3.1. Electrospinning

The preparation of the ES samples is detailed in Table 2.

Table 2. Comparison of the details of manufacturing using SNES and HSES.

Sample	Preparation Method	Applied Solvent	Dissolved PVPVA64 and CAR (99:1) in 10 mL of Solvent (g)	Flow Rate (mL/h)	Productivity for Dried Material (g/h)
PVPVA64 +1% CAR SNES	Single-needle electrospinning	96% EtOH	4.00	6	1.8
PVPVA64 +1% CAR HSES	High-speed electrospinning	96% EtOH	4.00	750	225

Single-needle electrospinning (SNES) is the basic method for preparing NASD; however, its production rate (few grams of product an hour) is way too limited for industrial purposes and applications. Our results fell in line with these assessments since our fiber production with SNES was only 1.8 g per hour. On the other hand, HSES offered a much higher output rate resulting in 225 g of fiber production per hour. In both cases, 96% ethanol was adopted as the solvent since it is accepted by the Pharmacopeia. Using this new technology, it was possible to increase our productivity 125-fold in regard to the dried product. It is encouraging that the output could have been further increased, but in this case, it was only a secondary objective.

3.2. Fiber Morphology

Once the ES materials were obtained their morphology were investigated with SEM. The images are shown in Figure 2. Upon inspecting them the average diameter was 1.02 ± 1.00 μm and 0.80 ± 0.31 μm for the HSES and SNES samples, respectively. However, the HSES sample contained more beads indicating that further research is required to reach optimal morphology. This outcome is likely the result of the fiber-forming technology. No crystalline objects were visible in either case, suggesting their amorphous states.

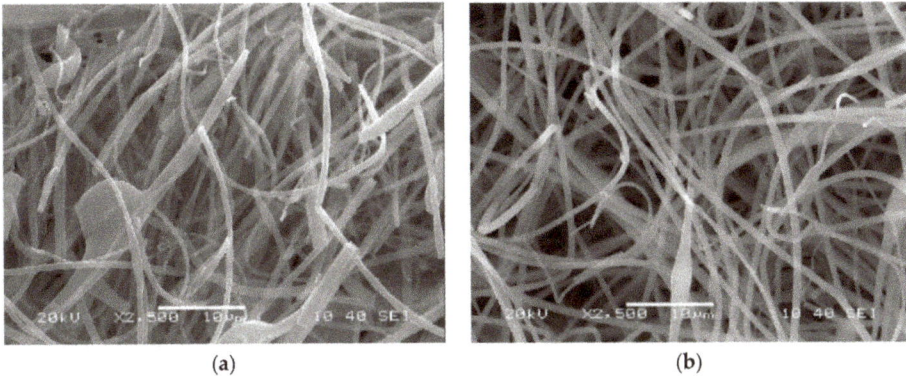

Figure 2. Scanning electron microscopic images of PVPVA64 + 1% CAR fibers prepared by high-speed electrospinning (**a**) and single-needle electrospinning (**b**).

3.3. Differential Scanning Calorimetry

To examine the physical state of carvedilol in the electrospun samples, differential scanning calorimetry measurements were carried out. Physical mixture and pure polymer were used as reference.

The DSC curves are detailed in Figure 3.

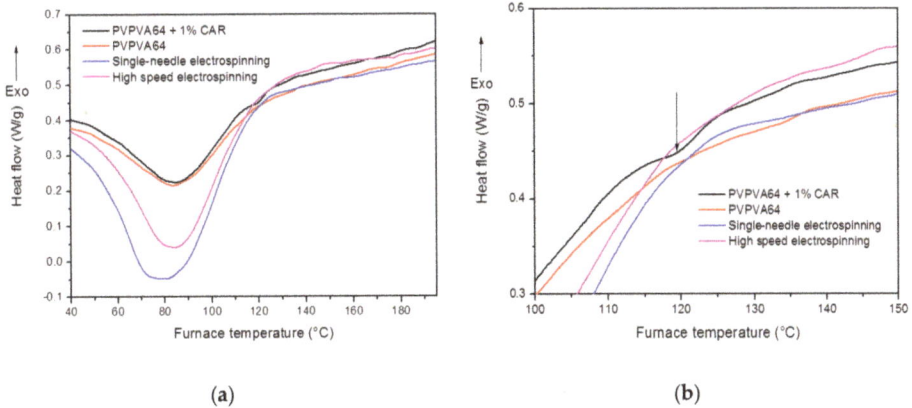

Figure 3. (**a**,**b**) Differential scanning calorimetry (DSC) thermograms of PVPVA64, PVPVA64 + 1% CAR physical mixture and fibers prepared by single-needle and high-speed electrospinning.

According to the thermograms, no endotherm melting peaks of API origin were observable in the electrospun fibers and only a very slight curvature was detected at 120 degrees Celsius in the physical mixture (3.b). Based on these results, we can assume that this faint signal comes from the minimal amount of crystalline carvedilol melting in the aforementioned sample.

These data further indicate that total amorphization was achieved in both the scaled up (HSES) and regular (SNES) ES samples. The wide endotherm peaks at lower temperatures are related to water evaporation.

3.4. Tableting

Once the ES products proved to be amorphous, a direct compression (DC) technology was developed to compress them. DC technology is the safest, easiest and most economical way to produce tablets since it takes the least amount of toll on the ingredients through simple and short homogenization steps [47].

However, in order to successfully apply the technology, proper tableting materials are needed. For our purposes, as they are briefly summarized in Table 1, an amorphous lactose with exceptional flowability called Flowlac was co-processed with microcrystalline cellulose (with low water content < 1.5%). The application of this MCC subtype was preferable since ES products are hygroscopic. The adoption of both materials was desirable since (as it was described in our previous work [48]) the electrospun samples can adhere to their surfaces. Ultimately, this phenomenon sets the foundation to achieve proper homogenization.

Croscarmellose sodium, specifically developed for manufacturing tablets was used as the superdisintegrant. These agents provide superior disintegration properties compared to regular disintegrants while maintaining a low-dose (1–4%) in the formulation [49]. Lastly, Sodium stearyl fumarate (Pruv), was adopted to lubricate the tablets. It is a hydrophilic agent, that has advantages compared to magnesium stearate such as less sensitivity to over-lubrication [50].

For the DC technology only plastic bags, a high-shear mixer, and a tablet rotary press were required. Only the HSES samples were compressed into tablets since the production of sufficient amounts of ingredients by SNES would have taken days to fabricate. Overall, 6 batches were produced 4 of which contained ES product. Two were manually homogenized in plastic bags emulating industrial container homogenization and the other two were homogenized in an HSM. The final two batches contained crystalline carvedilol serving as reference. One was homogenized in LSM conditions and the other by HSM. The batch characteristics are detailed in Table 3.

Table 3. Batch characteristics and their IPC results (A and B are repetitions of the same technology).

Characteristics	LSM Reference	HSM Reference	LSM HSES Batch A	LSM HSES Batch B	HSM HSES Batch A	HSM HSES Batch B
API type	Crystalline CAR	Crystalline CAR	Electrospun CAR	Electrospun CAR	Electrospun CAR	Electrospun CAR
Method of homogenization	Manual (LSM)	High-shear (HSM)	Manual (LSM)	Manual (LSM)	High-shear (HSM)	High-shear (HSM)
Weight (mg)	99.9 ± 0.5	99.2 ± 0.7	99.2 ± 0.8	100.2 ± 0.7	100.9 ± 1.0	99.8 ± 1.1
Thickness (mm)	3.08 ± 0.44	3.02 ± 0.54	3.06 ± 0.69	3.04 ± 0.57	3.05 ± 0.60	3.03 ± 0.52
Hardness (N)	64.3 ± 7.62	69.2 ± 6.22	60.6 ± 5.67	63.8 ± 7.51	68.6 ± 5.11	62.7 ± 6.71
Diameter (mm)	5.97 ± 0.19	5.95 ± 0.22	5.97 ± 0.27	5.98 ± 0.17	5.99 ± 0.29	5.97 ± 0.21
Friability (%)	0.21	0.31	0.39	0.25	0.20	0.27
Disintegration (s)	84	95	103	119	138	125

The HSM suitable for executing multiple technological steps, such as homogenization, granulation, and drying, was expected to work well with the ES product [51]. Once the homogenizations were completed, the mixtures were compressed into tablets using a tablet rotary press without any problems. IPC tests were carried out to evaluate the oral dosage forms. The summary of the results is detailed in Table 3.

According to the IPC results, all batches had roughly the same properties without any unacceptable data. Friability was well below the 1% limit, while disintegration [52] was easily achieved within 30 min both criteria set by the Pharmacopeias.

3.5. Content Uniformity

The measured average API contents and their homogeneity are detailed in Table 4. The batches containing crystalline carvedilol yielded expected results with acceptable API content and high RSD values. These results can be linked to the low quantity of API (250 mg) applied and to the fact that the average particle size of crystalline carvedilol is quite large, that makes its proper homogenization quite difficult in such a small dose. This phenomenon could not be solved even in the HSM since SD and RSD values were still too high, 4.65 and 5.13 respectively. Out of the ES samples, the batches homogenized in HSM proved to be much better than the LSM tablets homogenized in plastic bags under low-shear conditions. To differentiate between the samples, additional measurements were carried out.

Table 4. UV-Vis results.

Sample Number	Carvedilol %					
	LSM Reference	HSM Reference	LSM ES A	LSM ES B	HSM ES A	HSM ES B
Average	98.76	97.68	94.19	93.21	97.63	96.71
SD (%)	7.43	4.65	9.50	6.80	2.04	2.49
RSD	7.52	5.13	10.08	7.30	2.09	2.58

3.6. Raman Mapping Results

To evaluate the homogeneity differences between LSM and HSM ES tablets, Raman maps were taken of the aforementioned solid dosage forms. Raman mapping is a non-destructive analytical method enabling API homogeneity measurements in pharmaceuticals [53]. Analyses were conducted on individual tablet surfaces, one from each batch.

Since directly searching for the API at such a low-dose (50 µg) with Raman spectrometry is a very challenging task, an indirect method was applied. Given the fact, that the API is molecularly dispersed in the PVPVA64 polymer matrix [54], we can assume that the homogeneity of the API is related to the homogeneity of the polymer. Consequently, the maps were taken accordingly. These results are shown in Figure 4.

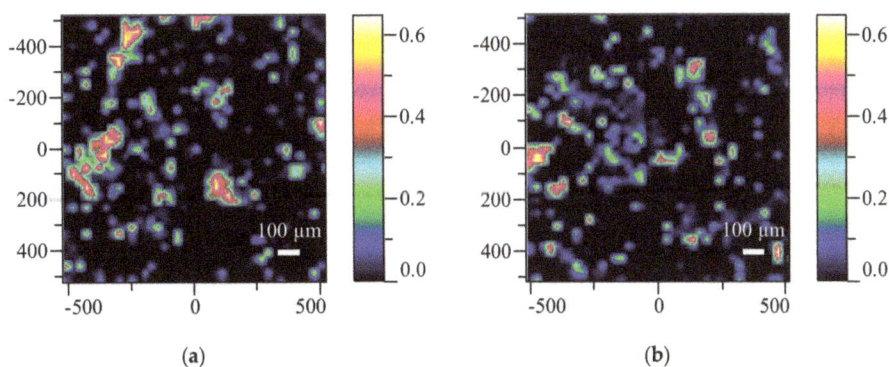

Figure 4. Raman maps of LSM (a) and HSM (b) ES tablets (colorful images show the distribution of the PVPVA64 polymer).

Upon inspecting the maps, the distribution of API could be indirectly investigated, but only slight differences were detected within the standalone tablets. This result indicates, that the API containing polymer is evenly distributed in the single solid dosage forms. However, this still does not explain the large inhomogeneity deviations discovered by the CU measurement, which is a result of evaluating multiple tablets at once.

3.7. Sieve Analysis

Since the analysis of single tablets did not clarify the deviations between the LSM and HSM, sieve analysis was chosen as an alternative method. A total weight of 25 g (the equivalent of 250 tablets) of LSM and HSM final powder mixtures along with the pure fibers were analyzed, whose results are detailed in Table 5. Both LSM and HSM tablets are mainly (more than 90%) made up of lactose and microcrystalline cellulose tableting materials, whose average particle sizes are 150 and 130 μm respectively.

Table 5. Sieve analysis results (the mixtures contain 5% ES material).

Sieve Size (μm)	Pure ES Material (g)	LSM Final Powder Mixture (g)	HSM Final Powder Mixture (g)
355	13.80	0.22	0.02
180	1.61	5.02	5.41
90	1.03	9.22	9.35
sub 90	8.56	10.54	10.22

According to the weighed sieve fractions, HSM homogenization was able to decrease the 355 μm portion by more than ten times compared to LSM mixing. This is crucial since the bulk of the pure electrospun materials was recovered on this sieve and, more importantly for complete homogenization, particle sizes should be as close to each other as possible to avoid segregation [55]. Based on these results, the high-performance impeller and chopper blades present in the HSM can further reduce the average particle sizes (due to high shear forces) of the fibrous materials, thus superior mixing of materials can be realized. These aforementioned fractions were also evaluated by Raman spectroscopy to look for traces of electrospun material. The spectra are shown in Figure 5.

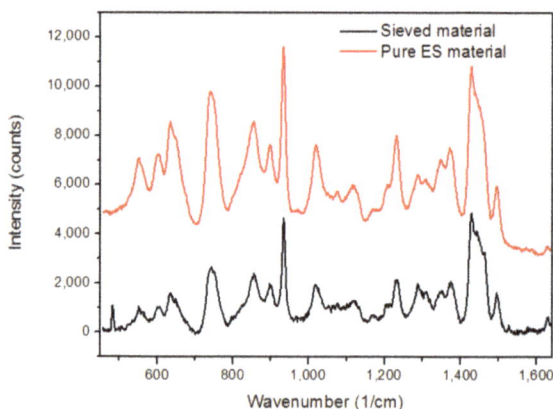

Figure 5. Raman spectra pure ES (red) and sieved (black) material.

It is clear that the spectrum of the sieved material is almost identical to the spectrum of the starting ES material ultimately proving that the API containing polymer was detected in the sieved mixture. In the end, this resulted in higher inhomogeneity among LSM tablets compared to HSM tablets. This outcome can be linked to Table 4 where the high SD and RSD values of the LSM tablets validate these findings.

Pharmaceutics **2018**, *10*, 114

Based on these results it is clear that a greater sample size was needed to be evaluated in order to identify the causes of homogeneity differences observed between the mixing methods. By implementing sieve analysis, the equivalent of 250 tablets could be screened, which enables broader examination compared to single tablet Raman mapping.

This outcome proves that the high-shear mixer coupled with the direct compression technology should be the first method of choice when proper homogenization of electrospun samples is required.

4. Conclusions

A low-dose, highly homogenous tablet formulation made from drug-loaded electrospun fibers was demonstrated by applying HSM homogenization. Carvedilol, an antihypertensive drug was used as the model API, while PVPVA64 was adopted as the matrix forming polymer. Electrospinning was carried out by HSES with increased productivity, while the SNES technology was applied as the reference. Homogenizations were made in plastic bags (LSM) and in an HSM, while tableting was performed by a tablet rotary press. Tablet batches containing crystalline carvedilol served as reference. Sieve analysis was used to study the particle size distribution in the final LSM and HSM powder mixtures. API content and homogeneity were measured by UV-Vis spectrometry, while the latter was also studied by Raman mapping.

HSM homogenization seems to be the preferred method of choice for preparing highly homogenous tablets containing electrospun NASDs. Their RSD values were much lower than their LSM counterparts. It is encouraging that this was achievable, despite setting a low API dose (50 µg) for the tablets. The technology can be scaled up easily, which could be truly beneficial for both academic researchers at universities and pharmaceutical technologists in the industry.

Author Contributions: G.F. designed and accomplished the experiments, like electrospinning and homogenization. A.F. performed and evaluated the Raman mapping measurements. A.B. carried out the SEM analysis, while B.F. performed and evaluated the fiber diameter measurements. E.B., B.D., and B.S. evaluated the results. Z.K.N. and G.M. finalized the manuscript.

Acknowledgments: This project was supported by the New Széchenyi Plan (project ID: TÁMOP-4.2.1/B-09/1/KMR-2010-0002), OTKA grant KH 124541, PD 116122, PD-121051, GINOP-2.1.1-15-2015-00541, ÚNKP-17-4-I and ÚNKP-17-4-II New National Excellence Program of the Ministry of Human Capacities, BME-KKP and the János Bolyai Research Scholarship of the Hungarian Academy of Sciences. This work was supported by the National Research, Development and Innovation in the frame of FIEK_16-1-2016-0007 (Higher Education and Industrial Cooperation Center) project.

Conflicts of Interest: The authors declare no conflict of interest.

References

1. Lieberman, H.A.; Lachman, L. *Pharmaceutical Dosage Forms: Tablets*; M. Dekker: New York, NY, USA, 1981.
2. Muselik, J.; Franc, A.; Dolezel, P.; Gonec, R.; Krondlova, A.; Lukasova, I. Influence of process parameters on content uniformity of a low dose active pharmaceutical ingredient in a tablet formulation according to GMP. *Acta Pharm.* **2014**, *64*, 355–367. [CrossRef] [PubMed]
3. US Pharmacopeia. Uniformity of Dosage Units/Content Uniformity. Available online: http://www.drugfuture. com/Pharmacopoeia/usp35/PDF/0420-0423%20[905]%20UNIFORMITY%20OF%20DOSAGE%20UNITS.pdf (accessed on 8 February 2017).
4. Baghel, S.; Cathcart, H.; O'Reilly, N.J. Polymeric amorphous solid dispersions: A review of amorphization, crystallization, stabilization, solid-state characterization, and aqueous solubilization of biopharmaceutical classification system class II drugs. *J. Pharm. Sci.* **2016**, *105*, 2527–2544. [CrossRef] [PubMed]
5. Paudel, A.; Worku, Z.A.; Meeus, J.; Guns, S.; Van den Mooter, G. Manufacturing of solid dispersions of poorly water soluble drugs by spray drying: Formulation and process considerations. *Int. J. Pharm.* **2013**, *453*, 253–284. [CrossRef] [PubMed]
6. Patil, H.; Tiwari, R.V.; Repka, M.A. Hot-melt extrusion: From theory to application in pharmaceutical formulation. *AAPS Pharm. Sci. Technol.* **2016**, *17*, 20–42. [CrossRef] [PubMed]

7. BioPharm. FDA Approves First Spray-Dried Biologic. Available online: http://www.biopharminternational. com/fda-approves-first-spray-dried-biologic (accessed on 7 May 2017).
8. Review, A.P. Recent Innovations in Pharmaceutical Hot Melt Extrusion. Available online: https://www.americanpharmaceuticalreview.com/Featured-Articles/179317-Recent-Innovations-in-Pharmaceutical-Hot-Melt-Extrusion/ (accessed on 4 June 2017).
9. Sosnik, A.; Seremeta, K.P. Advantages and challenges of the spray-drying technology for the production of pure drug particles and drug-loaded polymeric carriers. *Adv. Colloid Interface Sci.* **2015**, *223*, 40–54. [CrossRef] [PubMed]
10. Crowley, M.M.; Zhang, F.; Repka, M.A.; Thumma, S.; Upadhye, S.B.; Kumar Battu, S.; McGinity, J.W.; Martin, C. Pharmaceutical applications of hot-melt extrusion: Part I. *Drug Dev. Ind. Pharm.* **2007**, *33*, 909–926. [CrossRef] [PubMed]
11. Lee, S.L.; O'Connor, T.F.; Yang, X.; Cruz, C.N.; Chatterjee, S.; Madurawe, R.D.; Moore, C.M.V.; Yu, L.X.; Woodcock, J. Modernizing pharmaceutical manufacturing: From batch to continuous production. *J. Pharm. Innov.* **2015**, *10*, 191–199. [CrossRef]
12. Poechlauer, P.; Manley, J.; Broxterman, R.; Gregertsen, B.; Ridemark, M. Continuous processing in the manufacture of active pharmaceutical ingredients and finished dosage forms: An industry perspective. *Org. Process Res. Dev.* **2012**, *16*, 1586–1590. [CrossRef]
13. Vertex. FDA Approves Orkambi™ (Lumacaftor/Ivacaftor)—The First Medicine to Treat the Underlying Cause of Cystic Fibrosis for People Ages 12 and Older with Two Copies of the F508del Mutation. Available online: http://investors.vrtx.com/releasedetail.cfm?releaseid=920512 (accessed on 8 June 2017).
14. Pharmtech. EMA Approves Janssen Drug Made via Continuous Manufacturing. Available online: http://www.pharmtech.com/ema-approves-janssen-drug-made-continuous-manufacturing (accessed on 7 July 2017).
15. Pharmtech. Vertex Receives FDA Approval for Continuously Manufactured Drug Product. Available online: http://www.pharmtech.com/vertex-receives-fda-approval-continuously-manufactured-drug-product (accessed on 4 July 2017).
16. Lukáš, D.; Sarkar, A.; Martinová, L.; Vodsed' álková, K.; Lubasová, D.; Chaloupek, J.; Pokorný, P.; Mikeš, P.; Chvojka, J.; Komárek, M. Physical principles of electrospinning (electrospinning as a nano-scale technology of the twenty-first century). *Text. Prog.* **2009**, *41*, 59–140. [CrossRef]
17. Hutmacher, D.W.; Dalton, P.D. Melt electrospinning. *Chem. Asian J.* **2011**, *6*, 44–56. [CrossRef] [PubMed]
18. Reneker, D.H.; Yarin, A.L. Electrospinning jets and polymer nanofibers. *Polymer* **2008**, *49*, 2387–2425. [CrossRef]
19. Hu, X.; Liu, S.; Zhou, G.; Huang, Y.; Xie, Z.; Jing, X. Electrospinning of polymeric nanofibers for drug delivery applications. *J. Control. Release* **2014**, *185*, 12–21. [CrossRef] [PubMed]
20. Wang, Q.; Yu, D.-G.; Zhang, L.-L.; Liu, X.-K.; Deng, Y.-C.; Zhao, M. Electrospun hypromellose-based hydrophilic composites for rapid dissolution of poorly water-soluble drug. *Carbohydr. Polym.* **2017**, *174*, 617–625. [CrossRef] [PubMed]
21. Vuddanda, P.R.; Mathew, A.P.; Velaga, S. Electrospun nanofiber mats for ultrafast release of ondansetron. *React. Funct. Polym.* **2016**, *99*, 65–72. [CrossRef]
22. Illangakoon, U.E.; Gill, H.; Shearman, G.C.; Parhizkar, M.; Mahalingam, S.; Chatterton, N.P.; Williams, G.R. Fast dissolving paracetamol/caffeine nanofibers prepared by electrospinning. *Int. J. Pharm.* **2014**, *477*, 369–379. [CrossRef] [PubMed]
23. Lopez, F.L.; Shearman, G.C.; Gaisford, S.; Williams, G.R. Amorphous formulations of indomethacin and griseofulvin prepared by electrospinning. *Mol. Pharm.* **2014**, *11*, 4327–4338. [CrossRef] [PubMed]
24. Balogh, A.; Farkas, B.; Domokos, A.; Farkas, A.; Démuth, B.; Borbás, E.; Nagy, B.; Marosi, G.; Nagy, Z.K. Controlled-release solid dispersions of eudragit® FS 100 and poorly soluble spironolactone prepared by electrospinning and melt extrusion. *Eur. Polym. J.* **2017**, *95*, 406–417. [CrossRef]
25. Hamori, M.; Yoshimatsu, S.; Hukuchi, Y.; Shimizu, Y.; Fukushima, K.; Sugioka, N.; Nishimura, A.; Shibata, N. Preparation and pharmaceutical evaluation of nano-fiber matrix supported drug delivery system using the solvent-based electrospinning method. *Int. J. Pharm.* **2014**, *464*, 243–251. [CrossRef] [PubMed]
26. Shen, X.; Yu, D.; Zhu, L.; Branford-White, C.; White, K.; Chatterton, N.P. Electrospun diclofenac sodium loaded eudragit® l 100-55 nanofibers for colon-targeted drug delivery. *Int. J. Pharm.* **2011**, *408*, 200–207. [CrossRef] [PubMed]

27. Karthikeyan, K.; Guhathakarta, S.; Rajaram, R.; Korrapati, P.S. Electrospun zein/eudragit nanofibers based dual drug delivery system for the simultaneous delivery of aceclofenac and pantoprazole. *Int. J. Pharm.* **2012**, *438*, 117–122. [CrossRef] [PubMed]

28. Sill, T.J.; von Recum, H.A. Electrospinning: Applications in drug delivery and tissue engineering. *Biomaterials* **2008**, *29*, 1989–2006. [CrossRef] [PubMed]

29. Xue, J.; Xie, J.; Liu, W.; Xia, Y. Electrospun nanofibers: New concepts, materials, and applications. *Acc. Chem. Res.* **2017**, *50*, 1976–1987. [CrossRef] [PubMed]

30. Agarwal, S.; Wendorff, J.H.; Greiner, A. Use of electrospinning technique for biomedical applications. *Polymer* **2008**, *49*, 5603–5621. [CrossRef]

31. Nagy, Z.K.; Balogh, A.; Demuth, B.; Pataki, H.; Vigh, T.; Szabo, B.; Molnar, K.; Schmidt, B.T.; Horak, P.; Marosi, G.; et al. High speed electrospinning for scaled-up production of amorphous solid dispersion of itraconazole. *Int. J. Pharm.* **2015**, *480*, 137–142. [CrossRef] [PubMed]

32. Williams, G.R.; Chatterton, N.P.; Nazir, T.; Yu, D.G.; Zhu, L.M.; Branford-White, C.J. Electrospun nanofibers in drug delivery: Recent developments and perspectives. *Ther. Deliv.* **2012**, *3*, 515–533. [CrossRef] [PubMed]

33. Ignatious, F.; Sun, L.; Lee, C.P.; Baldoni, J. Electrospun nanofibers in oral drug delivery. *Pharm. Res.* **2010**, *27*, 576–588. [CrossRef] [PubMed]

34. Lukas, D.; Sarkar, A.; Pokorny, P. Self-organization of jets in electrospinning from free liquid surface: A generalized approach. *J. Appl. Phys.* **2008**, *103*, 084309. [CrossRef]

35. Sebe, I.; Szabó, B.; Nagy, Z.K.; Szabó, D.; Zsidai, L.; Kocsis, B.; Zelkó, R. Polymer structure and antimicrobial activity of polyvinylpyrrolidone-based iodine nanofibers prepared with high-speed rotary spinning technique. *Int. J. Pharm.* **2013**, *458*, 99–103. [CrossRef] [PubMed]

36. Raimi-Abraham, B.T.; Mahalingam, S.; Davies, P.J.; Edirisinghe, M.; Craig, D.Q.M. Development and characterization of amorphous nanofiber drug dispersions prepared using pressurized gyration. *Mol. Pharm.* **2015**, *12*, 3851–3861. [CrossRef] [PubMed]

37. Zhang, S.; Karaca, B.; Vanoosten, S.; Yuca, E.; Mahalingam, S.; Edirisinghe, M.; Tamerler, C. Coupling infusion and gyration for the nanoscale assembly of functional polymer nanofibers integrated with genetically engineered proteins. *Macromol. Rapid Commun.* **1322**, *36*, 1322–1328. [CrossRef] [PubMed]

38. Hong, X.; Mahalingam, S.; Edirisinghe, M. Simultaneous application of pressure-infusion-gyration to generate polymeric nanofibers. *Macromol. Mater. Eng.* **2017**, *302*, 1600564. [CrossRef]

39. Heseltine Phoebe, L.; Ahmed, J.; Edirisinghe, M. Developments in pressurized gyration for the mass production of polymeric fibers. *Macromol. Mater. Eng.* **2018**, 1800218. [CrossRef]

40. Hamori, M.; Nagano, K.; Kakimoto, S.; Naruhashi, K.; Kiriyama, A.; Nishimura, A.; Shibata, N. Preparation and pharmaceutical evaluation of acetaminophen nano-fiber tablets: Application of a solvent-based electrospinning method for tableting. *Biomed. Pharmacother.* **2016**, *78*, 14–22. [CrossRef] [PubMed]

41. Demuth, B.; Farkas, A.; Balogh, A.; Bartosiewicz, K.; Kallai-Szabo, B.; Bertels, J.; Vigh, T.; Mensch, J.; Verreck, G.; Van Assche, I.; et al. Lubricant-induced crystallization of itraconazole from tablets made of electrospun amorphous solid dispersion. *J. Pharm. Sci.* **2016**, *105*, 2982–2988. [CrossRef] [PubMed]

42. Poller, B.; Strachan, C.; Broadbent, R.; Walker, G.F. A minitablet formulation made from electrospun nanofibers. *Eur. J. Pharm. Biopharm.* **2017**, *114*, 213–220. [CrossRef] [PubMed]

43. Demuth, B.; Nagy, Z.K.; Balogh, A.; Vigh, T.; Marosi, G.; Verreck, G.; Van Assche, I.; Brewster, M.E. Downstream processing of polymer-based amorphous solid dispersions to generate tablet formulations. *Int. J. Pharm.* **2015**, *486*, 268–286. [CrossRef] [PubMed]

44. Vigh, T.; Démuth, B.; Balogh, A.; Galata, D.L.; Van Assche, I.; Mackie, C.; Vialpando, M.; Van Hove, B.; Psathas, P.; Borbás, E.; et al. Oral bioavailability enhancement of flubendazole by developing nanofibrous solid dosage forms. *Drug Dev. Ind. Pharm.* **2017**, *43*, 1126–1133. [CrossRef] [PubMed]

45. US Pharmacopeia. Tablet Friability. Available online: https://www.usp.org/sites/default/files/usp/document/harmonization/gen-chapter/g06_pf_ira_32_2_2006.pdf (accessed on 7 August 2017).

46. Balogh, A.; Farkas, B.; Farago, K.; Farkas, A.; Wagner, I.; Van Assche, I.; Verreck, G.; Nagy, Z.K.; Marosi, G. Melt-blown and electrospun drug-loaded polymer fiber mats for dissolution enhancement: A comparative study. *J. Pharm. Sci.* **2015**, *104*, 1767–1776. [CrossRef] [PubMed]

47. Pharmtech. Direct Compression Versus Granulation. Available online: http://www.pharmtech.com/direct-compression-versus-granulation (accessed on 7 September 2017).

48. Démuth, B.; Farkas, A.; Szabó, B.; Balogh, A.; Nagy, B.; Vágó, E.; Vigh, T.; Tinke, A.P.; Kazsu, Z.; Demeter, Á.; et al. Development and tableting of directly compressible powder from electrospun nanofibrous amorphous solid dispersion. *Adv. Powder Technol.* **2017**, *28*, 1554–1563. [CrossRef]

49. Battu, S.K.; Repka, M.A.; Majumdar, S.; Rao, Y.M. Formulation and evaluation of rapidly disintegrating fenoverine tablets: Effect of superdisintegrants. *Drug Dev. Ind. Pharm.* **2007**, *33*, 1225–1232. [CrossRef] [PubMed]

50. Shah, N.H.; Stiel, D.; Weiss, M.; Infeld, M.H.; Malick, A.W. Evaluation of two new tablet lubricants-sodium stearyl fumarate and glyceryl behenate. Measurement of physical parameters (compaction, ejection and residual forces) in the tableting process and the effect on the dissolution rate. *Drug Dev. Ind. Pharm.* **1986**, *12*, 1329–1346. [CrossRef]

51. Pharmaapproach. High-Shear Granulator. Available online: http://pharmapproach.com/high-shear-granulator/ (accessed on 1 August 2017).

52. EMA. Ich Topic q4b Annex 5 Disintegration Test General Chapter. Available online: http://www.ema.europa.eu/docs/en_GB/document_library/Scientific_guideline/2009/09/WC500003292.pdf (accessed on 2 September 2017).

53. Gordon, K.C.; McGoverin, C.M. Raman mapping of pharmaceuticals. *Int. J. Pharm.* **2011**, *417*, 151–162. [CrossRef] [PubMed]

54. Vo, C.L.-N.; Park, C.; Lee, B.-J. Current trends and future perspectives of solid dispersions containing poorly water-soluble drugs. *Eur. J. Pharm. Biopharm.* **2013**, *85*, 799–813. [CrossRef] [PubMed]

55. Williams, J.C. The segregation of particulate materials. A review. *Powder Technol.* **1976**, *15*, 245–251. [CrossRef]

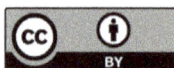

pharmaceutics

MDPI

Article

Enhanced Transepithelial Permeation of Gallic Acid and (−)-Epigallocatechin Gallate across Human Intestinal Caco-2 Cells Using Electrospun Xanthan Nanofibers

Adele Faralli, Elhamalsadat Shekarforoush, Ana C. Mendes and Ioannis S. Chronakis *

Nano-BioScience Research Group, DTU-Food, Technical University of Denmark, Kemitorvet, B202, 2800 Kgs. Lyngby, Denmark; adele.faralli@gmail.com (A.F.); elham.shekar@gmail.com (E.S.); anac@food.dtu.dk (A.C.M.)
* Correspondence: ioach@food.dtu.dk; Tel.: +45-4020-6413

Received: 17 December 2018; Accepted: 20 March 2019; Published: 1 April 2019

Abstract: Electrospun xanthan polysaccharide nanofibers (X) were developed as an encapsulation and delivery system of the poorly absorbed polyphenol compounds, gallic acid (GA) and (−)-epigallocatechin gallate (EGCG). Scanning electron microscopy was used to characterize the electrospun nanofibers, and controlled release studies were performed at pH 6.5 and 7.4 in saline buffer, suggesting that the release of polyphenols from xanthan nanofibers follows a non-Fickian mechanism. Furthermore, the X-GA and X-EGCG nanofibers were incubated with Caco-2 cells, and the cell viability, transepithelial transport, and permeability properties across cell monolayers were investigated. Increases of GA and EGCG permeabilities were observed when the polyphenols were loaded into xanthan nanofibers, compared to the free compounds. The observed in vitro permeability enhancement of GA and EGCG was induced by the presence of the polysaccharide nanofibers, which successfully inhibited efflux transporters, as well as by opening tight junctions.

Keywords: xanthan gum; electrospinning; gallic acid; (−)-epigallocatechin gallate; permeability

1. Introduction

Polyphenols are the most abundant antioxidants in our diet and they are receiving increasing interest due to the established association between the intake of a polyphenol-rich diet and the prevention of various diseases [1,2]. Because of their antioxidant [3], antimutagenic [4], and anticarcinogenic properties [5,6], polyphenols have recently attracted research interest towards the study of their metabolism and absorption mechanisms across the gut barrier [7].

Polyphenols are categorized according to the chemical structure of their carbon skeleton, and the most abundant classes in our diet are phenolic acids and flavonoids. The most encountered phenolic acids are caffeic acid, ferulic acid, and gallic acid (GA). The latter, also known as 3,4,5-trihydroxybenzoic acid, is one of the main endogenous phenolic acids found in plants, mostly in tea leaves [8]. GA, also found in vegetables, grapes, and pomegranates, is a potent non-enzymatic antioxidant and has a natural antitumor activity against lung, prostate, colon, gastric, and breast cancer and human pre-myelocytic leukemia [9–12]. It has been reported that the in vitro treatment of lung and human cervical cancer cells with GA concentrations in the micromolar range induces cell death associated with the depletion of glutathione (GSH) as well as reactive oxygen species (ROS) level changes [13,14]. The physiological impact and efficiency of GA is strictly dependent on its bioavailability, biochemical integrity, and successful interaction with target tissues. Many studies have demonstrated that only small amounts of orally administered GA are absorbed through the intestine due to its low permeability, poor water solubility, and chemical instability. The GA instability in the gastrointestinal tract is promoted by endogenous enzymes, interfering nutrients, and oxidative reactions that lead to a considerable loss in its activity [15]. It is also reported that the phenol concentrations needed to result in an in vitro efficiency are higher than the moderate in vivo levels, and gastrointestinal permeation is supported only by passive diffusion [15]. Moreover, previous studies found that after oral administration of *Phyllanthi* tannin fraction at a dose of 6 g/kg in rats, the maximum concentration of absorbed GA was less than 10.47 µg/mL [16]. In vitro investigations have also been conducted with Caco-2 cell monolayers, in order to evaluate the transepithelial transport of pure GA across the cellular barrier, and the apparent permeability coefficient, P_{app}, under a proton gradient was about 0.20×10^{-6} cm/s [8].

Flavonoids, the most abundant polyphenols in our diet together with phenolic acids, can be divided into several classes, and catechins are the main flavonols found in tea [1]. The major tea catechins are (−)-epigallocatechin gallate (EGCG), (−)-epicatechin gallate (ECG), (−)-epicatechin (EC), and (−)-epigallocatechin (EGC) [17]. These natural compounds have demonstrated various health-beneficial properties, including antioxidant, anti-inflammatory, and anticancer effects, both in animals and humans [18,19]. Indeed, an inverse association between tea consumption and colorectal cancer frequency as well as gastric cancer has been identified [20,21]. An increasing interest towards EGCG has led to an extensive investigation of the beneficial properties of this natural molecule in the cosmetic, nutritional, and pharmaceutical fields. However, like GA, EGCG has a poor oral bioavailability and poor biochemical stability. In fact, EGCG has a low lipophilicity (octanol/water partition coefficient of 0.86 ± 0.03), thus limiting its intrinsic permeability across the intestinal epithelium [19]. Several studies have instead demonstrated a high and specific accumulation of tea flavonoids in epithelial Caco-2 cells or epithelial cells along the aerodigestive tract [17,22,23], which have been recognized as major sites for biological activity of flavonoids. In the Caco-2 cell model, apical uptake transporters and efflux pumps, such as the multidrug resistance-associated proteins, MRP1 and MRP2, and P-glycoprotein have been identified to play a major role in cellular accumulation of catechins [17,19,24,25].

In the light of these considerations, the oral administration of GA and EGCG requires a formulation strategy able to protect and maintain their structural integrity, increase their bioavailability and water solubility, and deliver them to target tissues. Among the existing delivery and stabilization approaches, the encapsulation of sensitive compounds is considered the most effective strategy for improving the oral bioavailability and shelf-life of compounds [15,26,27]. Nowadays, a plethora of encapsulation techniques are commonly used in oral delivery systems, and carrier systems for phenolic acids and flavonoids encapsulation have found feasible approaches to overcome both enzymatic degradation and membrane permeation issues [7,19]. The encapsulation of EGCG in a niosomal formulation results in a significantly enhanced bioactive absorption, stronger chemical stability, and lower toxicity compared with the free EGCG [19]. The in vitro apparent permeability, P_{app}, of EGCG niosome across Caco-2 cell monolayers was found to be $1.42 \pm 0.24 \times 10^{-6}$ cm/s, almost 2-fold more as free EGCG ($P_{app} = 0.88 \pm 0.09 \times 10^{-6}$ cm/s). Furthermore, GA-loaded mesoporous silica nanoparticles (MSNs-GA) were easily internalized into Caco-2 cells without any deleterious effect on cell viability, and preserving the same antitumor properties of free GA [7]. In addition, the topical and transdermal delivery of GA loaded into poly(L-lactic acid) fiber mats resulted in a preserved radical scavenging activity of the released phenolic acid [28]. GA has also been encapsulated within electrospun fibers as delivery carriers using the protein zein [29], cellulose acetate [30], and polylactic acid (PLA) nanofibers, including GA-cyclodextrin complexes [31]. The encapsulation and release of EGCG loaded into electrospun nanofibers has also been investigated using zein nanofibers [32], hyaluronic acid/ lactic-*co*-glycolic acid fibers (HA/PLGA, core/shell) [33], PLGA nanofibers [34,35], cellulose electrospun nanofibrous mats coated with bilayers of chitosan and EGCG [36], and electrospun hydroxypropyl methylcellulose nanofibers [37].

In our previous study, electrospun xanthan-chitosan nanofibers loaded with curcumin, as a model hydrophobic bioactive, were incubated with Caco-2 cells and the transepithelial transport and permeability properties across cell monolayers were assessed. A 3.4-fold increase of curcumin permeability was detected in the presence of xanthan-chitosan nanofibers, in comparison with free-curcumin [38,39]. Moreover, electrospun xanthan nanofibers developed from a solution of xanthan dissolved in formic acid, remained intact and morphologically stable over a wide pH range in saline buffers [40]. In the present study, electrospun xanthan nanofibers were assessed as an encapsulation and delivery system of the two polyphenols, GA and EGCG. The xanthan-GA and xanthan-EGCG loaded nanofibers were incubated with Caco-2 cells, and the transepithelial transport and permeability of GA and EGCG across the cell monolayers were investigated.

2. Materials and Methods

2.1. Materials

The human colon adenocarcinoma cell line, Caco-2 [Caco-2] (ATCC® HTB-37™), was obtained from the American Type Culture Collection (Rockville, MD, USA). Dulbecco's modified Eagle's medium (DMEM) high glucose (4.5 g/L), L-glutamine (200 mM), nonessential amino acids (100X), penicillin-streptomycin (10,000 U/mL and 10 mg/mL in 0.9% sodium chloride, respectively), trypsin-EDTA (10X), Dulbecco's Phosphate Buffered Saline 1X without calcium chloride and magnesium chloride (indicated in the text as PBS), fluorescein sodium salt (FLUO), lucifer yellow dilithium salt (LY), methanesulfonic acid, MES (1 M; pH 5.5–6.7), 4-(2-hydroxyethyl)-1-piperazineethanesulfonic acid solution, HEPES (1 M; pH 7.0–7.6), gallic acid (GA), and (−)-epigallocatechin gallate (EGCG) were purchased from Sigma Aldrich (Brøndby, Denmark). Tissue culture 12-well plates and 12-mm polycarbonate cell culture inserts with an area of 1.12 cm^2 and a pore size of 0.4 μm were purchased from Corning Costar® Corporation. Fetal bovine serum (FBS) and Hanks' balanced salt solution (HBSS) with calcium and magnesium and without phenol red were obtained from Thermo Fisher Scientific (Roskilde, Denmark). CellTiter 96® AQueous One Solution Cell Proliferation Assay (MTS) was purchased from Promega Biotech AB (Nacka, Sweden). Xanthan gum (Cosphaderm X-34) from *Xanthomonas campestris* was kindly provided by Cosphatec GmbH (Drehbahn, Hamburg, Germany) [40].

2.2. Fabrication of Electrospun Nanofibers

Xanthan was dissolved in formic acid at a final concentration of 2.5% *w/v* under vigorous stirring overnight at room temperature. Subsequently, GA and EGCG were added to the polysaccharide solution and further stirred for 30 min. The electrospinning setup consisted of a high voltage generator (ES50P-10W, Gamma High Voltage Research, Inc., Ormond Beach, FL, USA) to provide a voltage of 20 kV, and a syringe pump (New Era Pump Systems, Inc., Farmingdale, NY, USA) to feed the xanthan solution at a flow rate of 0.01 mL/min using a 21 G needle gauge. Xanthan fibers were collected on a steel plate covered with an aluminum foil perpendicularly placed at 8 cm from the end of the needle. The electrospinning process was carried out at ambient conditions (20°C and around 20% relative humidity).

2.3. Morphology and FTIR Characterisation of the Nanofibers

The morphology of electrospun X, X-GA, and X-EGCG nanofibers was studied using a Phenom Pro scanning electron microscope (SEM) (Phenom World, Thermo Fisher Scientific, Eindhoven, The Netherlands). For SEM analysis, a small piece of nanofibers web was attached on SEM specimen stubs by a double-sided adhesive tape. The average fiber diameter of nanofibers was calculated using image J analysis software (National Institutes of Health, Bethesda, MD, USA) measured at 100 different points for each image.

Fourier transform infrared (FTIR) spectroscopy analysis of X, X-GA, X-EGCG nanofibers, GA, and EGCG was analyzed using a Perkin Elmer Spectrum 100 spectrometer (Perkin Elmer, Waltham, MA, USA) based on a universal attenuated total reflectance (ATR) sensor. Four scans for each sample were accumulated at 20 °C at a resolution of 1 cm^{-1}. The infrared peaks were identified with a Spectrum™ 10 software using a 1% transmittance (T) peak threshold.

2.4. In Vitro Release of Gallic Acid and (−)-Epigallocatechin Gallate from Electrospun Nanofibers

The amount of GA and EGCG loaded into xanthan nanofibers was evaluated by immersing the nanofibers in equal volumes of complete growth medium (DMEM-FBS) or HBSS at pH 6.5 or pH 7.4. Briefly, 1.0 mg of X-GA and X-EGCG fibers were immersed in 2 mL pre-warmed medium in a 48-well plate, and the release of molecules from nanofibers was conducted at 37 °C for 8 h. The withdrawn aliquots were analyzed by RP-HPLC with detection of GA and EGCG at 255 nm and 270 nm, respectively (see also Section 2.10). The cumulative amount of each compound released from nanofibers was then considered as the maximum releasable GA and EGCG from the nanofiber formulation under those conditions. All data are expressed as mean ± SD of three independent experiments.

2.5. Caco-2 Cell Culture and Subculture

Caco-2 cells were routinely seeded at a concentration of 1.0×10^5 cells/mL in T-75 cm^2 flasks and incubated at 37 °C in a humidified atmosphere of 5% CO_2. The complete cell medium, here indicated as DMEM-FBS, consisted of high glucose DMEM containing 10% heat-inactivated FBS, 2 mM L-glutamine, 1% nonessential amino acids, 100 U/mL penicillin, and 100 μg/mL streptomycin. The medium was renewed every second day until cells reached approximately 90% confluence. Cells were passaged at a subcultivation ratio of 1:4 by treatment with 0.25% trypsin—0.53 mM EDTA solution for 10 min at 37 °C. After trypsinization, the cells were suspended in complete growth medium and centrifuged for 5 min at 1000 rpm. After supernatant removal, the pellet was suspended in the growth medium and cell concentration was determined with an ORFLO Moxi Z Mini Automated Cell Counter using Type S cassette (Biofrontier Technology, Bukit, Singapore). All Caco-2 cells were used between passages 9–15.

2.6. Compounds and Electrospun Nanofibers Tested with Caco-2 Cell Monolayers

Xanthan (X), gallic acid-loaded xanthan (X-GA), and (−)-epigallocatechin gallate-loaded xanthan (X-EGCG) nanofibers were produced by electrospinning a solution of the mixed compounds dissolved in formic acid. These nanofibers were tested with Caco-2 cell monolayers to evaluate their toxicity and apparent permeability coefficient (P_{app}) after GA and EGCG release from nanofibers and as free compounds. Before testing nanofiber mats with Caco-2 cells, the collected fibers were kept under an air stream for 3 days allowing complete formic acid evaporation. Besides GA and EGCG, the transepithelial transport of fluorescein (FLUO) and Lucifer yellow (LY) across Caco-2 cell monolayers were also investigated as markers for intestinal epithelial permeability and integrity.

2.7. Caco-2 Cell Viability Assay

The in vitro Caco-2 cell viability after treatment with free GA, free EGCG, xanthan nanofibers (X), GA-loaded xanthan nanofibers (X-GA), and EGCG-loaded xanthan nanofibers was evaluated by using the MTS [3-(4,5-dimethylthiazol-2-yl)-5-(3-carboxymethoxyphenyl)-2-(4-sulfophenyl)-2H-tetrazolium inner salt] colorimetric bioassay. Different concentrations of free GA and EGCG ranging from 1 μM to 1 mM were prepared in PBS and sterile-filtered with a 0.22 μm pore size. Furthermore, increasing amounts of dried X, X-GA, and X-EGCG nanofibers were peeled off from the aluminum foils and incubated with cells. In a 48-well plate, 1.5×10^5 cells/mL were seeded in a complete growth medium and incubated for 2 days at 37 °C in a humidified atmosphere of 5% CO_2. Then, the monolayers were washed with PBS and the complete medium was renewed. Caco-2 cells were incubated with free GA and free EGCG solutions, X nanofibers, X-GA nanofibers, X-EGCG nanofibers, and PBS as a control. The plates were incubated for 24 h at 37 °C in a humidified atmosphere of 5% CO_2. The following day, all supernatants, including those with suspended nanofibers, were removed, cells were washed with PBS, and the medium was renewed. 40 μL of pre-warmed MTS solution was added to each well under dark conditions. After 3 h incubation at 37 °C, the absorbance of the reduced MTS (formazan product) was recorded at 490 nm through a well plate reader (Wallac 1420 Victor2 Multilabel Counter, Perkin Elmer, Waltham, MA, USA).

2.8. Transepithelial Transport

The transepithelial transport of free fluorescein (FLUO), free lucifer yellow (LY), free gallic acid (GA), free (−)-epigallocatechin gallate (EGCG), free gallic acid in the presence of empty xanthan nanofibers (X + GA), free (−)-epigallocatechin gallate in the presence of empty xanthan nanofibers (X + EGCG), gallic acid-loaded xanthan nanofibers (X-GA), and (−)-epigallocatechin gallate-loaded xanthan nanofibers (X-EGCG) across Caco-2 cell monolayers were investigated according to the protocol reported by Hubatsch et al. [41]. The transport experiments were performed in both apical-to-basolateral (AB, absorptive) and basolateral-to-apical (BA, secretory) directions, under a proton gradient. In fact, to mimic the acidic microclimate of the small intestine, apical and basolateral pH of around 6.5 and 7.4 were used, respectively. Briefly, 1.0×10^5 cells/insert were seeded onto pre-wetted 12-mm polycarbonate cell culture inserts with an area of 1.12 cm^2 and a pore size of 0.4 μm. The apical and basolateral compartments were filled with 0.5 mL and 1.5 mL complete medium, respectively. The Caco-2 cells were incubated onto the filters overnight at 37 °C in a humidified atmosphere of 5% CO_2. The day after, the growth medium was replaced in both compartments and the plates were incubated for 21 days at 37 °C in a humidified atmosphere of 5% CO_2, renewing the complete growth medium every second day. For the AB transport experiments, donor solutions of FLUO, LY, GA, and EGCG at a concentration of 11 mM, 9.57 mM, 1.1 mM, and 1.1 mM, respectively, were prepared in sterile-filter HBSS at pH 6.5 buffered with 10 mM MES. Again, donor solutions of FLUO, LY, GA, and EGCG at a concentration of 10.3 mM, 9 mM, 1.03 mM, and 1.03 mM, respectively, were prepared in sterile-filter HBSS at pH 7.4 buffered with 25 mM HEPES to evaluate their BA transport. A volume of 50 μL of each stock solution was added to the donor chamber (0.55 mL and 1.55 mL were the total volumes in A and B, respectively). The transport of GA and EGCG released from nanofibers and as free compounds in the presence of empty X nanofibers was also investigated. For the AB transport, 0.2 mg X-GA, 1.0 mg X-EGCG, 0.2 mg, and 1.0 mg X were used, and accordingly, 0.6 mg X-GA, 3.0 mg X-EGCG, 0.6 mg, and 3.0 mg X were incubated with cell monolayers to evaluate their BA transport. Prior to incubation of the nanofibers, the mats were peeled off from the aluminum foil and kept under an air stream for 3 days. After 21 days of cell growth, the complete DMEM medium was removed from the cell monolayers and replaced with HBSS at pH 6.5 and pH 7.4 at the apical and basolateral compartments, respectively. For the AB transport studies, 1.5 mL HBSS was used in the basolateral side and 0.55 mL of each donor solution and/or nanofibers were added to the apical side. Immediately, 200 μL aliquots were withdrawn from each donor compartment (time = 0). Aliquots from the acceptor side were then withdrawn at different time intervals, and the volume was replaced with fresh HBSS at pH 7.4 maintaining the well plates at 37 °C in a humidified atmosphere of 5% CO_2. A final aliquot from the donor chamber was taken as the last time point. BA transport studies were conducted using the same procedure and incubating 0.5 mL HBSS at pH 6.5 in the apical side and 1.55 mL of donor solution and/or nanofibers in the basolateral chamber. During the transport experiments, all cell media were pre-warmed at 37 °C. Each transport experiment was performed for a time interval of 8 h in triplicate (n = 3). After 8 h of transport studies and TEER measurements, both apical and basolateral chambers were washed twice with PBS and cell monolayers were detached from the insert membrane with 0.25% trypsin-0.53 mM EDTA solution for 10 min at 37 °C. The collected Caco-2 cell lysates were centrifuged for 5 min at 1000 rpm and supernatants were discarded. Furthermore, the semipermeable membranes were carefully removed from the insert using a scalpel and collected into Eppendorf tubes in 500 μL HBSS at pH 6.5 (apical conditions). Cell pellets were re-suspended in 500 μL HBSS at pH 6.5 and both cells and membranes were sonicated for 3 h using an ultrasonic bath (Branson Ultrasonic Corp., VWR, Søborg, Denmark). The collected samples were then centrifuged for 15 min at 10,000 rpm and supernatants were analyzed by HPLC (Thermo Fisher Scientific, Roskilde, Denmark). The same procedure was used to quantify the compound amounts adsorbed (X + GA and X + EGCG) or remaining encapsulated (X-GA and X-EGCG) in the nanofibers at the end of the transport experiments. The tested nanofibers were removed from the donor chamber and suspended in 500 μL of HBSS (pH 6.5 for AB transport and pH 7.4 for BA transport). After sonication and centrifugation, the molecules in the supernatants were quantified by HPLC.

2.9. Measurement of Transepithelial Electrical Resistance (TEER)

The transepithelial electrical resistance (TEER) was measured at 20 °C before and after permeability experiments with an epithelial volt-ohmmeter equipped with STX2 "chopstick" electrodes (EVOM2™, World Precision Instruments, Sarasota, FL, USA). Before measuring the resistance values of each well, the cell monolayers and the basolateral chamber were washed twice with pre-warmed HBSS at pH 6.5 and HBSS at pH 7.4, respectively. The resistance values of the semipermeable membrane without cells (R_{BLANK}) were recorded and subtracted from the resistance values obtained from the measurement of each cellular monolayer onto the semipermeable membrane (R_{TOTAL}). The specific cell resistance values (R_{TISSUE}) were calculated by:

$$R_{TISSUE} \ (\Omega) = R_{TOTAL} \ (\Omega) - R_{BLANK} \ (\Omega) \tag{1}$$

TEER values of cellular monolayers were expressed in $\Omega \times cm^2$ and calculated by:

$$TEER_{TISSUE} \ (\Omega \ cm^2) = R_{TISSUE} \ (\Omega) \times A_{MEMBRANE} \ (cm^2) \tag{2}$$

2.10. Quantification of Compounds

Donor solutions of FLUO, LY, GA, and EGCG were prepared and sterile-filtered in HBSS at pH 6.5 and pH 7.4 to perform transepithelial studies. Standard curves of GA and EGCG dissolved in HBSS at pH 6.5 and pH 7.4 were obtained by HPLC analysis. 200 µL samples withdrawn from the donor and acceptor compartments during transport experiments across cell monolayers were quantitatively analyzed using RP-HPLC (Thermo Fisher Scientific, Denmark). A C18 column (3.0 × 100 mm) and 0.5 mL/min flow rate were used. GA and EGCG were quantified with detection at 255 nm and 270 nm, respectively. FLUO and LY aliquots were instead analyzed by UV-vis spectrometry (Nanodrop One^C, Thermo Fisher Scientific, Denmark), recording their absorbance at 490 nm and 430 nm, respectively. The amount of each compound transported across the cell monolayers within a time interval of 8 h was calculated for both apical-to-basolateral (AB) and basolateral-to-apical (BA) directions. FLUO, LY, GA, and EGCG that remained entrapped within the cell monolayers, insert membranes and nanofibers were likewise quantified at the end of the permeability studies.

2.11. FLUO, LY, GA, and EGCG Distribution after Transport Experiments and Mass Balance

After transport experiments in both AB and BA directions, the amount of each compound collected at the apical and basolateral chambers was quantified. Donor concentrations at time = 0 ($C_{D,t=0\,h}$), donor and acceptor concentrations at time = 8 h ($C_{D,t=8\,h}$ and $C_{A,t=8\,h}$), compound concentrations remaining inside the cell monolayer at time = 8 h ($C_{Caco-2,t=8\,h}$), within membrane filters at time = 8 h ($C_{insert,t=8\,h}$), and adsorbed or remaining encapsulated in nanofibers at time = 8 h ($C_{fibers,t=8\,h}$) were experimentally measured. The mass balance of each compound was calculated as follows:

$$C_{D,t=0\,h} = C_{D,t=8\,h} + C_{A,t\,=\,8\,h} + C_{Caco-2,t=8\,h} + C_{insert,t=8\,h} + (C_{fibers,t=8\,h}) \tag{3}$$

Mass balance values of >90% were found for all tested compounds.

2.12. Calculation of the Apparent Permeability Coefficients, $P_{app,AB}$ and $P_{app,BA}$

The absorptive apparent permeability coefficient ($P_{app,AB}$) and the secretory apparent permeability coefficient ($P_{app,BA}$) were calculated by:

$$P_{app} = \frac{dC}{dt} * \frac{V}{A * C_0} \tag{4}$$

where, dC/dt (µM/s) is the rate of change in concentration on the acceptor chamber over time; V (cm^3) is the volume of the solution in the acceptor compartment; A (cm^2) is the area of the semipermeable membrane; and C_0 (μM) is the initial concentration in the donor chamber. The results of this study are expressed as mean ± SD of three independent experiments. Permeability directional ratio (PDR) is a measure of the compound polarization in Caco-2 cell monolayers, and was calculated by:

$$\text{PDR} = \frac{P_{app,BA}}{P_{app,AB}} \tag{5}$$

3. Results

3.1. Morphological and FTIR Characterization of Nanofibers

Uniform and randomly oriented xanthan nanofibers, with average diameters of 235 ± 49 nm, were obtained by electrospinning a 2.5% *w/v* xanthan solution in formic acid (Figure 1). The average diameter of electrospun X-GA and X-EGCG nanofibers was slightly increased to 327 ± 119 nm and 270 ± 95 nm, respectively, with the encapsulation of 2 mM of phenolic compounds.

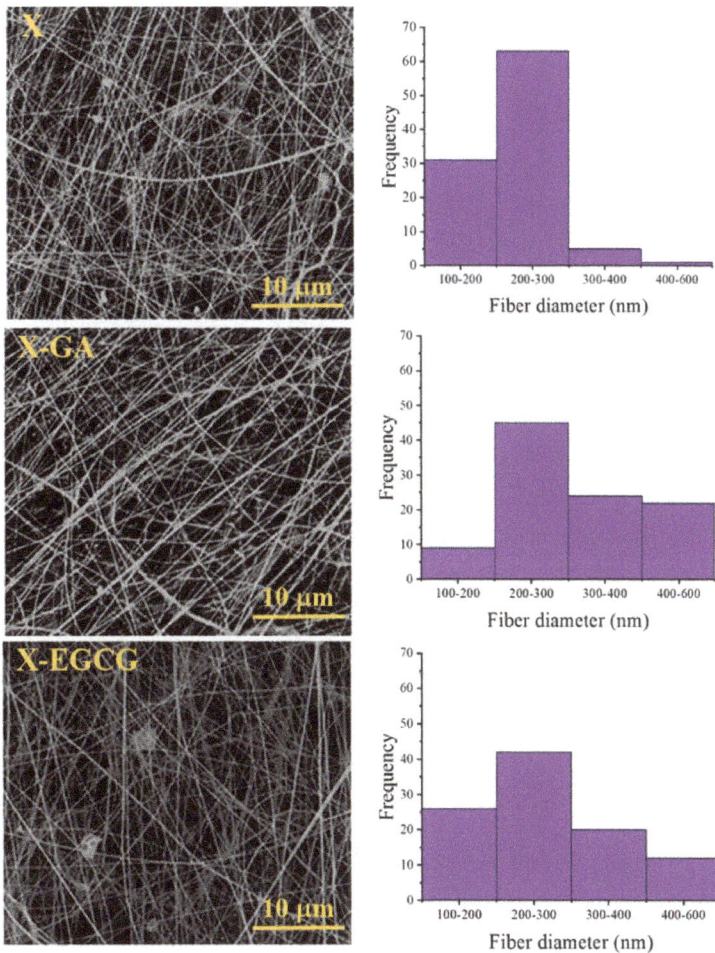

Figure 1. Morphological analysis by scanning electron microscopy (SEM) and average fiber diameter distributions of electrospun (upper) X nanofibers, (middle) X-GA, and (lower) X-EGCG nanofibers.

The FTIR spectra of X nanofibers, X-GA nanofibers, X-EGCG nanofibers, and GA and EGCG powders are shown in Figure 2. The FTIR spectrum of X nanofibers showed a characteristic broad peak in the region of 3500–3000 cm^{-1} due to O-H stretching, and a peak at around 2900 cm^{-1} due to the axial deformation of CH and CH_2 groups. In the region between 1800–1700 cm^{-1}, the stretching vibration of C=O was observed. In the region of 1200–1000 cm^{-1}, the O–H, C–O–C stretching of tertiary alcohols and esters, as well as the O–H stretching of primary alcohols was distinguished [40]. As discussed in the study by Shekarforoush et al. [40], the FTIR studies confirmed that an esterification reaction had taken place, where formic acid reacted with the pyruvic acid groups of xanthan. Hence, the esterification of pyruvic acid to pyruvyl formate induced a decrease of the negative charges of xanthan and stabilized the helical conformation of xanthan. Moreover, the FTIR spectra of X-GA and X-EGCG nanofibers are comparable to those of X without the bioactives. It is concluded that there are no physical or chemical interactions between the encapsulated GA, EGCG, and the X nanofibers matrix.

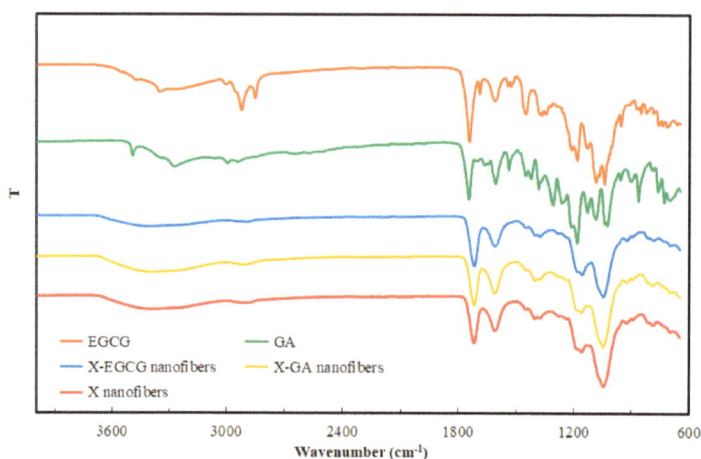

Figure 2. FTIR spectra of electrospun X, X-GA, X-EGCG nanofibers, GA, and EGCG.

3.2. In Vitro Release of GA and EGCG from Xanthan Nanofibers

The cumulative in vitro release of GA and EGCG from xanthan nanofibers was investigated by immersing the fibers in complete growth medium (DMEM-FBS), HBSS at pH 6.5 and HBSS at pH 7.4 (Figure 3). The total amount of GA and EGCG released from fibers was 69.01% and 70.53% in HBSS at pH 6.5, and 58.47% and 83.44% in HBSS at pH 7.4, respectively. Slightly different release values emerged from the immersion of fibers in the complete growth medium, which had an experimentally measured pH value of 7.28. Electrospun X, X-GA, and X-EGCG nanofibers remained intact in all release media and no morphological changes were observed during the experimental studies (data not shown). It is suggested that the presence of several salts in both DMEM-FBS and HBSS successfully prevented the dissolution of X, X-GA, and X-EGCG nanofibers.

The mechanism of GA and EGCG release from X nanofibers in pH 6.5 and 7.4 media were fitted by a Korsmeyer-Peppas kinetic model ($C = kt^n$), where, C is the amount of the compound released within the time, t; k is the rate constant; and n the release exponent. The constant value of k is usually related to the characteristics of the delivery system and drug; while n is the diffusion exponent, which characterizes the transport mechanism of the compound, and it depends on the type of transport, geometry, and polydispersity. The n values of the kinetic model in pH 6.5 and 7.4 media for the release of GA were 0.85 and 0.83, respectively. In the case of EGCG release, the n values in pH 6.5 and 7.4 media were 0.84 and 0.77, respectively. These results confirm that the release of the studied phenolic compounds is governed by the non-Fickian mechanism.

A)

B)

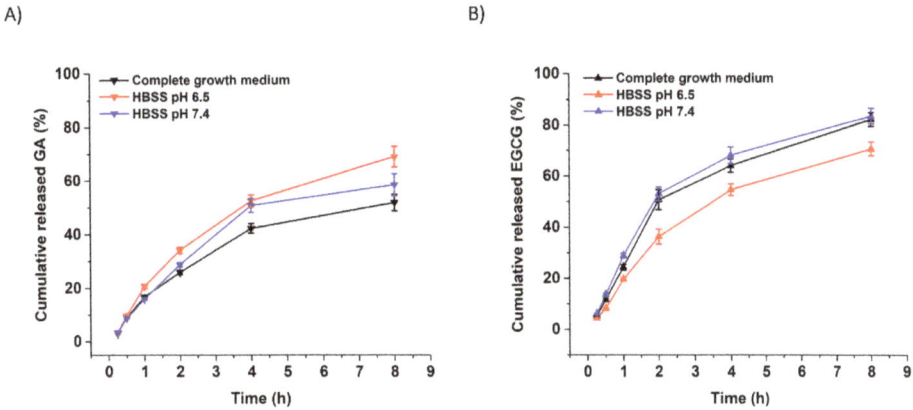

Figure 3. Cumulative in vitro release of GA (**A**) and EGCG (**B**) from xanthan nanofibers. All data were the mean ± SD of three independent experiments.

3.3. Effect of GA, EGCG, and Their Nanofiber Forms on Caco-2 Cell Viability

The viability of Caco-2 cells after 24 h treatment with free GA, EGCG, and PBS as the control was evaluated through MTS bioassay (Figure 4).

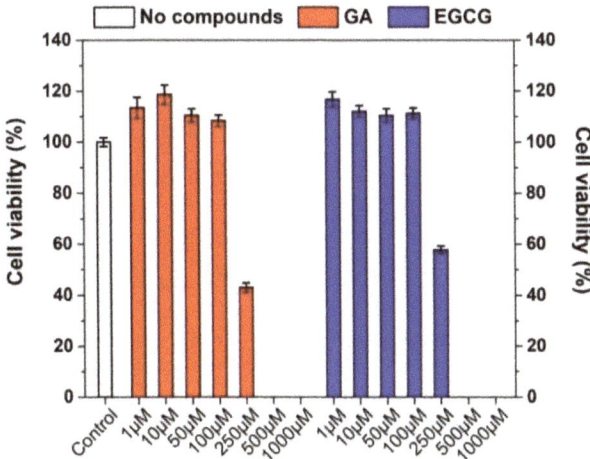

Figure 4. Viability bioassay of Caco-2 cells incubated with PBS (control, white bar) and increasing concentrations of free GA (red bars) and free EGCG (blue bars) diluted in PBS ranging from 1 μM to 1 mM. Data were the mean ± SD of four independent experiments.

When Caco-2 cells were incubated with free GA or EGCG in the concentration range between 1–100 μM, an increase in the cell viability was observed. By contrast, concentrations above 100 μM resulted in a drastically decreased cell viability, with a 50% or even higher cell mortality. The IC_{50} of free GA after 24 h incubation was estimated to be around 180 μM [7]. The concentration-dependent toxic effect of GA and EGCG was fundamental to perform transepithelial transport studies across proliferating cell monolayers. Indeed, the amount of X-GA and X-EGCG fibers was accordingly selected to obtain a final released GA and EGCG concentration lower or equal to 100 μM.

The viability of Caco-2 cells after 24 h treatment with increasing amounts of empty X, X-GA, and X-EGCG nanofibers was also investigated to establish the amount of fibers (in milligrams) to be used for transepithelial transport studies. As shown in Figure 5, the incubation of empty X fibers induced a directly proportional decrease of cell viability, reaching around 60% cell viability for 10 mg X nanofibers. However, this reduction was found to be more pronounced when cells were treated with X-GA and X-EGCG fibers. The release of GA from 2.0 mg X-GA fibers caused a cell mortality of around 70% and down until 98% for 5 mg X-GA fibers. The same effect was also confirmed after EGCG release from X-EGCG fibers, even though a 95% cell mortality was observed for 10 mg fibers. Consequently, the reduction of cell viability induced by X-GA and X-EGCG fibers was mainly attributed to GA and EGCG release, as confirmed in Figure 4, and partially caused by X nanofibers. Transepithelial transport studies were conducted incubating in 0.4 mg/mL X-GA (corresponding to 0.15 mM GA) and 1 mg/mL X-EGCG (corresponding to 0.051mM EGCG) in the donor chamber.

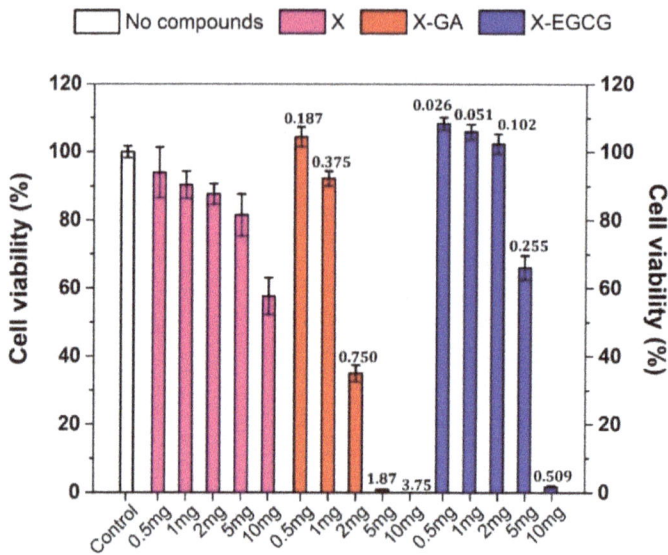

Figure 5. MTS viability bioassay of Caco-2 cells after 24 h incubation with complete growth medium (control, white bar) and increasing amounts of empty xanthan nanofibers (X, magenta bars), gallic acid-loaded xanthan nanofibers (X-GA, red bars), and (−)-epigallocatechin gallate-loaded xanthan nanofibers (X-EGCG, blue bars). The numbers reported on top of the red and blue bars represent the maximum releasable concentration (mM) of GA and EGCG in a 1.2 mL volume of complete growth medium. Data were the mean ± SD of four independent experiments.

3.4. Assessment of Cell Monolayers' Integrity

The cell monolayers' integrity is a fundamental determinant for the study of compound transport across the intestinal barrier, especially when passive transport through tight junctions is involved [42]. To ensure reliable in vitro permeability experiments across Caco-2 cell monolayers, the transport of non-radiolabeled markers, fluorescein (FLUO) and lucifer yellow (LY), and transepithelial electrical resistance measurement were conducted to quantitatively investigate the integrity of monolayers after 21 days growth on 12-mm polycarbonate inserts. The average TEER value for Caco-2 cell monolayers randomly chosen for transport studies was 370.74 ± 15.81 Ω cm^2. The TEER values of monolayers before and after transport of FLUO and LY were found in the range of 300–500 Ω cm^2 (Figure 6), indicating an "intermediate" tightness of the gastrointestinal epithelium [43].

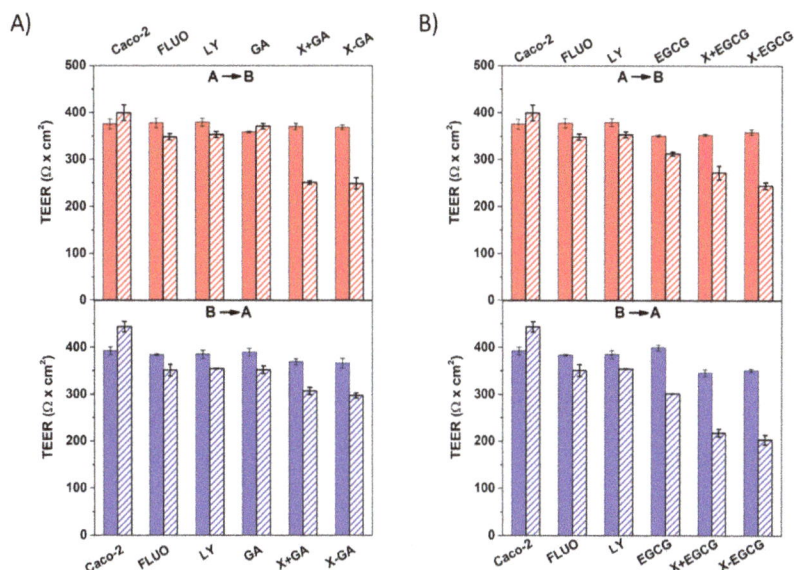

Figure 6. Transepithelial electrical resistance (TEER) measurements of cell monolayers before (full colored bars) and after (patterned bars) apical-to-basolateral (AB) and basolateral-to-apical (BA) studies for a time interval of 8 h. TEER values were recorded for GA, X + GA, and X-GA (**A**) and EGCG, X + EGCG, and X-EGCG (**B**). All data were the mean ± SD of three independent experiments.

The AB and BA transepithelial transports of FLUO and LY across Caco-2 monolayers under a proton gradient were investigated, resulting in a pH-dependent transport of FLUO. The apparent permeability coefficients of FLUO were $P_{app,AB} = 3.31 \times 10^{-6}$ cm/s and $P_{app,BA} = 2.01 \times 10^{-6}$ cm/s, whereas much lower values were observed from the LY transport: $P_{app,AB} = 1.13 \times 10^{-7}$ cm/s and $P_{app,BA} = 1.21 \times 10^{-7}$ cm/s (Figure 7C). Due to the lipoid nature of polarized epithelial cell layers, the transport of ions and hydrophilic compounds is restricted through the membrane. Indeed, hydrophilic LY was transported across epithelial cells solely via tight junctions, whereas the lipophilic FLUO permeated through transcellular transport [44–46]. Thus, from the TEER and permeability observations it was concluded that the integrity and tightness of epithelial cell monolayers were maintained after 21 days culturing.

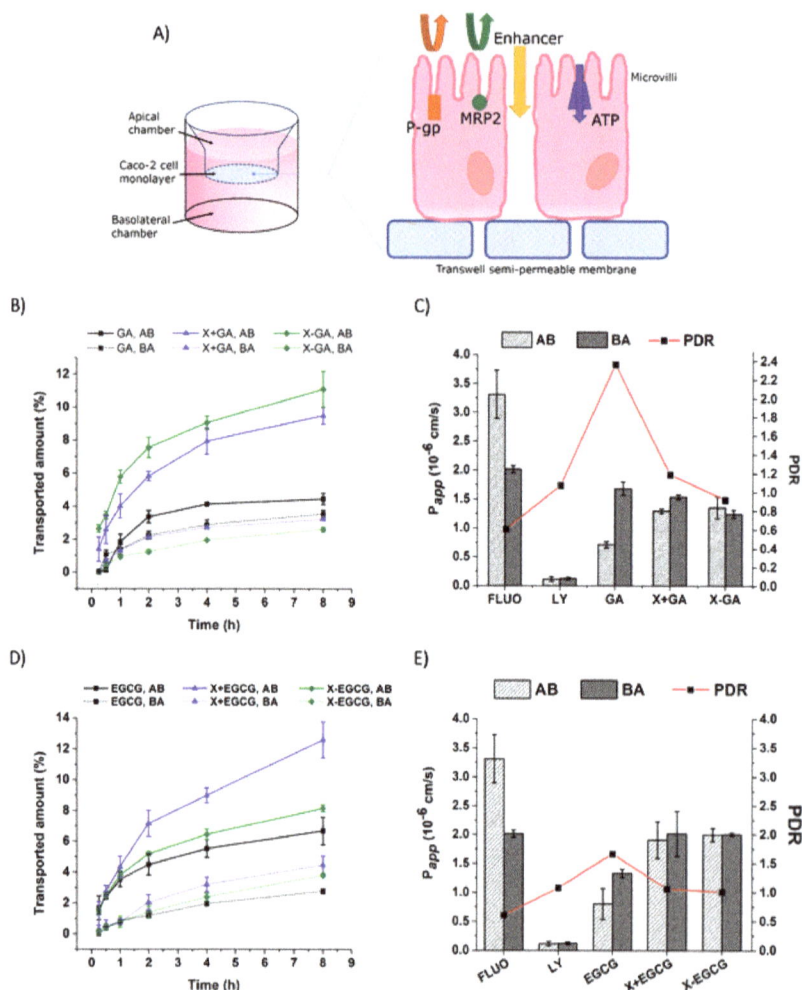

Figure 7. Transepithelial transport of GA and EGCG across Caco-2 monolayers. Illustration of the efflux transporters expressed on the apical membrane of epithelial cells (**A**). Transported amount of GA, X + GA, and X-GA (**B**), and EGCG, X + EGCG, and X-EGCG (**D**) in both AB and BA directions. Apparent permeability coefficient, P_{app}, and PDR of GA, X + GA and X-GA (**C**), and EGCG, X + EGCG, and X-EGCG (**E**). All data were the mean ± SD of three independent experiments.

3.5. Transepithelial Transport and Distribution of Free GA, EGCG, and Their Nanofiber Forms

The transported amounts of GA and EGCG, their apparent permeability coefficient, and their permeability directional ratio were assessed for both the AB and BA directions under a proton gradient. In addition, the compounds were incubated at the donor chamber in a free form (GA and EGCG), in a free form in the presence of empty xanthan nanofibers (X + GA and X + EGCG), and in the nanofiber forms (X-GA and X-EGCG). Figure 7 summarizes all the above-mentioned parameters. Firstly, the amounts of molecules transported in the acceptor chamber were higher in the AB direction than in the BA. Secondly, the addition of empty or loaded xanthan nanofibers enhanced the transport of GA and EGCG in the AB direction (Figure 7B–D). Indeed, the permeated amount of GA in the X + GA and X-GA formulations was 2-fold and 2.5-fold higher than that of free GA. The same results were obtained for the transported EGCG in the AB direction, but on the contrary, the X + EGCG form was the most effective (1.9-fold increase over the free EGCG). These results suggested that the permeation of the compounds was greatly enhanced by the presence of xanthan nanofibers, either as empty nanostructures or loaded with polyphenols. Accordingly, the apparent permeability coefficients of GA and EGCG incubated with nanofibers were at least 2-fold higher than those of the free compounds. Indeed, the GA and X-GA permeability values in the AB direction were $P_{app,AB} = 7.12 \times 10^{-7}$ cm/s and $P_{app,AB} = 1.96 \times 10^{-6}$ cm/s, respectively (Figure 7C). The same increase in permeability was detected also for the EGCG nanofiber form, where EGCG and X-EGCG had a $P_{app,AB} = 7.99 \times 10^{-7}$ cm/s and $P_{app,AB} = 1.99 \times 10^{-6}$ cm/s, respectively (Figure 7E). An increment of the apparent permeability coefficient values was also found in the BA direction, even though this was less pronounced than in the AB direction.

The fate of GA and EGCG during 8 h transepithelial transport in both AB and BA directions, was monitored by quantifying their concentration in the donor and acceptor compartments, in the cell lysate, insert membrane (filter), and within xanthan nanofibers (adsorbed or unreleased). Figure 8 shows the distribution of the tested compounds in the above-mentioned compartments. After 8 h experiment, most of the incubated compounds were still found in the donor chamber ($\geq 60\%$ of the concentration at time = 0 h), and only less than 20% were detected in the acceptor side. However, the yields of GA and EGCG recorded in A were higher when incubated with xanthan nanofibers than in its absence. Small amounts of GA and EGCG were also detected inside the epithelial monolayers (3% and 1.3%, respectively), and adsorbed to or unreleased from xanthan nanofibers (29% and 21%, respectively).

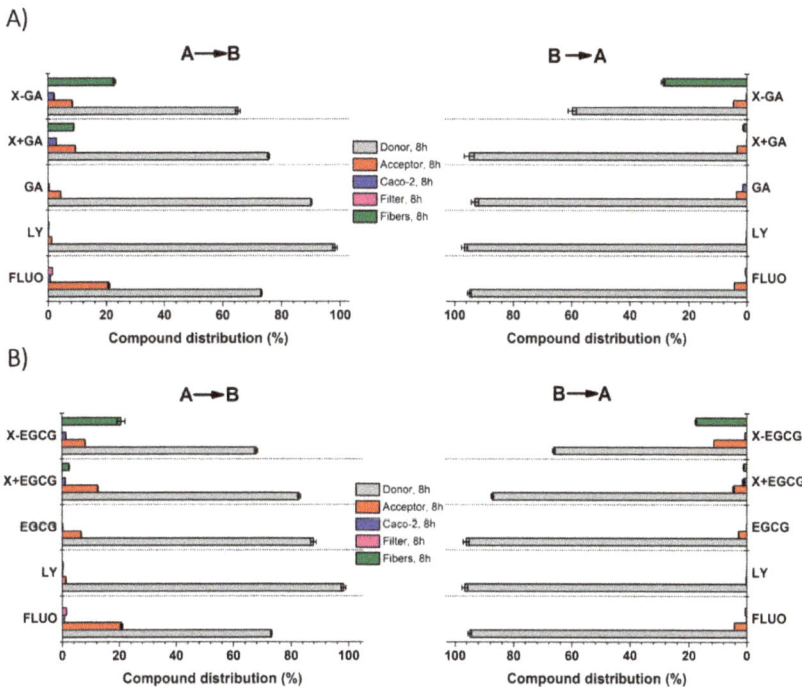

Figure 8. Quantification of GA (**A**) and EGCG (**B**) distribution in the donor side, acceptor side, cell lysate, membrane insert, and fibers after 8 h transepithelial transport in both AB and BA directions. All data are the mean ± SD of three independent experiments.

4. Discussion

In this study, human differentiated epithelial Caco-2 cells were chosen as an established in vitro cell model for the prediction of bioactive compounds' absorption and transport mechanism [47]. The Caco-2 cells possess many features, among which are their ability to slowly differentiate into monolayers forming microvilli and tight junctions at the apical side, and to express brush-border transporters and enzymes involved in the metabolism and transport of several substrates [41,48,49]. Therefore, transepithelial transport studies of GA and EGCG were performed across Caco-2 monolayers in the apical-to-basolateral and basolateral-to-apical directions under a proton gradient. The two polyphenols investigated in this study are characterized by a poor intestinal absorption due to their high hydrophilicity; in fact, they can hardly penetrate the cell membrane and only passive diffusion seems to be involved in their permeation [19].

The incubation of nanofibers with Caco-2 cells (24 h) revealed a proliferative effect in cell viability for amounts lower or equal to 0.5 mg X-GA and 2.0 mg X-EGCG; a drastic cell mortality was observed for doses above this range. In addition, the treatment of Caco-2 cells with increasing amounts of empty xanthan nanofibers resulted in a dose-dependent reduction of cell viability, close to 60% viability for 10.0 mg X incubated. However, the observed reduction in cell viability was expected to be less pronounced for transepithelial transport studies, since the cell monolayers were exposed to X, X-GA, and X-EGCG for 8 h rather than 24 h. The transepithelial transport of GA and EGCG in the acceptor compartment was successfully enhanced by the presence of xanthan, both as an empty nanostructure and as a nanocarrier, and the permeability coefficients were higher than those calculated for free compounds. In addition, the PDR values of free GA and free EGCG were both higher than 1.5 (2.4 and 1.7, respectively), suggesting that their transport is modulated by an active transport pathway, and more specifically by efflux. Several studies have described the mechanism and the efflux transporters involved in the unidirectional transport of GA and EGCG across the epithelial barrier [16,17,19,50,51]. Enterocytes express several transporters on the apical and basolateral membrane, which can actively transport a wide range of structurally diverse compounds into (influx) or out of (efflux) the cell. GA and EGCG, as depicted in Figure 7A, are actively transported outside cells through P-glycoprotein (P-gp), multidrug resistant protein 2 (MRP2), and the ATP binding cassette (ATP) transporters expressed on the apical membrane of Caco-2 monolayers [49,51]. These efflux pumps, therefore, restrict the influx of GA and EGCG into the acceptor chamber, rather promoting their efflux from enterocytes. Several efflux pump inhibitory compounds, such as indomethacin, verapamil, and MK-571 [16,19], have been thoroughly investigated, resulting in an increase in oral absorption. In this study, the calculated PDR values obtained for free GA and free EGCG transport were higher than 1.5, confirming their efflux from monolayers. However, the PDR values of X + GA, X-GA, X + EGCG, and X-EGCG were all lower than 1.5 (Figure 7C–E). Hence, the incubation of xanthan nanofibers in the donor compartment greatly improved the absorption of GA and EGCG across the epithelial barrier, suggesting an inhibitory effect of xanthan on efflux transporters.

The results presented in this study are congruent with our previous findings on the permeation across Caco-2 cells of a model protein (insulin) encapsulated within electrospun fish protein fibers [52]. Direct interactions between the fibers and the monolayer induced changes in the tight junctions, and thus, an increase in the permeation of insulin at local hot spots on the epithelial barrier was observed. Similarly, a 3.4-fold increase of curcumin permeability across Caco-2 cells was detected when the bioactive was encapsulated within xanthan-chitosan nanofibers, in comparison with free-curcumin [39].

5. Conclusions

Encapsulation and release of two poorly absorbed polyphenol compounds, GA and EGCG, using electrospun xanthan nanofibers were investigated. It was found that X, X-GA, and X-EGCG nanofibers remained stable in aqueous HBSS medium at different pH (6.5 and pH 7.4). The total amount of GA and EGCG released from xanthan nanofibers was 69.01% and 70.53% in HBSS at pH 6.5, and 58.47% and 83.44% in HBSS at pH 7.4, respectively. Moreover, the nanofibers were incubated with Caco-2 cells

Pharmaceutics **2019**, *11*, 155

and the cell viability, transepithelial transport, and GA and EGCG permeability properties across cell monolayers were investigated. At least a 2-fold increase of GA and EGCG permeability was observed in the presence of X-GA and X-EGCG nanofibers, in comparison with the free-phenolic compounds. Indeed, the polysaccharide nanofibers enhanced the GA and EGCG permeability by opening the tight junctions of Caco-2 monolayers, as well as inhibiting the efflux transporters. These findings are relevant for promoting the delivery not only of polyphenols, but also of other poorly absorbable bioactives and drugs.

Author Contributions: A.F. designed the experiments, A.F. and E.S. performed the experiments, A.F., A.C.M., I.S.C. analyzed the data and wrote the manuscript.

Funding: Part of this work was supported by the European Union funded project "Nano3Bio" (grant agreement no 613931).

Acknowledgments: The project was also supported by a PhD stipend (to Elhamalsadat Shekarforoush) from the Technical University of Denmark.

Conflicts of Interest: The authors declare no conflict of interest.

References

1. Scalbert, A.; Williamson, G. Dietary intake and bioavailability of polyphenols. *J. Nutr.* **2000**, *130*, 2073S–2085S. [CrossRef] [PubMed]
2. Kühnau, J. The flavonoids. A class of semi-essential food components: Their role in human nutrition. *World Rev. Nutr. Diet.* **1976**, *24*, 117–191.
3. Inoue, M.; Suzuki, R.; Koide, T.; Sakaguchi, N.; Ogihara, Y.; Yabu, Y. Antioxidant, gallic acid, induces apoptosis in HL-60RG cells. *Biochem. Biophys. Res. Commun.* **1994**, *204*, 898–904. [CrossRef] [PubMed]
4. Inoue, M.; Suzuki, R.; Sakaguchi, N.; Li, Z.; Takeda, T.; Ogihara, Y.; Jiang, B.Y.; Chen, Y. Selective induction of cell death in cancer cells by gallic acid. *Biol. Pharm. Bull.* **1995**, *18*, 1526–1530. [CrossRef]
5. Gali, H.U.; Perchellet, E.M.; Perchellet, J.P. Inhibition of tumor promoter-induced ornithine decarboxylase activity by tannic acid and other polyphenols in mouse epidermis in vivo. *Cancer Res.* **1991**, *51*, 2820–2825.
6. Gali, H.U.; Perchellet, E.M.; Klish, D.S.; Johnson, J.M.; Perchellet, J.P. Antitumor-promoting activities of hydrolyzable tannins in mouse skin. *Carcinogenesis* **1992**, *13*, 715–718. [CrossRef]
7. Rashidi, L.; Vasheghani-Farahani, E.; Soleimani, M.; Atashi, A.; Rostami, K.; Gangi, F.; Fallahpour, M.; Tahouri, M.T. A cellular uptake and cytotoxicity properties study of gallic acid-loaded mesoporous silica nanoparticles on Caco-2 cells. *J. Nanoparticle Res.* **2014**, *16*, 2285. [CrossRef]
8. Konishi, Y.; Kobayashi, S.; Shimizu, M. Transepithelial transport of *p*-coumaric acid and gallic acid in Caco-2 cell monolayers. *Biosci. Biotechnol. Biochem.* **2003**, *67*, 2317–2324. [CrossRef]
9. Huang, P.-J.; Hseu, Y.-C.; Lee, M.-S.; Senthil Kumar, K.J.; Wu, C.-R.; Hsu, L.-S.; Liao, J.-W.; Cheng, I.-S.; Kuo, Y.-T.; Huang, S.-Y.; et al. In vitro and in vivo activity of gallic acid and toona sinensis leaf extracts against HL-60 human premyelocytic leukemia. *Food Chem. Toxicol.* **2012**, *50*, 3489–3497. [CrossRef]
10. Inoue, M.; Sakaguchi, N.; Isuzugawa, K.; Tani, H.; Ogihara, Y. Role of reactive oxygen species in gallic acid-induced apoptosis. *Biol. Pharm. Bull.* **2000**, *23*, 1153–1157. [CrossRef]
11. Kaur, M.; Velmurugan, B.; Rajamanickam, S.; Agarwal, R.; Agarwal, C. Gallic acid, an active constituent of grape seed extract, exhibits anti-proliferative, pro-apoptotic and anti-tumorigenic effects against prostate carcinoma xenograft growth in nude mice. *Pharm. Res.* **2009**, *26*, 2133–2140. [CrossRef] [PubMed]
12. Pal, C.; Bindu, S.; Dey, S.; Alam, A.; Goyal, M.; Iqbal, M.S.; Maity, P.; Adhikari, S.S.; Bandyopadhyay, U. Gallic acid prevents nonsteroidal anti-inflammatory drug-induced gastropathy in rat by blocking oxidative stress and apoptosis. *Free Radic. Biol. Med.* **2010**, *49*, 258–267. [CrossRef]
13. You, B.R.; Park, W.H. Gallic acid-induced lung cancer cell death is related to glutathione depletion as well as reactive oxygen species increase. *Toxicol. Vitr.* **2010**, *24*, 1356–1362. [CrossRef]
14. You, B.R.; Moon, H.J.; Han, Y.H.; Park, W.H. Gallic acid inhibits the growth of HeLa cervical cancer cells via apoptosis and/or necrosis. *Food Chem. Toxicol.* **2010**, *48*, 1334–1340. [CrossRef] [PubMed]
15. Munin, A.; Edwards-Lévy, F. Encapsulation of natural polyphenolic compounds; a review. *Pharmaceutics* **2011**, *3*, 793–829. [CrossRef] [PubMed]

16. Mao, X.; Wu, L.-F.; Zhao, H.-J.; Liang, W.-Y.; Chen, W.-J.; Han, S.-X.; Qi, Q.; Cui, Y.-P.; Li, S.; Yang, G.-H.; et al. Transport of corilagin, gallic acid, and ellagic acid from fructus phyllanthi tannin fraction in Caco-2 cell monolayers. *Evid.-Based Complement. Alternat. Med.* **2016**, *2016*, 9205379. [CrossRef]

17. Vaidyanathan, J.B.; Walle, T. Cellular uptake and efflux of the tea flavonoid (−)epicatechin-3-gallate in the human intestinal cell line Caco-2. *J. Pharmacol. Exp. Ther.* **2003**, *307*, 745–752. [CrossRef]

18. Katiyar, S.; Mukhtar, H. Tea in chemoprevention of cancer. *Int. J. Oncol.* **1996**, *8*, 221–238. [CrossRef] [PubMed]

19. Song, Q.; Li, D.; Zhou, Y.; Yang, J.; Yang, W.; Zhou, G.; Wen, J. Enhanced uptake and transport of (+)-catechin and (−)-epigallocatechin gallate in niosomal formulation by human intestinal Caco-2 cells. *Int. J. Nanomed.* **2014**, *9*, 2157. [CrossRef]

20. Ji, B.T.; Chow, W.H.; Hsing, A.W.; McLaughlin, J.K.; Dai, Q.; Gao, Y.T.; Blot, W.J.; Fraumeni, J.F. Green tea consumption and the risk of pancreatic and colorectal cancers. *Int. J. Cancer* **1997**, *70*, 255–258. [CrossRef]

21. Su, J.; Arab, L. Tea consumption and the reduced risk of colon cancer—results from a national prospective cohort study. *Public Health Nutr.* **2002**, *5*, 419–425. [CrossRef] [PubMed]

22. Chow, H.H.; Cai, Y.; Alberts, D.S.; Hakim, I.; Dorr, R.; Shahi, F.; Crowell, J.A.; Yang, C.S.; Hara, Y. Phase I pharmacokinetic study of tea polyphenols following single-dose administration of epigallocatechin gallate and polyphenon E. *Cancer Epidemiol. Biomark. Prev.* **2001**, *10*, 53–58.

23. Warden, B.A.; Smith, L.S.; Beecher, G.R.; Balentine, D.A.; Clevidence, B.A. Catechins are bioavailable in men and women drinking black tea throughout the day. *J. Nutr.* **2001**, *131*, 1731–1737. [CrossRef]

24. Teng, Z.; Yuan, C.; Zhang, F.; Huan, M.; Cao, W.; Li, K.; Yang, J.; Cao, D.; Zhou, S.; Mei, Q. Intestinal absorption and first-pass metabolism of polyphenol compounds in rat and their transport dynamics in Caco-2 cells. *PLoS ONE* **2012**, *7*, e29647. [CrossRef] [PubMed]

25. Liu, L.; Guo, L.; Zhao, C.; Wu, X.; Wang, R.; Liu, C. Characterization of the intestinal absorption of seven flavonoids from the flowers of trollius chinensis using the Caco-2 cell monolayer model. *PLoS ONE* **2015**, *10*, e0119263. [CrossRef] [PubMed]

26. Dube, A.; Ng, K.; Nicolazzo, J.A.; Larson, I. Effective use of reducing agents and nanoparticle encapsulation in stabilizing catechins in alkaline solution. *Food Chem.* **2010**, *122*, 662–667. [CrossRef]

27. Caddeo, C.; Teskač, K.; Sinico, C.; Kristl, J. Effect of resveratrol incorporated in liposomes on proliferation and UV-B protection of cells. *Int. J. Pharm.* **2008**, *363*, 183–191. [CrossRef] [PubMed]

28. Chuysinuan, P.; Chimnoi, N.; Techasakul, S.; Supaphol, P. Gallic acid-loaded electrospun poly(L-lactic acid) fiber mats and their release characteristic. *Macromol. Chem. Phys.* **2009**, *210*, 814–822. [CrossRef]

29. Neo, Y.P.; Ray, S.; Jin, J.; Gizdavic-Nikolaidis, M.; Nieuwoudt, M.K.; Liu, D.; Quek, S.Y. Encapsulation of food grade antioxidant in natural biopolymer by electrospinning technique: A physicochemical study based on zein-gallic acid system. *Food Chem.* **2013**, *136*, 1013–1021. [CrossRef]

30. Phiriyawirut, M.; Phaechamud, T. Gallic acid-loaded cellulose acetate electrospun nanofibers: Thermal properties, mechanical properties, and drug release behavior. *Open J. Polym. Chem.* **2012**, *02*, 21–29. [CrossRef]

31. Aytac, Z.; Kusku, S.I.; Durgun, E.; Uyar, T. Encapsulation of gallic acid/cyclodextrin inclusion complex in electrospun polylactic acid nanofibers: Release behavior and antioxidant activity of gallic acid. *Mater. Sci. Eng. C* **2016**, *63*, 231–239. [CrossRef] [PubMed]

32. Li, Y.; Lim, L.-T.; Kakuda, Y. Electrospun zein fibers as carriers to stabilize (−)-epigallocatechin gallate. *J. Food Sci.* **2009**, *74*, C233–C240. [CrossRef]

33. Lee, E.J.; Lee, J.H.; Jin, L.; Jin, O.S.; Shin, Y.C.; Sang, J.O.; Lee, J.; Hyon, S.-H.; Han, D.-W. Hyaluronic acid/poly(lactic-co-glycolic acid) core/shell fiber meshes loaded with epigallocatechin-3-O-gallate as skin tissue engineering scaffolds. *J. Nanosci. Nanotechnol.* **2014**, *14*, 8458–8463. [CrossRef] [PubMed]

34. Lee, M.H.; Kwon, B.-J.; Koo, M.-A.; Jang, E.H.; Seon, G.M.; Park, J.-C. Exovascular application of epigallocatechin-3-O-gallate-releasing electrospun poly(L-lactide glycolic acid) fiber sheets to reduce intimal hyperplasia in injured abdominal aorta. *Biomed. Mater.* **2015**, *10*, 055010. [CrossRef]

35. Ho, L.J.; Cheol, S.Y.; Jun, Y.W.; Chul, P.J.; Hyu, H.S.; Wook, H.D. Epigallocatechin-3-O-gallate-loaded poly(lactic-co-glycolic acid) fibrous sheets as anti-adhesion barriers. *J. Biomed. Nanotechnol.* **2014**, *11*, 1461–1471. [CrossRef]

36. Tian, J.; Tu, H.; Shi, X.; Wang, X.; Deng, H.; Li, B.; Du, Y. Antimicrobial application of nanofibrous mats self-assembled with chitosan and epigallocatechin gallate. *Colloids Surf. B Biointerfaces* **2016**, *145*, 643–652. [CrossRef]

37. Ayca, A.; Gulum, S.; Serpil, S. Fabrication of gallic acid loaded hydroxypropyl methylcellulose nanofibers by electrospinning technique as active packaging material. *Carbohydr. Polym.* **2019**, *208*, 241–250. [CrossRef]
38. Shekarforoush, E.; Ajalloueian, F.; Zeng, G.; Mendes, A.C.; Chronakis, I.S. Electrospun xanthan-chitosan nanofibers as delivery carrier of hydrophobic bioactives. *Mater. Lett.* **2018**, *228*, 322–326. [CrossRef]
39. Faralli, A.; Shekarforoush, E.; Ajalloueian, F.; Mendes, A.C.; Chronakis, I.S. In vitro permeability enhancement of curcumin across Caco-2 cells monolayers using electrospun xanthan-chitosan nanofibers. *Carbohydr. Polym.* **2019**, *206*, 38–47. [CrossRef]
40. Shekarforoush, E.; Faralli, A.; Ndoni, S.; Mendes, A.C.; Chronakis, I.S. Electrospinning of xanthan polysaccharide. *Macromol. Mater. Eng.* **2017**, *302*, 1700067. [CrossRef]
41. Hubatsch, I.; Ragnarsson, E.G.E.; Artursson, P. Determination of drug permeability and prediction of drug absorption in Caco-2 monolayers. *Nat. Protoc.* **2007**, *2*, 2111–2119. [CrossRef] [PubMed]
42. Srinivasan, B.; Kolli, A.R.; Esch, M.B.; Abaci, H.E.; Shuler, M.L.; Hickman, J.J. TEER measurement techniques for in vitro barrier model systems. *J. Lab. Autom.* **2015**, *20*, 107–126. [CrossRef] [PubMed]
43. Amidon, G.L.; Lee, P.I.; Topp, E.M. *Transport Processes in Pharmaceutical Systems*; M. Dekker: New York, NY, USA, 2000; ISBN 9780824766108.
44. Högerle, M.L.; Winne, D. Drug absorption by the rat jejunum perfused in situ. Dissociation from the pH-partition theory and role of microclimate-pH and unstirred layer. *Naunyn. Schmiedebergs. Arch. Pharmacol.* **1983**, *322*, 249–255.
45. Bock, U.; Kolac, C.; Borchard, G.; Koch, K.; Fuchs, R.; Streichhan, P.; Lehr, C.M. Transport of proteolytic enzymes across Caco-2 cell monolayers. *Pharm. Res.* **1998**, *15*, 1393–1400. [CrossRef] [PubMed]
46. Konishi, Y.; Hagiwara, K.; Shimizu, M. Transepithelial transport of fluorescein in Caco-2 Cell monolayers and use of such transport in in vitro evaluation of phenolic acid availability. *Biosci. Biotechnol. Biochem.* **2002**, *66*, 2449–2457. [CrossRef] [PubMed]
47. Artursson, P.; Palm, K.; Luthman, K. Caco-2 monolayers in experimental and theoretical predictions of drug transport. *Adv. Drug Deliv. Rev.* **2001**, *46*, 27–43. [CrossRef]
48. Yee, S. In vitro permeability across Caco-2 cells (colonic) can predict in vivo (small intestinal) absorption in man—Fact or myth. *Pharm. Res.* **1997**, *14*, 763–766. [CrossRef] [PubMed]
49. Naruhashi, K.; Kurahashi, Y.; Fujita, Y.; Kawakita, E.; Yamasaki, Y.; Hattori, K.; Nishimura, A.; Shibata, N. Comparison of the expression and function of ATP binding cassette transporters in Caco-2 and T84 cells on stimulation by selected endogenous compounds and xenobiotics. *Drug Metab. Pharmacokinet.* **2011**, *26*, 145–153. [CrossRef] [PubMed]
50. Hoosain, F.G.; Choonara, Y.E.; Tomar, L.K.; Kumar, P.; Tyagi, C.; du Toit, L.C.; Pillay, V. Bypassing P-glycoprotein drug efflux mechanisms: Possible applications in pharmacoresistant schizophrenia therapy. *BioMed Res. Int.* **2015**, 484963. [CrossRef] [PubMed]
51. Werle, M. Expert review. Natural and synthetic polymers as inhibitors of drug efflux pumps. *Pharm. Res.* **2007**, *25*, 500–511. [CrossRef]
52. Stephansen, K.; García-Díaz, M.; Jessen, F.; Chronakis, I.S.; Nielsen, H.M. Bioactive protein-based nanofibers interact with intestinal biological components resulting in transepithelial permeation of a therapeutic protein. *Int. J. Pharm.* **2015**, *495*, 58–66. [CrossRef] [PubMed]

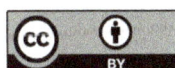

pharmaceutics

MDPI

Article

Gold Nanocage-Incorporated Poly(ε-Caprolactone) (PCL) Fibers for Chemophotothermal Synergistic Cancer Therapy

Ju Hyang Park [1], Hojun Seo [2], Da In Kim [1], Ji Hyun Choi [1], Jin Ho Son [1], Jongbok Kim [3], Geon Dae Moon [2,*] and Dong Choon Hyun [1,*]

[1] Department of Polymer Science and Engineering, Kyungpook National University, Daegu 41566, Korea; pjh99279@naver.com (J.H.P.); dada7230@naver.com (D.I.K.); jode1532@naver.com (J.H.C.); mlbask7@naver.com (J.H.S.)

[2] Dongnam Regional Division, Korea Institute of Industrial Technology, Busan 46938, Korea; dark911205@gmail.com

[3] Department of Materials Science and Engineering, Kumoh National Institute of Technology, Gumi, Gyeongbuk 39177, Korea; jb1956k@gmail.com

* Correspondence: gmoon@kitech.re.kr (G.D.M.); dong.hyun@knu.ac.kr (D.C.H.); Tel.: +82-53-950-5625 (D.C.H.)

Received: 29 November 2018; Accepted: 28 December 2018; Published: 1 February 2019

Abstract: This paper introduces a new fibrous system for synergistic cancer therapy, which consists of gold nanocage (AuNC)-loaded poly(ε-caprolactone) (PCL) fibers with encapsulation of a chemotherapeutic anticancer drug in their core and loading of a phase-changeable fatty acid in their sheath. Under on–off switching of near-infrared (NIR) light irradiation, the excellent photothermal ability and photostability of AuNCs allows repeated, significant heating of the fibers to a temperature available to hyperthermia. Simultaneously, the NIR light-induced heat generation enables the melting out of the loaded fatty acid, leading to a rapid release of the drug molecules from the fibers. The combination of this NIR light-triggered drug release with the repeated hyperthermia treatment exhibits excellent anticancer efficacy.

Keywords: PCL; electrospinning; combination therapy; photothermal therapy; NIR-triggered drug release

1. Introduction

Over the past several decades, considerable effort has been dedicated to the fabrication of polymeric fibers. These have a large surface area and high aspect ratio, and are applicable to a broad spectrum of applications, including air filtration, catalysis, energy harvesting and conversion, electronics, sensors, and in regenerative medicine [1–7]. Among many strategies that have been developed for the production of polymeric fibers, electrospinning has been extensively explored due to its merits such as simplicity, high efficiency, low cost, and high reproducibility [3]. More importantly, it allows a variety of functional molecules to be easily loaded into polymeric fibers [8], which has expanded the applicability of the fibers to the biomedical treatment of diseases through the delivery and even the controlled release of drugs [9].

Recently, the use of electrospun polymeric fibers in biomedical application has been directed towards the therapy of cancer, an intractable health issue worldwide. Such electrospun fibres possess unique features including high drug loading efficiency, good stability as a bulk material, and ease in temporal release of drugs [10–14]. In particular, their implantability at tumor sites or in the cavities remaining after surgical removal of solid tumors enables a localized release of chemotherapeutic drugs, which can maintain a low concentration of the systematic drugs while allowing their sufficient dosage locally [12]. However, the use of chemotherapeutic drugs can bring inevitably several problems such as drug resistance and toxicity in side effects [13,15,16]. Furthermore, it is difficult to sufficiently eliminate tumors using drugs only, even though they are useful for treating many types of cancers.

In addressing these issues, combination therapy, which uses the synergistic effects of two or more treatment modalities, has been developed for higher therapeutic efficacy. Photothermal therapy (PTT), in which an incident light is converted into heat for destroying cancer cells, has been used together with chemotherapy because it can induce a selective death of cancer cells [17,18]. As the combination strategy, until recently, electrospun polymeric fibers have been incorporated with both chemotherapeutic drugs and photothermal agents. As an exemplary case, smart electrospun fibers, which can potentially realize a synergistic effect of chemotherapy and PTT, were produced by Burdick and coworkers [19]. They encapsulated gold nanorods (AuNRs), as a photothermal agent, and drug molecules into poly(*N*-isopropylacrylamide-co-polyethylene glycol acrylate) (PNPA) fibers with thermosensitivity. Near-infrared (NIR) light-triggered release of the loaded drug occurred by an interplay of the photothermal effect of AuNRs with the temperature responsiveness of PNPA. Mao and coworkers fabricated Yb^{3+}/Er^{3+} co-doped $CaTiO_3$ nanofibers [12]. Increase in local temperature at the surface of the fibers by NIR light irradiation enhanced the vibration of poly(acrylic acid) (PAA) chains functionalized on the surface of the fibers, weakening an electrostatic bonding between the fibers and preloaded doxorubicin anticancer drug molecules. As a result, NIR light-triggered release of the drug was achieved. Recently, Kim and coworkers demonstrated the use of poly(ε-caprolactone) (PCL) fibers functionalized by NIR light-responsive polypyrrole (PPy) for synergistic cancer therapy [13]. Under an on–off operation of NIR light, the fibers allowed a precisely controlled release of paclitaxel anticancer drug together with a repeated application of NIR light-triggered hyperthermia, which exhibited excellent anticancer efficacy. Nevertheless, for their practical application in cancer therapy, the systems need to stop the undesirable drug release in non-triggered state and/or the loss of activity of chemotherapeutic drugs arising from the use of multi-stage physicochemical processes [20]. Alternatively, a system, consisting of PCL hollow fibers with entrapment of indocyanine green (ICG) in their sheath, was developed for combination therapy [21]. However, the use of ICG as a photothermal agent would make the repeated hyperthermia of the system difficult due to its loss of photothermal ability by photobleaching or chemical/thermal denaturation.

In this study, we introduce a PCL fibrous system incorporated with gold nanocages (AuNCs) that can function as a NIR light-absorbing photothermal agent with excellent stability. The incorporation of AuNCs enables a significant heating of the fibers upon exposure to NIR light. This NIR light-triggered heat generation can be repeatedly achieved through an on–off switching of NIR light irradiation, leading to a significant death of cancer cells by repeated hyperthermia treatment. Additional loading of the anticancer drug doxorubicin and a phase-changeable fatty acid to the fibres will enhance the anticancer activity of the system more through NIR light-triggered release of the drug in combination with hyperthermia.

2. Materials and Methods

2.1. Materials

The following chemicals were purchased from Sigma-Aldrich (St. Louis, MO, USA): PCL (Mn ≈ 45,000 Da), WST-1 solution, doxorubicin hydrochloride (DOX), Span 80, silver trifluoroacetate (CF_3COOAg), sodium hydrosulfide hydrate (NaHS), poly(vinylpyrrolidone) (PVP, Mw ≈ 55,000 Da), lauric acid (LA), stearic acid (SA), *O*-[2-(3-mercaptopropionylamino)ethyl]-*O*′-methylpolyethylene glycol (PEG-thiol, Mw ≈ 5000 Da), and gold (III) chloride trihydrate ($HAuCl_4 \cdot 3H_2O$). Ethylene glycol (EG) and sodium chloride (NaCl) were obtained from J.T. Baker (Phillipsburg, NJ, USA) and Duksan Chemical (Daegu, Korea), respectively. Human breast cancer SK-BR-3 cells and fibroblast (FB) cells were procured from Korea Cell Line Bank (KCLB, Seoul, Korea).

2.2. Preparation of Eutectic Mixture of Fatty Acids

We prepared a eutectic mixture of fatty acids with a melting point of 39 °C as previously reported [22]. Briefly, 0.8 g of LA and 0.2 g of SA were first put together in a glass vial (20 mL), followed by heating at 90 °C in nitrogen (N_2) atmosphere with magnetic stirring at 500 rpm. After 1 h, the fatty acid mixture was cooled down to 25 °C in ambient air.

2.3. Synthesis and Phase Transfer of AuNCs

First, EG (50 mL) was added to a 250 mL round bottom flask and then heated at 150 °C under magnetic stirring using a heating mantle, followed by the addition of a NaHS solution in EG (0.6 mL, 3 mM). After 4 min, 5 mL of a HCl solution in EG (3 mM) was added, followed by 12.5 mL of a PVP solution in EG (20 mg/mL). Then, 4 mL of CF_3COOAg solution in EG (282 mM) was additionally injected to synthesize silver nanocubes (AgNCs). After 30 min, the reaction was quenched in an ice-water bath, followed by centrifugation and washing with acetone and deionized (DI) water (18.2 MΩ). The resultant AgNCs were converted into AuNCs using a previously reported procedure with several minor modifications [23]. In a typical synthesis process, an aqueous solution of $HAuCl_4$ (0.75 mM) was prepared. A specific amount of the $HAuCl_4$ solution was then added dropwise into 5 mL of an aqueous solution of AgNCs (0.01 mg/mL) preheated to 90 °C. After 10–15 min, the sample was cooled down to 25 °C and a sufficient amount of NaCl was added to remove the AgCl precipitated in the synthesis. The sample was then centrifuged three times at 9000 rpm for 20 min. The collected AuNCs were re-dispersed in DI water and stored in the dark until further use.

To achieve phase transfer of the as-synthesized AuNCs from water phase to organic, their surface was modified. In order to accomplish this, 1 mg of the as-synthesized AuNCs was dispersed in 5 mL of DI water, followed by adding 1 mL of an aqueous solution of PEG-thiol (1 wt%) and 3 mL of chloroform. The solution mixture was mechanically agitated using a vortex mixer for 2 min, and thus the AuNCs were transferred from the water phase to the chloroform. The chloroform phase was then extracted, followed by centrifugation, washing with fresh chloroform, and drying in ambient air. The resultant sample was stored at 4 °C until further use.

2.4. Fabrication of Electrospun Fibers

To fabricate electrospun fibers, a water-in-oil (W/O) emulsion was first prepared. To accomplish this, a Span 80 solution in chloroform was made by dissolving 2 g of the surfactant in 38 g of the solvent. The solution was mixed with 200 µL of an aqueous solution containing DOX (3 mg) to generate a W/O emulsion using a high-speed mixer at a rotation rate of 15,000 rpm. The resultant W/O emulsion (3.5 g) was mixed with the eutectic mixture of fatty acids, the phase-transferred AuNCs, and PCL (1.5 g). The weight fraction of the eutectic mixture to PCL (f_{fatty}) was varied. Polymeric fibers loaded with AuNCs and DOX were produced by electrospinning the prepared W/O emulsion. For the electrospinning, the W/O emulsion was filled into a syringe (5 mL) with attachment to a stainless steel needle (22 gauge) and a voltage in the range of 6 and 8 kV was applied to the needle. The feed rate of the emulsion was fixed at 0.03 mL/h and an electrically grounded aluminum foil, placed 20 cm away from the needle, was used as a collector. Loading of DOX into the fibers was confirmed using a confocal laser scanning microscope (CLSM) (LSM700, Carl Zeiss, Oberkochen, Germany) and the amount of the loaded drug was quantified through UV–VIS spectral measurement (T60, PG Instrument, Leicestershire, United Kingdom), as previously reported [21].

2.5. NIR Light-Induced Heat Generation

The photothermal ability of the as-synthesized AuNCs and the phase-transferred AuNCs was characterized using a digital thermometer (Scilab Co., Daejeon, Korea). In a typical procedure, 0.5 mg of the particles was dispersed in 5 mL of dispersion medium (DI water for the former and chloroform for the latter). Each sample was exposed to 1 W/cm^2 NIR light with a wavelength of 808 nm (LASERLAB Co., Anyang, Korea) for 50 min. For checking the photothermal behavior of the AuNC-loaded fibers, a mesh made of 20 mg of the fibers with a dimension of 1 cm × 1 cm was first prepared, followed by exposing to NIR light irradiation (1 W/cm^2). The thermal infrared images and the temperature change were obtained with the use of a thermal infrared camera (G100EX, Avio, Tokyo, Japan).

2.6. Release of DOX from Fibers in Response to NIR Light Irradiation

To obtain the release profiles of DOX, we prepared 100 mg of AuNC-loaded PCL fibers encapsulating DOX, followed by immersing in 5 mL of phosphate-buffered saline (PBS) solution at pH 7.4. After incubation in a thermostat preheated to 37 °C for 4 h under mild agitation, NIR light irradiation (1 W/cm^2, 808 nm) was applied to the sample for 5 min to increase the temperature to 45 °C. After the treatment, the sample was re-incubated at 37 °C. At different time intervals, 1 mL of the solution was taken out and the concentration of DOX in it was characterized using UV–VIS spectrophotometry, as previously reported [21]. After characterization, the solution was poured back for further testing. For each time interval, three samples were tested.

2.7. Cell Viability Test

The cytotoxicity of NIR light irradiation (1 W/cm^2, 808 nm) was examined using a previously reported procedure [20]. Additionally, we investigated the cytotoxicity of phase-transferred AuNCs, which was achieved by introducing a solution of the particles (10 µL) in dimethyl sulfoxide with a certain concentration to the cells cultured through the aforementioned procedure. The sample without the treatment with the nanoparticles and NIR irradiation was used as a control. The cell viability was determined using WST-1 assay.

The biocompatibility of plain PCL fibers, AuNC-incorporated PCL fibers, AuNC-incorporated PCL fibers loaded with DOX, and AuNC-incorporated PCL fibers with loading of the fatty acid mixture and DOX was also tested using FB cells. Meshes with a dimension of 1 cm × 1 cm were first prepared from each type of fibers (20 mg) and then placed in each well of a 24-well cell culture plate. After their sterilization for 30 min under UV light irradiation, FB cells were cultured on the meshes as reported previously [20]. The anticancer activity of those fibers and PCL fibers loaded with the fatty acid mixture and DOX against SK-BR-3 cells was evaluated using a live/dead cell assay as well as a WST-1 assay. SK-BR-3 cells cultured on the meshes made of each type of fibers through the aforementioned procedure were subsequently treated with 1 W/cm^2 NIR light (5 min of exposure per treatment), followed by incubation at 37 °C for an additional 19–24 h according to the number of the exposure to conduct the WST-1 assay and the live/dead assay using a commercially available kit (Biotium, Fremont, CA, USA).

2.8. Characterization

Transmission electron microscope (TEM) analysis was performed on the fibers incorporated with AuNCs and the as-synthesized AuNCs using a HT7700 (Hitachi) operated at 75 kV. The morphology of the produced fibers was also investigated using a scanning electron microscope (SEM) (SU8220, Hitachi, Tokyo, Japan) with an accelerating voltage of 3 kV. Differential scanning calorimetry (DSC) measurement was conducted using DSC Q100 (TA Instrument, New Castle, DE, USA). Typically, samples with a weight of approximate 3 mg were used for scanning in the range of −70 and 250 °C at a scanning rate of 2 °C/min. X-ray diffraction (XRD) patterns were recorded in the range of 2θ = 10° to 90° using a Rigaku D/MAX II X-ray diffractometer with Cu K$_\alpha$ radiation.

2.9. Statistical Analysis

Student's *t*-test was used to examine the differences between two groups, and a one-way analysis of variance (ANOVA) with a Tukey's post hoc test was performed to examine the differences among four groups. $p < 0.01$ was considered to indicate a statistically significant difference.

3. Results and Discussion

NIR light, which has the minimum absorption by human blood and body tissues, is known to penetrate into soft tissues up to several inches in depth and to be converted into heat with a photothermal agent [24], which makes it advantageous for PTT. To achieve NIR light-induced cancer therapy, a NIR light-sensitive system was made of biocompatible/ biodegradable PCL fibers incorporated with AuNCs. The unique plasmonic property of AuNCs due to an interaction of light with their conduction band electrons allows photon energy to be efficiently converted into thermal energy [25]. When the generated heat increases the temperature of the system to a window available for hyperthermia (ca. 40–45 °C) [26], inactivation and eventual death of cancer cells will occur. Since AuNCs are non-susceptible to photobleaching and chemical/thermal denaturation [27], the hyperthermia can be repeatedly achieved.

AuNCs were synthesized using a galvanic replacement reaction between AgNCs (Figure S1, Supplementary Materials) and $HAuCl_4$. When a very small amount of $HAuCl_4$ solution was added to an aqueous solution of AgNCs, the replacement reaction was activated at a specific site on the surface of each AgNC, generating a hole (Figure 1A). As the reaction proceeded, the hole worked as an anode, oxidizing Ag atoms. Consequently, the released electrons moved to the surface of the AgNCs for reducing $HAuCl_4{}^-$, leading to an epitaxial growth of Au atoms on the AgNCs [28]. As the Au layer formed, the holes functioned as a site for the dissolution of Ag, transforming the AgNCs into a hollow structure (Figure 1B). When the amount of the $HAuCl_4$ solution was increased, the hollow interior would be larger in size, forming Au-Ag nanoboxes with a uniform wall (Figure 1C). The Ag atoms in the nanoboxes would be selectively removed with the further addition of $HAuCl_4$, eventually leading to the formation of AuNCs with a porous structure (Figure 1D).

Figure 1E shows UV-VIS–NIR extinction spectra for the samples of Figure 1A–D dispersed in DI water, indicating that their surface plasmon resonance (SPR) band was dependent on the amount of $HAuCl_4$ used. When a larger amount of $HAuCl_4$ was used, the extinction peak appeared at a longer wavelength. For example, the sample of Figure 1B exhibited an extinction peak at 575 nm, while the SPR peak for the solution of AuNCs (Figure 1D) was red-shifted to 790 nm in the NIR region. This shift in SPR band had a direct impact on the photothermal ability of the samples. Figure 1F shows the change in temperature of each sample during exposure to 1 W/cm^2 NIR light irradiation with a wavelength of 808 nm, indicating that the temperature of all the samples was increased by NIR light irradiation. However, the exact profiles differed. The sample of Figure 1A exhibited a temperature increase to 35 °C, while the increase in temperature up to 37 °C was seen in the sample of Figure 1B. The largest temperature rise was observed for the sample of Figure 1D because the SPR peak of this sample well matched the central wavelength of the laser source [29]. This result indicates that AuNCs could be a photothermal agent responding to NIR light.

For the fabrication of NIR light-sensitive fibrous system, loading of AuNCs into polymeric fibers is required. To accomplish this, the particles should be dispersed in organic media without aggregation. We phase-transferred the as-synthesized AuNCs from the aqueous phase to the organic using thiolated PEG as a transfer agent. PEG-thiol was first introduced to an aqueous solution containing the as-synthesized AuNCs, followed by chloroform. As shown in Figure 2A, the organic phase and the aqueous phase containing the particles were phase-separated because of their immiscibility. After vigorous agitation, most of the particles transferred from the water phase to the chloroform in 30 min (Figure 2B) [30]. This successful phase transfer was due to the surface modification caused by the strong affinity between the surface of AuNCs and the thiol group [30,31]. After extraction, centrifugation, and washing, the particles were re-dispersed in fresh chloroform to make a W/O emulsion for electrospinning (Figure 2C).

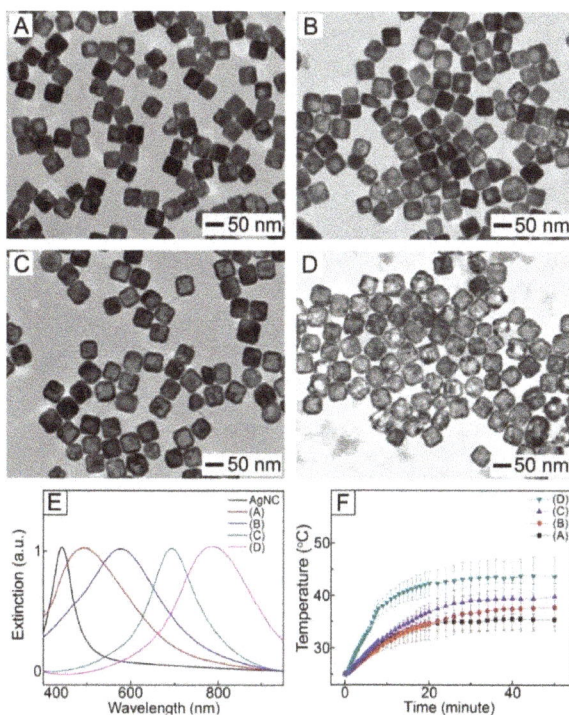

Figure 1. (**A–D**) TEM images of the particles obtained after the reaction of AgNCs with different amounts of HAuCl$_4$ solution: (**A**) 0.06, (**B**) 0.08, (**C**) 0.15 and (**D**) 0.2 mL. (**E**) UV–VIS–NIR extinction spectra for the particles of (**A–D**) in DI water. (**E**) UV–VIS–NIR extinction spectra for the particles of (**A–D**) and AgNCs in DI water. (**F**) Change in temperature for the particles of (**A–D**) in DI water with a concentration of 0.1 mg/mL under NIR light irradiation (1 W/cm^2, 808 nm).

Figure 2D shows UV–VIS–NIR extinction spectra for the as-synthesized AuNCs dispersed in DI water and the phase-transferred AuNCs dispersed in chloroform. No broadening of the SPR band was observed for the latter as compared with the former, which implies that aggregation among the AuNCs and change in their morphology did not happen during the phase transfer process. On the other hand, the phase transfer caused a red-shift in SPR band and the extinction peak moved to 815 nm in the NIR region, which was a result of change in the refractive index of the local environment surrounding the AuNCs [32].

We tested the photothermal conversion property of the phase-transferred AuNCs by exposing a solution of the phase-transferred particles in chloroform to NIR light irradiation. As shown in Figure 2E, the temperature of the sample increased in response to NIR light irradiation and its time-dependent temperature profile was similar to that of the aqueous solution of the as-synthesized AuNCs, which suggest that the photothermal ability of AuNCs was still kept after the phase transfer process. We also measured the optical property of the phase-transferred AuNCs after NIR light treatment. No change in the SPR band was observed after the treatment (Figure S2, Supplementary Materials), implying that the particles maintained their morphology without aggregation after NIR light irradiation. These results reveal that the phase-transferred AuNCs had excellent photostability.

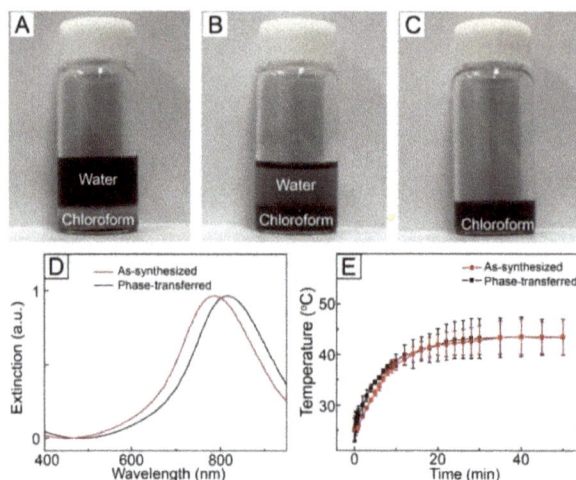

Figure 2. Photographs of AuNC solutions: (**A**) a mixture solution of AuNCs and PEG-thiol in a co-solvent of DI water and chloroform before vigorous agitation, (**B**) a mixture solution of AuNCs and PEG-thiol in a co-solvent of DI water and chloroform after vigorous agitation, and (**C**) a solution of phase-transferred AuNCs in chloroform. (**D**) UV–VIS–NIR extinction spectra for as-synthesized AuNCs in DI water and phase-transferred AuNCs in chloroform. (**E**) Time-dependent change in temperature for the as-synthesized AuNC solution in DI water and the phase-transferred AuNC solution in chloroform under NIR light irradiation (1 W/cm^2, 808 nm).

The phase-transferred AuNCs were dispersed in a W/O emulsion prepared for fabrication of NIR light-sensitive polymeric fibers. Figure 3A shows a SEM image of the fibers produced by electrospinning the W/O emulsion. The used W/O emulsion contained the phase-transferred AuNCs of 0.1 wt% without any inclusion of drug. The produced fibers had a smooth surface and their average diameter was 2.84 ± 0.12 μm. Figure 3B shows a TEM image of a single fiber of Figure 3A. It was found that a hollow interior, which can be a reservoir of hydrophilic drug, was formed in the core of the fiber, which was a result of a big difference in the surface energy between water droplet phase and chloroform one that were present within the W/O emulsion [21]. A magnified image of the region, marked by a black box, is shown in the inset, demonstrating that the phase-transferred AuNCs were well distributed within the fiber. Figure 3C shows XRD patterns for the phase-transferred AuNCs, plain PCL fibers, and the fibers of Figure 3A. The XRD pattern from the sample of Figure 3A contained the peaks generated by the AuNCs as well as those corresponding to the plain PCL fibers. This result also confirms that the nanoparticles were successfully loaded into the fibers.

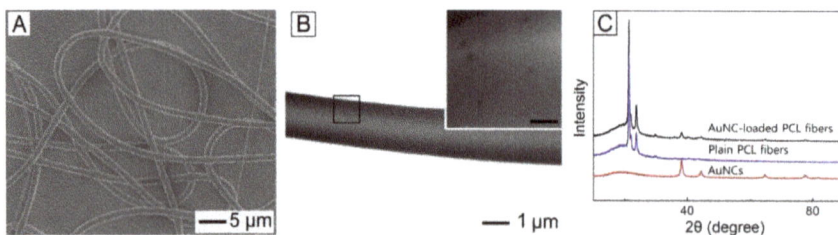

Figure 3. (**A**) SEM and (**B**) TEM images of PCL fibers loaded with AuNCs. The scale bar in the inset is 300 nm. (**C**) XRD patterns for AuNCs, plain PCL fibers, and AuNC-loaded PCL fibers.

To investigate a NIR light sensitivity of the fibers loaded with AuNCs, the fibres were exposed to NIR light irradiation and then their change in temperature observed. Figure 4A shows the time-lapse thermal infrared photographs of the fibers of Figure 3A under NIR light with a power density of 1 W/cm^2. When the fibers were exposed to NIR irradiation, a drastic change in color from blue to red was observed at the center of the images (marked with a white box) where the fibers were placed. This change in color implies that the temperature of the sample increased due to the loading of AuNCs with photothermal conversion capability. Change in the concentration of AuNCs in the W/O emulsion had an influence on the heat generation property of the fibers. As shown in Figure 4B, the sample without the inclusion of AuNCs exhibited no significant change in temperature under NIR light irradiation, whereas the use of the W/O emulsion with 0.01 wt% AuNCs allowed the temperature rise to 33 °C. When the concentration increased to 0.1 wt%, the temperature reached 45 °C. This result was because the higher concentration of AuNCs would lead to loading of the more amount of the particles into the fibers, which resulted in stronger heat generation.

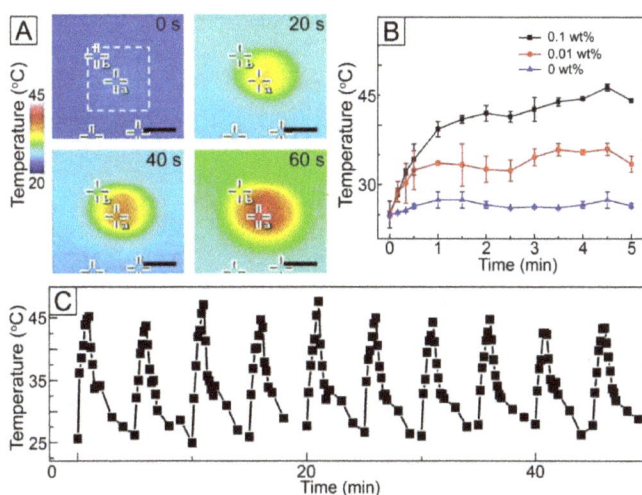

Figure 4. (**A**) Time-lapse thermal infrared images of AuNC-loaded fibers under NIR light irradiation (1 W/cm^2, 808 nm). The scale bar is 0.5 cm. (**B**) Change in temperature for the fibers, which were produced from the W/O emulsions with different concentration of AuNCs, under NIR light (1 W/cm^2, 808 nm). (**C**) Time-dependent temperature curve for AuNC-loaded fibers under on–off switching of NIR light (1 W/cm^2, 808 nm).

The NIR light-triggered heat generation could reversibly happen when NIR light irradiation was applied in an on–off manner, as shown in Figure 4C. The treatment with NIR light for 1 min changed the temperature of the sample of Figure 3A from 26 to 45 °C, and the temperature returned to 26 °C after the light remained off for 4 min. This NIR light-sensitive manner in temperature change was still kept when the light was switched on and off ten times under the same condition, which indicates that the fibers would be useful for repeated hyperthermia treatment.

We evaluated the anticancer ability of the fibers against SK-BR-3 cells. Before the evaluation, we checked the cytotoxicity of NIR light to the cells. Figure S3A (Supplementary Materials) shows the viability of SK-BR-3 cells after exposure to 1 W/cm^2 NIR light, determined using a WST-1 assay. The viability of the cells was >90% for all the conditions compared with the control without the treatment of NIR light. In addition, we tested the cytotoxicity of the phase-transferred AuNCs and the result reveals that the particles were biocompatible (Figure S3B, Supplementary Materials). These results suggest that their effects on the anticancer ability of the fibers were negligible.

Figure 5A shows the viabilities of SK-BR-3 cells treated with plain PCL fibers and AuNC-loaded PCL fibers of Figure 3A. Under no exposure to NIR light, both the samples exhibited cell viabilities >90%. A similar result was also observed with FB cells (Figure S4, Supplementary Materials). The high viabilities indicate that the fibers are biocompatible. On the other hand, when irradiated with NIR light, only the fibers loaded with AuNCs had a lower cell viability (78%). This decrease in cell viability was because the photothermal conversion generated by the loaded particles increased the temperature of the sample to 45 °C for hyperthermia, and consequently damaged the cells. However, many cells were still alive, even though they might be weakened.

This hyperthermia effect could be strengthened by increasing the number of cycles of NIR light irradiation. Figure 5B shows the cell viability with respect to the number of NIR light treatments, demonstrating that the value of viability decreased as the number of the treatments increased. Two cycles of NIR light treatment yielded a cell viability of 44%, while four cycles of the treatment reduced the value to 16%. This decrease in viability can be explained by the shock effect [33]. The repeated, rapid temperature change due to multiple cycles of on–off operation of NIR light irradiation could damage more the already weakened cells, resulting in more destruction of the cells. Live/dead assay also showed the decrease in cell viability. Figure 5C shows a CLS micrograph of SK-BR-3 cells treated with AuNC-loaded fibers under no NIR light, which exhibited only a bright green fluorescence. This result suggests that all the cancer cells were still alive. On the other hand, the red fluorescence became more visible as the number of cycles of NIR light treatment increased (Figure 5D–F), implying cell death was induced by the applications of NIR light-driven hyperthermia.

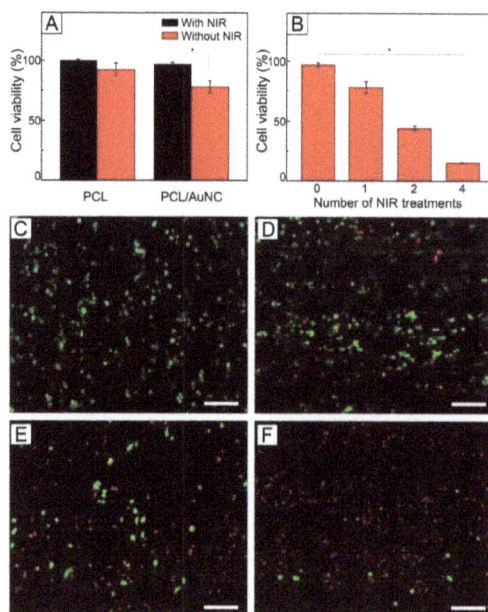

Figure 5. (**A**) Viability of SK-BR-3 cells treated with plain PCL and AuNC-loaded PCL fibers without and with NIR irradiation (1 W/cm², 808 nm). (**B**) Viability of SK-BR-3 cells treated with AuNC-loaded PCL fibers under on–off switching of NIR light irradiation (1 W/cm², 808 nm). * indicates $p < 0.01$. (**C–F**) CLS micrographs showing live (green) and dead (red) SK-BR-3 cells treated with AuNC-loaded PCL fibers under different numbers of cycles of 1 W/cm² NIR light irradiation: (**C**) Zero, (**D**) one, (**E**) two, and (**F**) four cycles. The scale bars are 100 µm.

However, the use of only NIR light-induced hyperthermia cannot achieve a satisfactory therapeutic efficacy because of the non-uniform distribution of heat generated within a tumor [13]. Furthermore, residual cancer cell survival after the treatment can cause metastasis or recurrence [20]. To improve the anticancer activity of the AuNC-loaded fibers, we additionally loaded a chemotherapeutic drug, DOX, into the fibers together with a biocompatible, phase-changeable fatty acid that could induce a NIR-light triggered release of the drug [21,22,26]. Figure 6A shows a SEM image of AuNC-loaded PCL fibers with the inclusion of the drug and the fatty acid mixture of LA and SA, which were produced by electrospinning a W/O emulsion containing DOX in the water phase and the fatty acid mixture (f_{fatty} = 0.05) in the oil phase. The average diameter of the fibers was 2.88 ± 0.14 μm, which was similar to that for the sample of Figure 3A. A cross-sectional SEM image is shown in the inset, demonstrating that the fibers had a hollow interior and a smooth surface. These results indicate that the addition of the fatty acid mixture and the drug did not affect the formation of fibers or their structure. Figure 6B–D show CLS images of the single fiber of Figure 6A. Red fluorescence generated from DOX is observed in the fluorescence image of Figure 6B, suggesting that the drug molecules were well loaded in the fibers. The merged image (Figure 6D) with its corresponding optical image (Figure 6C) clearly demonstrates that DOX was placed in the central region of the fiber. Taken together with the inset of Figure 6A, this result indicates that the drug molecules were encapsulated in the hollow core of the fibers.

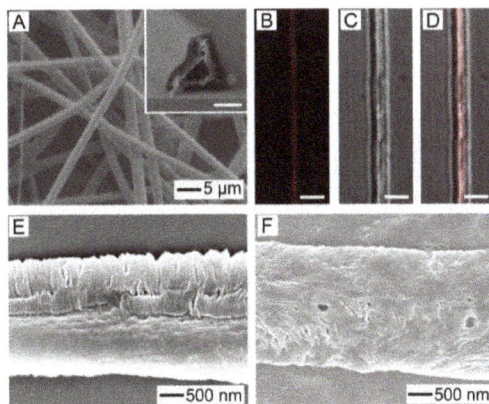

Figure 6. (**A**) SEM image of AuNC-loaded fibers containing the fatty acid mixture and DOX, which were produced using a W/O emulsion of f_{fatty} = 0.05. The inset scale is 1 μm. (**B–D**) CLS micrographs showing the fluorescence from DOX loaded in the as-spun fiber. The scales are 3 μm. (**E,F**) SEM images of AuNC-loaded fibers after exposure to 1 W/cm^2 NIR light. The fibers were made using W/O emulsions of: (**E**) f_{fatty} = 0.05 and (**F**) f_{fatty} = 0.1.

To check the inclusion of the fatty acid mixture into the fibers, DSC measurement was conducted. The fibers of Figure 6A exhibited two sharp peaks at 39 and 59 °C (Figure S5, Supplementary Materials), which corresponded to the melting points of the fatty acid mixture and PCL, respectively [22]. This result reveals the successful loading of the fatty acid mixture into the fibers. After introduction of 1 W/cm^2 NIR light irradiation to increase the temperature of the fibers to 45 °C, the peak at 39 °C given by the fatty acid mixture disappeared (Figure S5), indicating that the mixture was removed from the fibers. This removal was a result of NIR light-induced photothermal effect. Upon exposure to NIR light, a photothermal conversion was caused by the loaded AuNCs, increasing the local temperature of the sample above the melting point of the fatty acid mixture and melting out the mixture from the fibers. Consequently, small pores were generated in the sheath of the fibers, as shown in Figure 6E. The size and density of the formed pores increased with f_{fatty} (Figure 6F) because of the inclusion of the larger amount of the mixture in the fibers.

Figure 7A shows the release profiles of DOX from the fibers produced from the W/O emulsions with different values of f_{fatty}. The sample with no inclusion of the fatty acid mixture ($f_{fatty} = 0$) did not release the drug molecules over 4 h without NIR light treatment. A similar result was also observed for the fibers produced with the use of the W/O emulsion of $f_{fatty} = 0.05$ because the fatty acid mixture present in the solid state blocked the diffusion-out of the encapsulated drug molecules. When 1 W/cm^2 NIR light was irradiated for 5 min, the sample of $f_{fatty} = 0$ still did not release the drug molecules, whereas the fibers of $f_{fatty} = 0.05$ allowed the release of 33% DOX for 4 h since NIR light was irradiated. The release in the latter case resulted from the formation of the pores in response to NIR light, as visualized in Figure 6E. The formation of the pores caused by the melting out of the loaded fatty acid could increase the surface area of the fibers, allowing an easy uptake of the PBS buffer into the fibers and a generation of effective paths for the preloaded drug molecules to be released quickly [22]. This NIR light-triggered release could be controlled by varying the value of f_{fatty}. When f_{fatty} increased to 0.1, the release of 55% DOX was achieved over the same period. This difference was attributed to the larger size and density of the generated pores for the sample of $f_{fatty} = 0.1$ (Figure 7F), which increased surface area [21] and consequently led to the faster release of the drug.

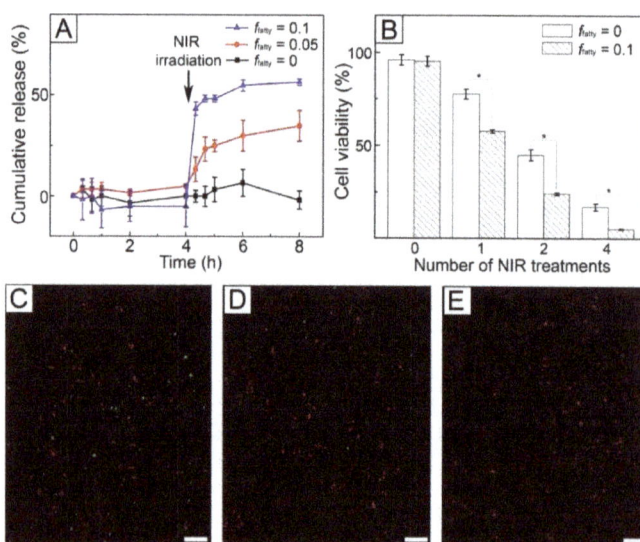

Figure 7. (**A**) Release profiles of DOX from AuNC-loaded fibers containing the fatty acid mixture and the drug. The cumulative release (%) percentage was defined as a ratio of the accumulated amount of released drug at a given time to the initial amount loaded. (**B**) Viability of SK-BR-3 cells treated with AuNC-loaded fibers containing the fatty acid mixture and DOX under different numbers of cycles of 1 W/cm^2 NIR light irradiation. The fibers were made using W/O emulsions of $f_{fatty} = 0$ and 0.1. * indicates $p < 0.01$. (**C–E**) CLS micrographs showing live (green) and dead (red) SK-BR-3 cells treated with the fibers of $f_{fatty} = 0.1$ under different numbers of cycles of 1 W/cm^2 NIR light irradiation: (**C**) one, (**D**) two, and (**E**) four cycles. The scale bars are 100 µm.

Figure 7B shows the viability of SK-BR-3 cells treated with the fibers of $f_{fatty} = 0$ and 0.1 in Figure 7A. When the fibers were not exposed to NIR light, the cell viabilities were above 90%. In the case of FB cells, the similar result was also observed (Figure S4). These results were because the fibers were biocompatible and the drug encapsulated in their core was not released, as indicated by the result of *in vitro* release in Figure 7A. When NIR light was irradiated, the cell viability was reduced for both the systems. However, their anticancer ability was different. The cell viability for the system with $f_{fatty} = 0$ was similar to that of Figure 5B because the loaded drug molecules were not released

(Figure 7A) and consequently only hyperthermia occurred. In the case of the system with f_{fatty} = 0.1, the cell viability decreased to 57% after one cycle of NIR light, which was lower than the value (77%) of the fibers with f_{fatty} = 0 with the use of only hyperthermia. This decrease in cell viability was due to the synergistic effect of the drug release and hyperthermia. The effect was much stronger with the increase of the number of cycles of NIR light treatment. Two cycles of NIR irradiation reduced the cell viability to 24%, and four cycles led to a cell viability of 4%. This cell death was also confirmed using a live/dead assay (Figure 7C–E), demonstrating that the majority of the cells were dead after four cycles of the treatment, as shown in Figure 7E.

4. Conclusions

A fibrous system for synergistic cancer therapy was successfully developed using a simple emulsion electrospinning technique. The system consisted of AuNC-incorporated PCL fibers encapsulating an anticancer drug, DOX, in their core and loading a phase-changeable fatty acid in their sheath. The excellent photothermal ability and photostability of AuNCs led to the repeated, significant heating of the fibers in response to on–off switching of NIR light irradiation. When the irradiation increased the temperature of the system to a window suitable for hyperthermia, the death of cancer cells was observed. The NIR light-induced heat generation also simultaneously allowed the release of the drug molecules through the pores in the fibers generated by the melting of the loaded fatty acid. The combination of this NIR light-triggered drug release with the repeated hyperthermia treatment exhibited excellent therapeutic efficacy in an in vitro model. Thus, the fibers have potential in synergistic cancer therapy with a combination of NIR-triggered hyperthermia and chemotherapy.

Supplementary Materials: The following are available online at http://www.mdpi.com/1999-4923/11/2/60/s1, Figure S1. TEM image of AgNCs used for synthesis of AuNCs. Figure S2. UV-vis-NIR extinction spectra for phase-transferred AuNCs in chloroform before and after exposure to NIR light for 50 min. Figure S3. Viability of SK-BR-3 cells treated with: A) NIR light and B) phase-transferred AuNCs. Figure S4. Viability of FB cells treated with plain PCL fibers, AuNC-incorporated PCL fibers, AuNC-incorporated PCL fibers loaded with DOX, and AuNC-incorporated PCL fibers with loading of the fatty acid mixture and DOX. Figure S5. DSC thermograms for AuNC-loaded fibers produced with a W/O emulsion of f_{fatty} =0.05 before and after NIR irradiation.

Author Contributions: G.D.M. and D.C.H. conceived and designed the experiments; J.H.P., H.S., D.I.K., J.H.C., and J.H.S. performed the experiments and analyzed the data; J.B.K. reviewed the data; J.H.P., G.D.M. and D.C.H. wrote the paper.

Funding: D.C.H. acknowledges the financial support from Basic Science Research Program (NRF-2018R1D1A1B07043878) through the National Research Foundation of Korea (NRF) funded by the Ministry of Education (MOE). G.D.M. acknowledges the support from the Korea Institute of Industrial Technology through Fundamental Research and Development (KITECH EO-18-00222).

Conflicts of Interest: The authors declare that they have no conflict of interest.

References

1. Kadam, V.V.; Wang, L.; Padhye, R. Electrospun nanofibre materials to filter air pollutants—A review. *J. Ind. Text.* **2018**, *47*, 2253–2280. [CrossRef]
2. Lu, P.; Qiao, B.; Lu, N.; Hyun, D.C.; Wang, J.; Kim, M.J.; Liu, J.; Xia, Y. Photochemical deposition of highly dispersed Pt nanoparticles on porous CeO_2 nanofibers for the water-gas shift reaction. *Adv. Funct. Mater.* **2015**, *25*, 4153–4162. [CrossRef]
3. Shi, X.; Zhou, W.; Ma, D.; Ma, Q.; Bridges, D.; Ma, Y.; Hu, A. Electrospinning of nanofibers and their applications for energy devices. *J. Nanomater.* **2015**. [CrossRef]
4. Lee, B.S.; Park, B.; Yang, H.S.; Han, J.W.; Choong, C.; Bae, J.; Lee, K.; Yu, W.-R.; Jeong, U.; Park, J.-J.; et al. Effects of substrate on piezoelectricity of electrospun poly(vinylidene fluoride)-nanofiber-based energy generators. *ACS Appl. Mater. Interfaces* **2014**, *6*, 3520–3527. [CrossRef] [PubMed]
5. Park, M.; Im, J.; Park, J.; Jeong, U. Micropatterned stretchable circuit and strain sensor fabricated by lithography on an electrospun nanofiber mat. *ACS Appl. Mater. Interfaces* **2013**, *5*, 8766–8771. [CrossRef] [PubMed]

6.   Park, M.; Im, J.; Shin, M.; Min, Y.; Park, J.; Cho, H.; Park, S.; Shim, M.-B.; Jeon, S.; Chung, D.-Y.; et al. Highly stretchable electric circuits from a composite material of silver nanoparticles and elastomeric fibers. *Nat. Nanotechnol.* **2012**, *7*, 803–809. [CrossRef] [PubMed]

7.   Braghirolli, D.I.; Steffens, D.; Pranke, P. Electrospinning for regenerative medicine: A review of the main topics. *Drug Discov. Today* **2014**, *19*, 743–753. [CrossRef]

8.   Yu, D.G.; Zhu, L.M.; White, K.; Branford-White, C. Electrospun nanofiber-based drug delivery systems. *Health* **2009**, *1*, 67–75. [CrossRef]

9.   Chen, M.; Li, Y.F.; Besenbacher, F. Electrospun nanofibers-mediated on-demand drug release. *Adv. Healthc. Mater.* **2014**, *3*, 1721–1732. [CrossRef]

10. Yang, G.; Wang, J.; Wang, Y.; Li, L.; Guo, X.; Zhou, S. Implantable active-targeting micelle-in-nanofiber device for efficient and safe cancer therapy. *ACS Nano* **2015**, *9*, 1161–1174. [CrossRef]

11. Zhang, J.; Wang, X.; Liu, T.; Liu, S.; Jing, X. Antitumor activity of electrospun polylactide nanofibers loaded with 5-fluorouracil and oxaliplatin against colorectal cancer. *Drug Deliv.* **2016**, *23*, 784–790. [CrossRef] [PubMed]

12. Liu, H.; Fu, Y.; Li, Y.; Ren, Z.; Li, X.; Han, G.; Mao, C. A fibrous localized drug delivery platform with NIR-triggered and optically monitored drug release. *Langmuir* **2016**, *32*, 9083–9090. [CrossRef] [PubMed]

13. Tiwari, A.P.; Hwang, T.I.; Oh, J.-M.; Maharjan, B.; Chun, S.; Kim, B.S.; Joshi, M.K.; Park, C.H.; Kim, C.S. pH/NIR-responsive polypyrrole-functionalized fibrous localized drug-delivery platform for synergistic cancer therapy. *ACS Appl. Mater. Interfaces* **2018**, *10*, 20256–20270. [CrossRef] [PubMed]

14. Chen, P.; Wu, Q.S.; Ding, Y.P.; Chu, M.; Huang, Z.M.; Hu, W. A controlled release system of titanocene dichloride by electrospun fiber and its antitumor activity in vitro. *Eur. J. Pharm. Biopharm.* **2010**, *76*, 413–420. [CrossRef] [PubMed]

15. Tran, T.H.; Nguyen, H.T.; Pham, T.T.; Choi, J.Y.; Choi, H.G.; Yong, C.S.; Kim, J.O. Development of a graphene oxide nanocarrier for dual-drug chemo-phototherapy to overcome drug resistance in cancer. *ACS Appl. Mater. Interfaces* **2015**, *7*, 28647–28655. [CrossRef] [PubMed]

16. Cheng, M.; Wang, H.; Zhang, Z.; Li, N.; Fang, X.; Xu, S. Gold nanorod-embedded electrospun fibrous membrane as a photothermal therapy platform. *ACS Appl. Mater. Interfaces* **2014**, *6*, 1569–1575. [CrossRef] [PubMed]

17. Hu, S.H.; Fang, R.H.; Chen, Y.W.; Liao, B.J.; Chen, I.W.; Chen, S.Y. Photoresponsive protein−graphene−protein hybrid capsules with dual targeted heat-triggered drug delivery approach for enhanced tumor therapy. *Adv. Funct. Mater.* **2014**, *24*, 4144–4155. [CrossRef]

18. Jian, W.H.; Yu, T.W.; Chen, C.J.; Huang, W.C.; Chiu, H.C.; Chiang, W.H. Indocyanine green-encapsulated hybrid polymeric nanomicelles for photothermal cancer therapy. *Langmuir* **2015**, *31*, 6202–6210. [CrossRef] [PubMed]

19. Ramanan, V.V.; Hribar, K.C.; Katz, J.S.; Burdick, J.A. Nanofiber–nanorod composites exhibiting light-induced reversible lower critical solution temperature transitions. *Nanotechnology* **2011**, *22*. [CrossRef]

20. Choi, J.H.; Seo, H.; Park, J.H.; Son, J.H.; Kim, D.I.; Kim, J.; Moon, G.D.; Hyun, D.C. Poly(D,L-lactic-co-glycolic acid) (PLGA) hollow fiber with segmental switchability of its chains sensitive to NIR light for synergistic cancer therapy. *Colloids Surf. B* **2019**, *173*, 258–265. [CrossRef]

21. Park, J.H.; Choi, J.H.; Son, J.H.; Hwang, S.J.; Seo, H.; Kang, I.K.; Park, M.; Kim, J.; Hyun, D.C. Poly(ε-caprolactone) (PCL) fibers incorporated with phase-changeable fatty acid and indocyanine green for NIR light-triggered, localized anti-cancer drug release. *Polymer* **2018**, *135*, 211–218. [CrossRef]

22. Park, J.H.; Ahn, H.; Kim, J.; Hyun, D.C. Phase-changeable fatty acid available for temperature-regulated drug release. *Macromol. Mater. Eng.* **2016**, *301*, 887–894. [CrossRef]

23. Skrabalak, S.E.; Au, L.; Li, X.; Xia, Y. Facile synthesis of Ag nanocubes and Au nanocages. *Nat. Protoc.* **2007**, *2*, 2182–2190. [CrossRef] [PubMed]

24. Riley, R.S.; Day, E.S. Gold nanoparticle-mediated photothermal therapy: Applications and opportunities for multimodal cancer treatment. *Wiley Interdiscip. Rev. Nanomed. Nanobiotechnol.* **2017**, *9*, e1449. [CrossRef] [PubMed]

25. Vats, M.; Mishra, S.K.; Baghini, M.S.; Chauhan, D.S.; Srivastava, R.; De, A. Near infrared fluorescence imaging in nano-therapeutics and photo-thermal evaluation. *Int. J. Mol. Sci.* **2017**, *18*, 924. [CrossRef] [PubMed]

Pharmaceutics **2019**, *11*, 60

26. Sun, T.; Zhang, Y.S.; Pang, B.; Hyun, D.C.; Yang, M.; Xia, Y. Engineered nanoparticles for drug delivery in cancer therapy. *Angew. Chem. Int. Ed.* **2014**, *53*, 12320–12364. [CrossRef] [PubMed]

27. Skrabalak, S.E.; Chen, J.; Sun, Y.; Lu, X.; Au, L.; Cobley, C.M.; Xia, Y. Gold nanocages: Synthesis, properties, and applications. *Acc. Chem. Res.* **2008**, *41*, 1587–1595. [CrossRef]

28. Sun, Y.; Xia, Y. Mechanistic study on the replacement reaction between silver nanostructures and chloroauric acid in aqueous medium. *J. Am. Chem. Soc.* **2004**, *126*, 3892–3901. [CrossRef]

29. Chen, J.; Wang, D.; Xi, J.; Au, L.; Siekkinen, A.; Warsen, A.; Li, W.-Y.; Zhang, H.; Xia, Y.; Li, X. Immuno gold nanocages with tailored optical properties for targeted photothermal destruction of cancer cells. *Nano Lett.* **2007**, *7*, 1318–1322. [CrossRef]

30. Alkilany, A.M.; Bani Yaseen, A.I.; Park, J.; Eller, J.R.; Murphy, C.J. Facile phase transfer of gold nanoparticles from aqueous solution to organic solvents with thiolated poly(ethylene glycol). *RSC Adv.* **2014**, *4*, 52676–52679. [CrossRef]

31. Liu, M.; Law, W.C.; Kopwitthaya, A.; Liu, X.; Swihart, M.T.; Prasad, P.N. Exploring the amphiphilicity of PEGylated gold nanorods: Mechanical phase transfer and self-assembly. *Chem. Commun.* **2013**, *49*, 9350–9352. [CrossRef] [PubMed]

32. Serrano-Montes, A.B.; Jimenez de Aberasturi, D.; Langer, J.; Giner-Casares, J.J.; Scarabelli, L.; Herrero, A.; Liz-Marzán, L.M. A general method for solvent exchange of plasmonic nanoparticles and self-assembly into SERS-active monolayers. *Langmuir* **2015**, *31*, 9205–9213. [CrossRef] [PubMed]

33. Huang, C.; Soenen, S.J.; Rejman, J.; Trekker, J.; Chengxun, L.; Lagae, L.; Ceelen, W.; Wilhelm, C.; Demeester, J.; De Smedt, S.C. Magnetic electrospun fibers for cancer therapy. *Adv. Funct. Mater.* **2012**, *22*, 2479–2486. [CrossRef]

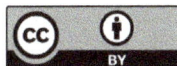

MDPI

St. Alban-Anlage 66

4052 Basel

Switzerland

Tel. +41 61 683 77 34

Fax +41 61 302 89 18

www.mdpi.com

Pharmaceutics Editorial Office

E-mail: pharmaceutics@mdpi.com

www.mdpi.com/journal/pharmaceutics

www.ingramcontent.com/pod-product-compliance
Lightning Source LLC
Chambersburg PA
CBHW051854210326
41597CB00033B/5895